Lecture Notes in Electrical Engineering

Volume 96

Subhas Chandra Mukhopadhyay

New Developments in Sensing Technology for Structural Health Monitoring

Springer

Prof. Subhas Chandra Mukhopadhyay
Massey University
12 Woodgate Court
Palmerston North
New Zealand
E-mail: S.C.Mukhopadhyay@massey.ac.nz

ISBN 978-3-642-21098-3 e-ISBN 978-3-642-21099-0

DOI 10.1007/978-3-642-21099-0

Lecture Notes in Electrical Engineering ISSN 1876-1100

Library of Congress Control Number: 2011928067

Typeset & Coverdesign: Scientific Publishing Services Pvt. Ltd., Chennai, India.

Printed on acid-free paper

9 8 7 6 5 4 3 2 1

springer.com

Guest Editorial

In recent times several incidents of bridge/buildings collapse took place in different parts of the world. After these accidents it has become paramount importance of early detection of the health of structures and the sensors must have intelligent features to detect the problem. It is expected that the special issue have provided many new ideas of detection and inspection of the health of structures which are very important for human being and society. There is an urgent need to design, develop, fabricate of different types of sensors and sensing technology based on non-invasive techniques to determine the integrity of a material, component or structure or quantitatively measure some characteristics of the systems to prevent catastrophic failure. So in short the fabricated sensor systems should be able to inspect or measure without doing any harm or damage of the system. Not only the monitoring of structural health the applications of the developed sensing systems are necessary at almost any stage in the production or the life cycle of a component in many years such as civil engineering, metal industry, transportation, power stations, inspection of pipes and piping systems in industrial plants, fatigue estimation in aircraft surface and other parts and in many other areas.

Many different sensing techniques available with different characteristics are available for these inspection areas. The following are the most commonly used: Magnetic, Ultrasonic, Acoustic, Radiography, Eddy current and X-ray. The sensors to be used entirely depend entirely on the specific application.

The proposed Special Issue has focussed on the different aspects of sensing technology, i.e. high reliability, adaptability, recalibration, information processing, data fusion, validation and integration of novel and high performance sensors specifically aims to use to inspect mechanical health of structure and similar applications.

The book, on one hand, illustrates theoretical aspects and applications, and it displays new criteria in characterizing raw data of SHM, at the other hand. Characterization is a key issue since it allows to know the performances of devices and systems described in the book by showing some statistics and result representation. The book contains 15 contributions from experts working on the topic and under different approaches and aspects; these co-ordinated approaches are the true richness of the book. The editor gracefully thanks the contributors for contribution included in this special issue. The editor hopes this special issue will be a very useful for readers with experience who can breathe fresh life into their research.

Subhas Chandra Mukhopadhyay, Guest Editor
School of Engineering and Advanced Technology (SEAT),
Massey University (Turitea Campus)
Palmerston North, New Zealand
S.C.Mukhopadhyay@massey.ac.nz

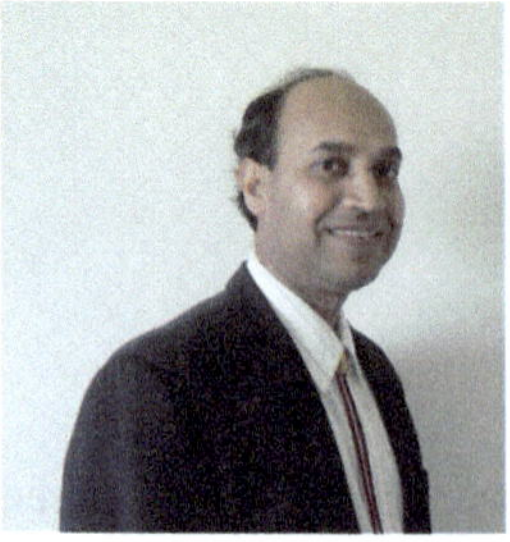

Dr. Subhas Chandra Mukhopadhyay graduated from the Department of Electrical Engineering, Jadavpur University, Calcutta, India in 1987 with a Gold medal and received the Master of Electrical Engineering degree from Indian Institute of Science, Bangalore, India in 1989. He obtained the PhD (Eng.) degree from Jadavpur University, India in 1994 and Doctor of Engineering degree from Kanazawa University, Japan in 2000.

During 1989-90 he worked almost 2 years in the research and development department of Crompton Greaves Ltd., India. In 1990 he joined as a Lecturer in the Electrical Engineering department, Jadavpur University, India and was promoted to Senior Lecturer of the same department in 1995.

Obtaining Monbusho fellowship he went to Japan in 1995. He worked with Kanazawa University, Japan as researcher and Assistant professor till September 2000.

In September 2000 he joined as Senior Lecturer in the Institute of Information Sciences and Technology, Massey University, New Zealand where he is working currently as an Associate professor. His fields of interest include Sensors and Sensing Technology, Electromagnetics, control, electrical machines and numerical field calculation etc.

He has authored over 200 papers in different international journals and conferences, edited nine conference proceedings. He has also edited eight special issues of international journals as guest editor and ten books with Springer-Verlag.

He is a **Fellow** of IEEE (USA), a **Fellow** of IET (UK), an associate editor of IEEE Sensors journal and IEEE Transactions on Instrumentation and Measurements. He is in the editorial board of e-Journal on Non-Destructive Testing, Sensors and Transducers, Transactions on Systems, Signals and Devices (TSSD), Journal on the Patents on Electrical Engineering, Journal of Sensors. He is the co-Editor-in-chief of the International Journal on Smart Sensing and Intelligent Systems (www.s2is.org). He is in the technical programme committee of IEEE Sensors conference, IEEE IMTC conference and IEEE DELTA conference and numerous other conferences. He was the Technical Programme Chair of ICARA 2004, ICARA 2006 and ICARA 2009. He was the General chair/co-chair of ICST 2005, ICST 2007, IEEE ROSE 2007, IEEE EPSA 2008, ICST 2008, IEEE Sensors 2008, ICST 2010 and IEEE Sensors 2010. He has organized the IEEE Sensors conference 2009 at Christchurch, New Zealand during October 25 to 28, 2009 as General Chair.

He is the **Chair** of the IEEE Instrumentation and Measurement Society New Zealand Chapter.

He is a **Distinguished Lecturer** of the IEEE Sensors Council.

Contents

Sensors and Technologies for Structural Health Monitoring: A Review

S.C. Mukhopadhyay[1] and I. Ihara[2]

[1] School of Engineering and Advanced Technology
Massey University, Palmerston North, New Zealand
S.C.Mukhopadhyay@massey.ac.nz
[2] Department of Mechanical Engineering
Nagaoka University of Technology, Nagaoka, Japan
ihara@mech.nagaokaut.ac.jp

Abstract. Incidents such as building and bridge collapse are on rise in many parts of the world without little apparent warning. Due to the increase number of incidents it has become of increasingly paramount importance to develop methods detecting the degradation or damage that result in these events. Thus, buildings and critical infrastructure could be monitored, much like a patient in a hospital, for signs of degradation or impending disability or collapse. The sensors are very important to know the state of the health of the structures and technologies are like human brains to analyze the abnormal situation. This chapter will provide a review of different available sensors and technologies to be used for monitoring the health of structures.

1 Introduction and Literature Review

Intelligent sensors and technologies that are able to take a potentially diverse array of data and create a picture of the structure's condition will help to determine the early detection of damage from natural hazards or other events. Thus, the sensors must have access to or contain intelligent features to detect the problem. It is therefore important to know wide varieties of sensors and technologies for Structural Health Monitoring (SHM) which can be deployed for the detection and inspection of structures to increase their safety and reliability. The reported sensor and technologies should be able to inspect or measure without doing any harm or damage of the structure. They should also be robust to poor signal-to-noise ratio compared to the level of damage they are trying to detect in these critical infrastructures. Finally, they need to be highly reliable and operate without input for long periods of time, potentially over years.

A lot of research articles have been reported on monitoring health of structures. A structural health monitoring system based on wireless sensor nodes equipped with inexpensive strain gauges has been proposed [1]. Due to the deployment of multi-hop technique the performance of the system is not limited. Strain gauges are very popular in SHM as they are inexpensive, easy to install and having good sensitivity to detect potential danger or collapse of a building or structure. The developed system has been tested with simulated structure.

S.C. Mukhopadhyay (Ed.): New Developments in Sensing Technology for SHM, LNEE 96, pp. 1–14.
springerlink.com

MEMS inertial sensors [2] including an acceleration sensor and an angular velocity sensor (gyroscope) can be used as a popular device for monitoring the health of structure due to their miniaturized size, low cost, mass production and three-dimensional detection.

An impedance measurement system for lead zirconate titanate (PZT) ceramics based SHM has been reported in [3]. The PZT sensors are inexpensive, small, light weight, require low power, less sensitive to temperature variation and provide a linear response under low electric field.

The importance of monitoring health of aerospace structure using optical sensors was considered more than a decade back as was reported by Foote and Read [4]. It states that with the help of a smart sensor network, the stress and strains induced in the aircraft and possible degradation occurred since last inspection can be known clearly.

Fibre optic accelerometer based monitoring of civil engineering infrastructure and damage detection of concrete slab has been reported by Kim and Feng [5]. The sensor system integrates Moire fringe phenomenon with fibre optics to achieve accurate and reliable measurement.

Fibre optic sensors emerged as an important technology to evaluate structural integrity [6]. The strain along the fibre length provides distributed information about mechanical state of the structure.

Bo-lin et. al., [7] have described some works and applications of new sensors such as optical fibre sensors, piezoelectric sensors, MEMS sensors, wireless sensing system etc. for aircraft structural health monitoring. The experimental works have been carried out in laboratory conditions and some more works are required to integrate the sensors to the structures effectively, determination of optimum number of sensors and their location and enhancement of the reliability of the sensors in order to survive the rugged environments.

In [8] a structural health monitoring system using wireless sensor network consisting of 17 sensor nodes, a base station and a processing computer has been implemented. The acceleration data synchronously sampled from each sensor node are transported to a data processing computer through a base station. A time division multiple access (TDMA) approach has been proposed to reduce the packet collision and energy consumption.

The experimental works on the design and implementation of an innovative technological framework for monitoring critical structures in Italy has been reported [9]. The use of wireless sensors networks allowed for a pervasive observation over the sites of interest to minimize the potential damages that natural phenomenon may cause to architectural or engineering works. The temperature, relative humidity, linear strain and 3-axis acceleration sensors are used for the measurement of observed parameters.

A SHM flexible testbed system has been developed for detecting high-velocity impacts in the skin of a structure [10]. The system is a large sensor network containing about two hundred nodes, each of which contains multiple sensors. The testbed is used for studying wide range of SHM applications.

The configurations of a novel wireless system for infrastructure health monitoring has been proposed and developed with a special attention to the low frequency characteristics of the wireless transmission [11].

Sensors deployed for monitoring bridges, buildings etc. always face a constraint from energy consideration. A novel wireless sensor system has been presented in [12] that harvests vibrations of the bridge created by passing traffic, which is converted into usable energy by means of a linear electromagnetic generator. In the particular design [12], harvesting of power up to 12.5 mW in the resonant mode with an excitation frequency of 3.1 Hz has been reported.

A field study of monitoring the ambient vibration using 60 accelerometers interfaced with 30 wireless sensor nodes operating within one or two simultaneously star topology network has been reported [13]. It is envisioned that the reported system can address short-term and long-term management and condition assessment needs for highway bridges.

In [14], a novel sensor network architecture for SHM has been presented. The system is based on contactless sensors that make use of near-field coupling to both sense the structure displacement and deploy a local communication network.

A simple custom-built gages based detection of cracks in critical structural elements and its design, implementation and experimental evaluation of a WSN for real-time SHM has been reported [15]. The paper [15] has shown that a variety of low-cost, off-the-shelf data acquisition/communication devices can be used to support remote monitoring by a control centre. The assessment of the developed system done for a full-scale three-story reinforced concrete building that was tested under lateral forces emulating forces induced by earthquakes.

P.F.dC. Antunes et. al., [16] have reported the implementation of an optical accelerometer unit based on fiber Bragg gratings, suitable to monitor structures with frequencies up to 45 Hz. The developed system has been used to estimate the eigenfrequencies of a steel foot bridge structure of total length of 300 m.

Bragg grating-based optical fiber sensors integrated into carbon fiber polymer reinforcement (CFPR) rod have been used to measure strains in concrete structures [17]. It has been concluded from experimental results that the effective strain measurement can be obtained from the different sensors mounted along the rod. From the results it can be concluded that in-situ monitoring of strains in different engineering structure is possible.

In [18] comparative test results between the performance of electrical resistance strain gauges (ERSG) and fiber-optic sensors (FOS) based on in-fiber Bragg grating technology for monitoring health of structures are reported. The results have shown a close comparison of the data obtained between different methods of strain measurement.

Micro-Opto-Electro-Mechanical Systems (MOEMS) acoustic sensors have been employed to detect acoustic emissions (AE) for Structural Health Monitoring (SHM) [19].

Acoustic sensing cantilevers (~ 200 x 100 x 50 μm) with variable frequency response, directionality and dynamic range have been fabricated in large quantity using a novel non-silicon process. The packaged sensors are low-cost, easy-to-install and ElectroMagnetic Interference (EMI) free during operation. The acoustic sensors' broadband sensitivity is demonstrated by standard structural break tests.

A wireless embedded system that performs active ultrasonic SHM has been reported in [20]. The proposed Shimmer platform is an autonomous, battery-less system, powered by an energy harvester, which uses 16 piezoelectric sensors/actuators attached to the structure surface for SHM analysis. The collected data (4MB) are analyzed by the on-board DSP and the result is transmitted using the 6LoWPAN protocol with IEEE802.15.4 transceiver working at 915MHz. The significant challenge is running such intense analysis on the collected data with only energy harvesting as a power source.

Sensors used for monitoring the health of structures are critical and their damage will create important issues in SHM. Y. Matsushiba and H. Nishi have proposed data-distributed fault-tolerant sensor network system for a SHM system [21-22]. The proposed system consists of three functions, PING (Packet InterNet Groper) based Network Monitoring function (PNM), backup node selecting function (BNS) and socket communication function. The proposed system has been implemented on PCs and has been practically evaluated in a laboratory environment on test bed system.

The inherent limitations of WSN such as low-bandwidth wireless communication, limited resources on wireless sensors nodes need to be addressed for a successful SHM system. A multi-scale strategy in WSNs for SHM has been proposed in [23]. The approach, called the Auto-Correlation Function and Cross-Correlation Function (ACF-CCF), utilizes the autocorrelation function of individual sensor node to detect the existence of damage and the cross-correlation function of designated node pairs to obtain damage location.

The signal processing issues related to SHM have been described in [24]. The key components of the SHM process include data acquisition and normalization, feature extraction and information condensation and statistical model development.

Piezoelectric based distributed sensors are embedded to investigate the deformation and deflection of the buried pipes due to unexpected and external loadings [25]. The vibration and frequency response of a modeled pipeline integrated with piezoelectric sensors has been investigated to identify, locate and quantify the structural performance of the system.

The requirements of sensors for monitoring the health of structures are to be cheap, replaceable, durable, low-power requirements and on-site artificial intelligence which will be useful to distinguish the abnormal behavior from normal one. The damage detection techniques should be developed which can recognize when damage has occurred and provide direction to the location of the damage [26].

The SHiMmer, a wireless platform for sensing and actuation that combines localized processing with energy harvesting to provide long-lived structural health monitoring has been reported in [27]. It has been reported that with the use of super-capacitor the life-cycle of the node has been significantly extended.

The development of an integrated structural health monitoring and reporting (SHMR) system for use on Navy aircraft has been discussed in [28]. Wireless sensors included strain gauges, accelerometers and thermocouples and wired sensors included gyroscopes, accelerometers and magnetometers have been used. The data from an embedded Global Positioning System (GPS) provided position, velocity and precise timing information.

The authors have reported the development of an all-digital excitation and sensing techniques to reduce the size of the hardware and power requirements of the system used for SHM [29].

For an energy harvesting WSN, it is important for the task scheduler to adapt the task complexity and maximize the accuracy of the tasks within the constraints of limited energy reserves. A task scheduler has been proposed for the sensing systems for SHM [30]. It is based on a Linear Regression Model embedded with Dynamic Voltage and Frequency Scaling (DVFS) functionality.

The feasibility of using electrical reflectometry method for fault location on concrete anchors has been explored in [31]. Concrete dams and other large civil structures utilize steel cable anchors to improve strength and stability. Reflectometry methods are suitable to determine the location of faults and quantization of possible deterioration on concrete anchors.

To employ WSN for SHM application, system requirements are need to be considered. In [32] the system requirements posed by SHM applications have been considered to assess potential candidates for the protocols in WSN for SHM. The authors have concluded that none of the commonly available protocols satisfy all the requirements associated with SHM systems. So there is a necessity to modify the existing protocols or it may be good to design an entirely new protocol to completely satisfy the requirements of WSN for SHM applications.

T. Harms, S. Sedigh and F. Bastianini [33] have described a complete overview of emerging wireless sensor networks for autonomous SHM systems, their application, the power use and sources needed to support autonomy and the type of communication that allows remote monitoring.

A proper analysis of raw data from sensors is very important to conclude the real and accurate prediction of health of structures. Many algorithms are proposed for the analysis. Ling Yu et.al., [34, 35] have proposed a Principal Component Analysis (PCA) based and an Ant Colony Optimization (ACO) based algorithm techniques to apply in SHM systems.

The authors have summarized the most important measurement results of standard POF (Polymer Optical Fiber) and PF GI POF (PerFluorinated Graded-Index Polymer Optical Fiber), their strain and external disturbances with respect to their applicability of SHM [36].

The authors have presented an algorithm [37] for real-time SHM during earthquake events using only acceleration measurements and infrequently measured displacement motivated by global positioning system. The developed algorithm has identified a nonlinear baseline model including hysteretic dynamics and permanent deformation using convex integral-based fitting methods and piecewise linear least squares fitting.

The authors [38] have presented a prototype wireless system for the detection of active fatigue cracks in aging railway bridges in real-time. The system is based on a small low-cost sensor node, called an AEPod, that has four acoustic emission (AE) channels and a strain channel for sensing, as well as the capability to communicate in a wireless fashion with other nodes and a base station.

A new type of passive wireless sensor based on resonant RF cavities has been reported [39]. The significant problems in the installation and long term use of wired sensors have been eliminated. The resonant frequency is being modulated by a measurand. A probe inside the cavity couples RF signals from the cavity to an externally attached antenna. The sensor can then be interrogated remotely using microwave pulse-echo techniques.

A wireless, multisensory inspection system for nondestructive evaluation of materials has been described [40].

2 Characteristics of Sensors for Monitoring Health of Structures

The sensors are the fundamental element for monitoring the health of structures. There are different types of sensors available and to be chosen depending on the applications. A few sensors such as strain gauges, accelerometers, temperature, acoustic emission sensors are very commonly used sensors used for monitoring the health of structures. Nowadays, the fibre optic based sensor systems are becoming very popular due to their different advantages compared to other sensors. The selection of sensors, cost, number of sensors and their placements, protection against mechanical and chemical damage, reduction of noise, and the collection of more representative data are the few things considered for the sensors used for health monitoring. The sensitivity of sensors to moisture and humidity is another concern, especially when long-term measurement is planned, particularly in a harsh environment. Special provisions are often needed to protect the sensors in order to obtain acceptable measurements. Since the sensors are planned to be used for a long duration, the energy harvesting may also need to be considered. The sensors considered for health monitoring of structures are usually smart wireless sensors as wired sensors may not be a cheap and simple option for this type of applications. The sensors along with signal conditioning in combination with a microcontroller/microprocessor all come in the same package and can be defined as smart sensors or smart wireless sensors. Usually the smart sensors have the ability to compensate for random errors, can adapt to changes in the environment, can adjust non-linearities to give a linear output, have the provision of self-calibration and self-diagnosis of fault. The smart sensors have their own standard, IEEE 1451 so that they can be used in a 'plug-and-play' manner. The following characteristics are very important for the selection of sensors used for monitoring the health of structures.

a) Range

It is defined as the limits between which the inputs of the sensor can vary. It is very important for the sensors used for health monitoring of structures as the maximum input applied to the sensor may be unknown in many instances. The sensors should not be damaged at that abnormal condition.

b) Sensitivity

The sensors used for health monitoring should be sensitive enough to give correct information on the effect of the input signal. The sensitivity is the relationship between output and input and is also used to indicate about the change of output to inputs other than being measured, such as environmental parameter changes. It is desirable that the sensitivity of the sensors to the environmental parameter changes is ideally zero or should be very small so that it can be easily negligible.

c) Accuracy

It is a measure of the closeness of the actual output to the ideal output of the sensor. It is an indication of the extent by which the measurement is wrong. It is the summation of all the possible errors that are likely to occur and it also depends on the calibration method. The accuracy may be represented either in absolute value or may be in percentage of the full range output.

d) Stability

The sensors used for SHM are in service continuously over many years. The sensors should be stable enough to give the same output for a constant input over a period of time. With respect to stability, a term 'drift' is used to describe the change in output that occurs over time. It is expressed as a percentage of the full range output.

e) Repeatability

This is very important for any sensors especially for the sensors used for SHM. It is the ability to give the same amount of output for repeated applications to the same amount of input. It is also termed as 'reproducibility'. The error is usually expressed as a percentage of the full range output:

$$\text{Repeatability} = \frac{\text{Maximum Output (for an input) - Minimum Output (for the same input)}}{\text{Full Range}} * 100$$

It is expected that the repeatability of the sensors used for SHM should be better than 0.01%.

f) Static and dynamic characteristics

While the sensors are used for SHM, the static and dynamic characteristics of the sensors such as rise time, time constant and settling time should be looked into for selection. In some situation the slow response of the sensors may not be very critical for SHM applications. While the sensors are subjected to a dynamic input condition, the response should be free from hysteresis.

g) Energy Harvesting

The sensors employed for SHM are used for many years. So it may be a good idea to investigate some kind of energy harvesting option so that the sensors will be self-sufficient.

h) Compensation due to change of temperature and other environmental parameters

The responses of the sensors are usually affected due to change of ambient temperature, humidity and other environmental parameters. To reduce the effect of the external influences, adequate compensation schemes must be included in the signal conditioning part of the sensors.

3 Analyzing Techniques for SHM

The sensors raw data are analyzed to derive the information of the status of the health of the structures. Usually the sensors are wireless sensors distributed over a large area. The raw data can be collected from the sensors through wireless communication and all data can be gathered in the central processor situated at a far distant. For the transmission of data, a comparison has been made between a single-hop data transmission and multi-hop data transmission [1]. It has been shown that the throughput of a single source node decreases as the number of hops increase. This is due to the interference from 2- or 3-hop nodes, even though the radio range is only one hop [1].

One of the requirements of employing WSN for SHM is that the amount of wireless communication required by the algorithm to be as minimum as possible to save energy and decrease packet loss rate [22]. The sensor node should be light weight. Moreover, the resource consuming algorithms are not suitable to be implemented in smart sensor nodes. The whole software design should be such that is should be able to accommodate energy saving strategies like wakeup and sleep scheduling. The algorithm should be developed to minimize false-positive and false-negative indication of damage. The software should be able to detect damage at an early stage and should also provide the location of the damage. A combination of ACF (Auto-correlation function) and CCF (Cross-correlation function) can be useful for SHM. If there is any damage in the structure, the ACF of the obtained time series will be different from those obtained from the undamaged structure. It is expected that the ACF is sensitive to damage but not to input/environmental changes. If the ACF algorithm provides indication of damage then the CCF is used to locate the damage. The sensor nodes deployed on the structure are divided as node pairs. Each node pair covers an area of the structure where the node pair is located. If damage occurs in that area, the dynamic relationship of the two nodes in the node pair will be changed. The CCF of the two nodes will be altered correspondingly.

To obtain correct information from optical fibre based strain sensors a considerable effort in signal de-multiplexing is required to realize practical systems [4]. The strain measurements were made separately recording the wavelength of the maxima in reflection from each Bragg grating. Two forms of electronically tunable optical filters were developed as de-multiplexing systems.

One method which is very useful in SHM analysis is distributed processing – network intelligence [10]. The intelligent sensing network must produce intelligent responses to the sensed environment and it should be on-line. The response should be produced by self-organization: it is emergent behavior of the system. The SHM problem involves multiple inter-related hierarchical sub-tasks (e.g. damage detection, evaluation, diagnosis, prognosis and repair). The approach assumes that single cells may make fast and automatic responses to critical emergencies, while collection of cells may solve more complex hierarchical tasks including [10]:

i) Self-calibration and discrimination between component and sensor failures;
ii) Formation of a dynamic artificial neural network, characterizing the nature of possible damage and producing a self-organizing diagnosis;
iii) Self-scheduling of secondary inspections, maintenance or corrective actions based on information from the network while issuing warnings;
iv) Direction of recovery resources, human or robotic, to the repair site [10].

Determining desirable and quantitative information from the raw data observed by SHM may be equivalent to solving an inverse problem. Optimization procedures are often used to solve such inverse problem because optimum values are easier to obtain the exact values, and good enough for practical use.

Ant Colony Optimization (ACO) algorithms has been proposed to be sued for SHM analysis [10, 35, 36]. The algorithms use the ability of agents to interact indirectly through changes in their environment by depositing pheromones and forming a pheromone trail. A form of autocatalytic behavior – allelomimesis: the probability with which an ant chooses a trail increases the number of ants that choose the same path in the past has also been employed. In the algorithm, ants are implemented as communication packets, policies are implemented via appropriate message passing, cells are responsible for interpreting received packets or sending packets. Since ants cannot move into the cells with broken communication links, they are supposed to find the shortest paths around them using positively reinforced pheromone trails. In general, the ACO approach attempts to solve an optimization problem by iterating the following two steps:

i) Candidate solutions are constructed in a probabilistic way by using a probability distribution over the search space,
ii) the candidate solutions are used to modify the probability distribution in a way that is deemed to bias future sampling towards high quality solutions.

An adaptive sensing approach based monitoring can be effective method of SHM [13]. The strain sensors can be used as the primary asset for health indication through schedules-based experimental load ratings to assess structural deterioration and determine up-to-date structural capacity. During the intermediate periods between load ratings, sensor can monitor continuously to detect any anomalies to indicate any external failure triggering events. The approach is well suited to wireless network based instrumentation as the system demands are within the power and bandwidth limitations. During the majority of time, vibration would be monitored locally by the sensor nodes to maintain ultralow- power consumption.

For successful SHM, fault tolerant sensor network for SHM has to be developed [21, 22, 24]. To implement this, distributed and data shared sensor network is indispensable. It is difficult to implement complex data sharing method in sensor network system due to its limited processing power and network bandwidth. The simple and effective data sharing method for fault-tolerance is inter-sharing of sampled data among sensor nodes. This sharing method may be influenced by the topology of the sensor network system which can be changed dynamically by both faulty nodes and link disconnections. The sensor node sends data to server at a regular or specific time. If the data backup timing is synchronized with the time when sensor node sends data to server, network throughput and processing load of sensor node will be increased rapidly according to the growth of data sharing throughput. Backup or data sharing node can be selected from all nodes of the sensor network. This means that the latency and throughput of backup is changeable by the distance between original node and backup node. If backup node is close to original node, synchronized backup is preferable. Thus, backup rate or timing should be controlled by the distance.

It is not easy to measure damage directly from the sensors' data obtained in SHM [23]. Many parameters must be measured throughout the structure and should be utilized to assess the health of the structure. It is important to know the type, number and placement of sensors on the structure, which are problem dependent. The following methods of analysis are quite common in relation to SHM:

a) Normalization: It is applied to account for changes in structural response due to environmental conditions or structural loads which are not associated with any structural damage. Some parameters, such as elastic modules of a structure, being temperature- dependent may have a significant effect on the dynamic of the structure. Normalization is required to ensure that the changes in the dynamics of the structure are due to change in temperature or any other environmental parameters, and is not interpreted as damage. Gain normalization is utilized by dividing the response by its peak amplitude or standard deviation. Once the effects of environmental changes are compensated, the remaining changes in the measured response are a direct result of changes in the structural state. Normalization is closely related to calibration. It is defined as the transformation of sensor output to a nominal value based on a known input and specified environmental conditions. Calibration does not, however, account for any effects the environment may have on a structure's dynamics.

b) Feature Extraction: It is the process of computing metrics from sensor signals that have the potential to discriminate among the structural states to be identified. Desirable features are ones that are responsive to the structural damage states, yet insensitive to other factors. In many situations, the features are generated from simulation analysis.

c) Dimensionality Reduction: To simplify the problem, only a selected number of features are used. The feature selection is the process of finding a subset of the original features. It can be categorized into filter methods and wrapper methods. In a filter method, relevant features are determined solely based on attributes computed from the data. But, for the wrapper approaches, it is determined based on how well a subset of features performs when used in a classifier. Another method of dimensional reduction is to project the original feature space into a lower dimensional space. Principal Component Analysis (PCA) is commonly used for that. It is the optimum projection in the sense of capturing the maximum data variance for any specified number of basis vectors.

The Collaborative Damage Event Detection (CBED) method is quite useful in SHM [22]. In this method, each note continuously collects measured responses and checks the existence of any abrupt changes, which is assumed to be the indication of damage. In the case of abrupt responses, it communicates with neighbors to confirm the existence of damage. Usually damage on structures is accumulated slowly and doesn't incur abrupt changes. It is also difficult to distinguish the change caused by the real damage from the one caused by environmental conditions (noise or input change) and is prone to giving false positive alarms.

4 Conclusions

This paper has reviewed some technical literature on the subject of sensors and technologies used for monitoring the health of structures. The subject is gaining importance in recent times and new sensors cum technologies are reported continuously. It is a very demanding and complex area and a lot of issues are to be considered for a perfect solution. The fabricated sensor systems should be able to inspect or measure without doing any harm or damage of the system. They should also be robust to poor signal-to-noise ratio compared to the level of damage they are trying to detect in the critical infrastructure. Finally, they need to be highly reliable and operate without input for long periods of time, potentially over years. It is expected that the interest in this field is ensured by the constant supply of emerging modalities, techniques and engineering solutions, as well as an increasing need from aging structures, many of the basic concepts and strategies have already matured and now offer opportunities to build upon.

References

[1] Choi, H., Choi, S., Cha, H.: Structural Health Monitoring System Based on Strain Gauge Enabled Wireless Sensor Node. In: Proceedings of the Fifth International Conference on Netwroked Sensing Systems, Kanazawa, Japan, June 17-19, pp. 211–214 (2008)

[2] Maenaka, K.: MEMS Inertial Sensors and Their Applications. In: Proceedings of the Fifth International Conference on Netwroked Sensing Systems, Kanazawa, Japan, June 17-19, pp. 71–73 (2008)

[3] Baptista, F.G., Filho, J.V.: 'A New Impedance Measurement System for PZT-Based Structural Health Monitoring. IEEE Transactions on Instrumentation and Measurements 58(10), 3602–3608 (2009)
[4] Foote, P.D., Read, I.: Optical Sensors for Aerospace Structural Monitoring. IEE Colloquium on Optical Techniques for Structural Monitoring, 2/1–2/6 (April 28, 1995)
[5] Kim, D.H., Feng, M.Q.: Real-Time Structural Health Monitoring Using a Novel Fiber-Optic Accelerometer System. IEEE Sensors Journal 7(4), 536–543 (2007)
[6] Michie, W.C., Thursby, G., Walsh, D., Culshaw, B., Konstantaki, M.: Distributed Sensing of Physical and Chemical Parameters for Structural Monitoring. IEE Colloquium on Optical Techniques for Structural Monitoring , 9/1–9/6 (April 28, 1995)
[7] Bo-lin, S., Bi-feng, S., Fei, C.: New Sensors Technologies in Aircraft Structural Health Monitoring. In: Proceedings of the 2008 International Conference on Condition Monitoring and Diagnosis, Beijing, China, April 21-24, pp. 1–4 (2008)
[8] Niu, J., Deng, Z., Zhou, F., Cao, Z., Liu, Z., Zhu, F.: A Structural Health Monitoring System Using Wireless Sensor Network". In: Proceedings of the 5th International Conference on Wireless Communication, Networking and Mobile Computing, Beijing, China, September 24-26, pp. 1–4 (2009)
[9] Anastasi, G., Lo Re, G., Ortolani, M.: WSNs for Structural Health Monitoring of Historical Buildings. In: Proceedings of the 2nd Human Systems Interactions 2009, Catania, Italy, May 21-23, pp. 574–579 (2009)
[10] Hedley, M., Hoschke, N., Johnson, M., Lewis, C., Murdoch, A., Price, D., Prokopenko, M., Scott, A., Wang, P., Farmer, A.: Sensor Network for Structural Health Monitoring. In: Proceedings of the 2004 Intelligent Sensors, Sensor Networks and Information Processing Conference, Melbourne, Australia, December 14-17, pp. 361–366 (2004)
[11] Wang, D.H., Liao, W.H.: Instrumentation of a Wireless Transmission System for Health Monitoring of Large Infrastructures. In: Proceedings of the 2001 IEEE Instrumentation and Measurements Technology Conference 2001, Budapest, Hungary, May 21-23, pp. 634–639 (2001)
[12] Sazonov, E., Li, H., Curry, D., Pillay, P.: Self-Powered Sensors for Monitoring of Highway Bridges. IEEE Sensors Journal 9(11), 1422–1429 (2009)
[13] Whelan, M.J., Gangone, M.V., Janoyan, K.D.: Highway Bridge Assessment Using an Adaptive Real-Time Wireless Sensor Network. IEEE Sensors Journal 9(11), 1405–1413 (2009)
[14] Merlino, P., Abramo, A.: An Integrated Sensing/Communication Architecture for Structural Health Monitoring. IEEE Sensors Journal 9(11), 1397–1404 (2009)
[15] Chin, J.C., Rautenberg, J.F., Ma, C.Y.T., Pujol, S., Yau, D.K.Y.: An Experimental Low-Cost, Low-Data-Rate Rapid Structural Assessment Network. IEEE Sensors Journal 9(11), 1361–1369 (2009)
[16] da Costa Antunes, P.F., et al.: Optical Fiber Accelerometer System for Structural Dynamic Monitoring. IEEE Sensors Journal 9(11), 1347–1354 (2009)
[17] Kerrouche, A., Boyle, W.J.O., Sun, T., Grattan, K.T.V., Schmidt, J.W., Taljsten, B.: Strain Measurement Using Embedded Fiber Bragg Grating Sensors Inside an Anchored Carbon Fiber Polymer Reinforcement Prestressing Rod for Structural Monitoring. IEEE Sensors Journal 9(11), 1456–1461 (2009)

[18] Grattan, S.K.T., Taylor, S.E., Sun, T., Basheer, P.A.M., Grattan, K.T.V.: In Situ Cross-Calibration of In-Fiber Bragg Grating and Electrical Resistance Strain Gauges for Structural Monitoring Using an Extensometer. IEEE Sensors Journal 9(11), 1355–1360 (2009)

[19] Zhang, Y., Tsai, J., Li, G.P., Feng, M.Q., Bachman, M.: MOEMS Acoustic Sensors for Structural Health Monitoring. In: Proceedings of IEEE Sensors Conference, Waikaloa, Hawaii, November 1-4, pp. 2311–2315 (2010)

[20] Dondi, D., Di Pompeo, A., Tenti, C., Simunić Rosing, T.: Shimmer: a Wireless Harvesting Embedded System for Active Ultrasonic Structural Health Monitoring. In: Proceedings of IEEE Sensors Conference, Waikaloa, Hawaii, November 1-4, pp. 2325–2328 (2010)

[21] Matsushiba, Y., Nishi, H.: Structural Health Monitoring System Considering Fault-tolerance. In: Proceedings of the IEEE International Conference on Industrial Informatics (INDIN 2008), Daejeon, Korea, July 13-16, pp. 330–335 (2008)

[22] Matsushiba, Y., Nishi, H.: Effective Data Sharing System for Fault Tolerant Structural Health Monitoring System. In: Proceedings of the 11th IEEE International Workshop on Advanced Motion Control, Nagaoka, Japan, March 21-24, pp. 76–81 (2010)

[23] Liu, X., Cao, J., Xu, Y., Wu, H., Liu, Y.: A Multi-Scale Strategy in Wireless Sensor Networks for Structural Health Monitoring. In: Proceedings of the 5th International Conference on Intelligent Sensors, Sensor Networks and Information Processing, Melbourne, Australia, December 7-10, pp. 361–366 (2009)

[24] DeSimio, M.P., Olson, S.E., Montes de Oca, J.A., Derriso, M.M.: Signal Processing Issues Related to Structural Health Monitoring. In: Proceedings of the 41st Asilomar Conference on Signals, Systems and Computers, Pacific Grove, California, USA, November 4-7, pp. 843–847 (2007)

[25] Dezfouli, S., Zabihollah, A.: Structural Health Monitoring of Buried Pipelines under Static Dislocation and Vibration. In: 2010 IEEE/ASME International Conference on Mechatronics and Embedded Systems and Applications, July 15-17. IEEE Computer Society Press, Los Alamitos (2010), doi:10.1109/MESA.2010.5552052.

[26] Shrive, N.G.: Intelligent Structural Health Monitoring: a Civil Engineering Perspective. In: Proceedings of the 2005 IEEE International Conference on Systems, Man and Cybernetics, October 10-12, pp. 1973–1977. IEEE Computer Society Press, Los Alamitos (2005), IEEE DOI: 10.1109/ICSNC.2005.1571436

[27] Musiani, D., Lin, K., Simunic Rosing, T.: Active Sensing Platform for Wireless Structural Health Monitoring. In: Proceedings of the 2007 International Conference on Information Processing in Sensors Network, ISNP 2007, Cambridge, Massachusetts, USA, April 25-27, pp. 390–399 (2007)

[28] Arms, S.W., Galbreath, J.H., Townsend, C.P., Churchill, D.L., Corneau, B., Ketchan, R.P., Pham, N.: Energy Harvesting Wireless Sensors and Networked Timing Synchronization for Aircraft Structural Health Monitoring. In: Proceedings of the 1st International Conference on Wireless Communication, Vehicular Technology, Information Theory and Aerospace & Electronic Systems Technology (Wireless VITAE), Aalborg, Denmark, May 17-20, pp. 16–20 (2009)

[29] Kim, J., Grisso, B.L., Ha, D.S., Inman, D.J.: An All-Digital Low-Power Structural Health Monitoring System. In: Proceedings of the 2007 IEEE Conference on Technologies for Homeland Security, Woburn, MA, USA, May 16-17, pp. 123–128 (2007)

[30] Ravinagarajan, A., Dondi, D., Simunic Rosing, T.: DVFS Based Task Scheduling in a Harvesting WSN for Structural Health Monitoring. In: Proceedings of the 2010 Conference on Design, Automation and Test in Europe, Dresden, Germany, March 8-12, pp. 1518–1523 (2010)
[31] Furse, C., Smith, P., Diamond, M.: Feasibility of Reflectometry for Nondestructive Evaluation of Prestressed Concrete Anchors. IEEE Sensors Journal 9(11), 1322–1329 (2009)
[32] Wijetunge, S., Gunawardana, U., Liyanapathirana, R.: Wireless Sensors networks for Structural Health Monitoring: Considerations for Communication Protocol Design. In: Proceedings of the 17th International Conference on telecommunication, Doga, Qatar, April 4-7, pp. 694–699 (2010)
[33] Harms, T., Sedigh, S., Bastianini, F.: Structural Health Monitoring of Bridges Using Wireless Sensor Networks. IEEE Instrumentation and Measurement Magazine, 14–18 (December 2010)
[34] Yu, L., Zhu, J.H., Chen, L.J.: Parametric Study on PCA-based Algorithm for Structural Health Monitoring. In: Proceedings of the 2010 Prognostic & System Health Management Conference (PHM 2010), Macau, January 12-14 (2010) paper: MU3072
[35] Yu, L., Xu, P.: An ACO-based Algorithm for Structural Health Monitoring. In: Proceedings of the 2010 Prognostic & System Health Management Conference (PHM 2010), Macau, January 12-14 (2010) paper: MU3053
[36] Liehr, S., Lenke, P., Wendt, M., Krebber, K., Seeger, M., Thiele, E., Metschies, H., Gebreselassie, B., Munich, J.C.: Polymer Optical Fiber Sensors for Distributed Strain Measurement and Application in Structural Health Monitoring. IEEE Sensors Journal 9(11), 1330–1338 (2009)
[37] Hann, C.E., Singh-Levett, I., Deam, B.L., Mander, J.B., Chase, J.G.: Real-Time System Identification of a Nonleaner Four-Story Steel Frame Structure – Application to Structural Health Monitoring. IEEE Sensors Journal 9(11), 1339–1346 (2009)
[38] Ledeczi, A., Hay, T., Volgyesi, P., Hay, D.R., Nadas, A., Jayaraman, S.: Wireless Acoustic Emission Sensor Network for Structural Health Monitoring. IEEE Sensors Journal 9(11), 1370–1377 (2009)
[39] Thomson, D.J., Card, D., Bridges, G.E.: RF Cavity Passive Wireless Sensors with Time-Domain Gating-Based Interrogation for SHM of Civil Structures. IEEE Sensors Journal 9(11), 1430–1438 (2009)
[40] Friedrich, M., Dobie, G., Chan, C.C., Pierce, S.G., Galbraith, W., Marshall, S., Hayword, G.: Miniature Mobile Sensor Platforms for Condition Monitoring of Structures. IEEE Sensors Journal 9(11), 1439–1448 (2009)

Self-sustaining Wireless Acoustic Emission Sensor System for Bridge Monitoring

Ákos Lédeczi[1], Péter Völgyesi[1], Eric Barth[1], András Nádas[1], Alexander Pedchenko[1], Thomas Hay[2], and Subash Jayaraman[2]

[1] Vanderbilt University,
Nashville, TN, USA
akos.ledeczi@vanderbilt.edu
[2] Waves in Solids LLC
State College,
PA, USA
thomhay@wavesinsolids.com

Abstract. A novel approach to structural monitoring of bridges is presented. Acoustic emission sensing has been constrained to hardwired systems up till now because the processing of high bandwidth sensor data on multiple channels requires a lot of energy. The presented prototype wireless system for the real-time detection of active fatigue cracks in bridges overcomes this problem by utilizing a low-power Flash FPGA for signal processing, a novel vibration energy harvester and a sophisticated sleep scheduler.

1 Introduction

There are close to 33,000 steel railroad bridges and 600,000 highway bridges in the United States, over 30% of which are structurally deficient or functionally obsolete [1]. Currently, highway bridges in the U.S. are mostly inspected visually [2]. Such inspection only detects an estimated 3.9 percent of existing fatigue cracks [3] Most bridges that people utilize every day were built at least 50 years ago, and were not designed to withstand today's demanding traffic loads.

One of the most comprehensive bridge testing methods is based on acoustic emissions (AE). AE are the stress waves produced by the sudden internal stress redistribution of the materials caused by the changes in the internal structure. Possible causes include crack initiation and growth, crack opening and closure, and dislocation movement among others. Most of the sources of AE are damage-related; thus, the detection and monitoring of these emissions are commonly used to predict material failure [13]. When load is applied to a fracture-critical member with an existing fatigue crack, stress concentration around the crack tip can eventually cause brittle fracture. Acoustic emission is generated from growing fatigue cracks when a fracture-critical member is stressed. The growing fatigue crack generates a stress wave that travels through the member and can be detected by an AE sensor as well as accurately localized by multiple such sensors using a Time Difference of Arrival (TDOA) method.

S.C. Mukhopadhyay (Ed.): New Developments in Sensing Technology for SHM, LNEE 96, pp. 15–39.
springerlink.com

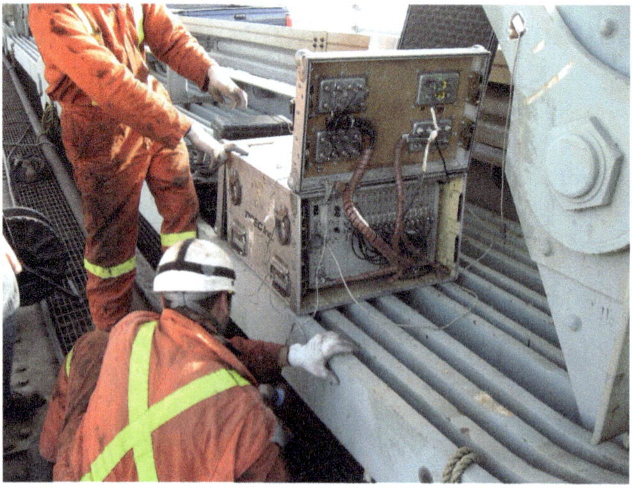

Fig. 1 Wired Bridge Testing

Current AE measurement systems based on hardwired centralized data collection are expensive, power hungry and heavy. This is because AE are high frequency signals and the speed of sound in steel is over 3000 m/s. Hence, detection, feature extraction and accurate source localization requires over 1 MHz sampling rates on multiple channels. Figure 1 shows a typical data collection unit during an inspection. The system is powered by a 1000 Watt power generator and requires long cables (30-200ft) to reach the fracture-critical bridge components where the AE sensors are installed. Just setting up the system takes several hours. Moreover, the expensive equipment needs to be protected against theft and vandalism. Today these systems are used for the occasional inspection of a few selected bridges. However, the importance of real time detection of damage in a critical structural component at an early stage was recently evident in the case of the Oakland Bay Bridge. During retrofitting of the bridge for improved seismic performance, an unexpected crack of dangerous proportions was accidentally discovered on September 7, 2009, prompting complete closure of the bridge due to safety reasons. The bridge could be opened to traffic only after the unscheduled expensive replacement of the affected component was completed. Timely detection of the damage before assuming dangerous proportions would have allowed convenient scheduling of strengthening or replacement of the affected component at significantly lesser cost. This event underscores the obvious need for a cost-effective system that is able to continuously and autonomously monitor the structural health of bridges.

The current state-of-the-art is illustrated by the replacement of the collapsed I-35W Mississippi River Bridge in Minneapolis, Minnesota. The new bridge has an integrated monitoring system that is completely wired both for power and communication [4]. The main reason a current system must be wired is the lack of self sustainability. Current energy harvesting and power management techniques are insufficient to sustain prolonged sensing and monitoring especially if wireless communication is utilized which is notoriously power-hungry. While the cost of a wired system is negligible compared to that of a new bridge, retrofitting the thousands of existing bridges with miles of cables each is cost-prohibitive.

The main requirements for a bridge monitoring system then are as follows. A single structure needs to be instrumented with a high number of sensors to cover all critical components. All system components need to rely on energy harvesting since the availability of power near the sensors cannot be assumed and long-term unsupervised operation is desired. Sensor nodes distributed across the bridge need to communicate wirelessly since wiring long bridges is not economical. The system needs to be able to communicate with a central monitoring center to report on the status of the bridge. Finally, the system needs to be low cost to enable instrumentation of a large number of bridges.

The remainder of this paper presents the prototype system that meets these requirements enabling the continuous monitoring of railways bridges. We also present out ongoing work toward extending the technology to highway bridges. The next sections will provide a detailed description of the sensor node requirements and design. This is followed by a short description of the signal processing algorithms. The main enabler of the extended operation of the system is a novel vibration energy harvesting technique that is introduced in the subsequent section. Then an overview of the overall system architecture and operation is presented, followed by a summary of the wireless network protocols and offline data evaluation methodology. The paper then concludes with initial test results and our planned future work.

2 Sensor Node

A fatigue crack generates an acoustic emission event through the rapid release of elastic energy with each step in the crack growth process. To measure such a phenomenon, an array of three or more acoustic emission sensors are placed on the fracture critical bridge member. Measuring the time of arrival of AE events then enables the localization of the active flaw within the array using standard Time Difference of Arrival (TDoA) techniques. Acoustic emission signal features may be used to estimate fatigue crack growth rates. Useful AE signal features include amplitude, rise-time, counts, signal duration, and energy.

Since an AE event is very short (< 1 msec), it contains a substantial amount of frequency information to assist in signal interpretation, and the speed of sound in steel is can range from 2500 to 5850 m/sec, the AE signal needs to be sampled at a high rate, typically at 2-3 MHz to enable feature extraction and source localization. Sampling and especially signal processing at this rate on multiple channels is the most significant design driver of a battery-powered device.

Low-power DSP chips simply do not have the horse power needed in this application. In fact, the only choice that can meet the requirements is an FPGA-based solution. However, FPGAs are not low-power thus mandating some kind of power management. Traditional FPGAs do not support sleep modes; if you power them down, you lose all configuration information. Also, initializing an FPGA incurs a current spike. However, the new flash-based FPGAs overcome these limitations. In sleep mode, their power consumption is practically zero, yet they can wake up in 1 microsecond while conserving their configuration and state. Furthermore, the power consumption in active mode is also reduced significantly. On the down side, flash-based FPGAs are not as powerful as state of the art SRAM-based FPGAs

To support the continuous operation of the node for months as opposed to hours on a single charge, the device needs to sleep most of the time. The question is then how and when to wake it up? Using one of the AE channels as a "sentry" is suboptimal since it is power hungry. This could be improved by having one such channel per system as opposed to per node, and alternate the sentry nodes, but then a relatively complex scheme needs to be implemented that wakes up the rest of the nodes using the radio. Again, the radios cannot be listening continuously either, since that is also notoriously power hungry even with low-power radios. Furthermore, having an AE event on one channel (of one node) may mean that we have already missed the same event on the other channels of the same node (and possibly all other nodes).

Instead, we employ an application-specific method that fits railway bridge monitoring especially well. AE events are only expected when a train passes over the bridge. If we can detect an oncoming train in time, we can wake up the network. As the train enters the bridge, stresses shall be applied to the bridge's fracture critical members. A strain sensor, therefore, will detect a train approaching the sensor network provided the strain is of sufficient magnitude. In our prototype, a strain gage channel is employed that is slowly sampled (typically at 1 Hz). The strain data are checked by a low-power duty-cycled microcontroller and if elevated values are observed, it wakes up the rest of the board including the AE channels and the FPGA.

While this technique works well for railway bridges, it is not applicable to highway bridges with almost continuous traffic. We are working on an adaptive algorithm that will decide when to turn on the AE channels based on a correlation of past AE events with other sensor modalities. It will try to listen to the AE channels as much as possible given the current battery charge level and the recharge rate from the energy harvester. When significant AE events are observed, it will store other sensor values that preceded these events. The algorithm will be then able to recognize common patterns and continuously adapt its triggering mechanism for the AE channels.

AE sensors come in two flavors: with or without pre-amplification. Pre-amplification is very useful since the typical AE signals are just a few microvolts. However, the preamps need excitation voltage 5V or higher. To conserve power, we opted to support AE sensors with no pre-amplifiers. To compensate for the missing sensor gain, this mandates programmable gain on the node with up to 100 dB amplification.

In addition to AE sensing and processing, the second critical requirement of the sensor node is wireless communication capability. The critical design drivers are again low-power and low cost. Many Wireless Sensor Networks (WSN)

applications have similar requirements. A few examples include military applications [6], environmental monitoring [7] or precision agriculture [8]. The most widely adopted hardware platform in this domain is IEEE 802.15.4 compliant radio nodes operating in the 2.4GHz range. Typical products provide a few hundred meter communication range, 50 mW power consumption and 250 kbps raw data rate.

Sensor Node Architecture

The first generation prototype design is illustrated in Figure 2. The four AE channels can be sampled at up to 3 MHz each. However, the resolution of the selected ADC is 12 bits, not the traditional 16 bits. At this sampling rate, higher resolution would have meant a much more complex ADC chip making the board more complicated and expensive. Data from the strain gage is used to correlate stress on the monitored structure to AE from an active fatigue crack, hence, it is connected to the FPGA. The sampling rate is a fixed 100 Hz and a 16-bit ADC is utilized. The channel has a fixed low-pass filter for anti-aliasing. The channel's equally important task is to wake up the board as trains approach, so the analog

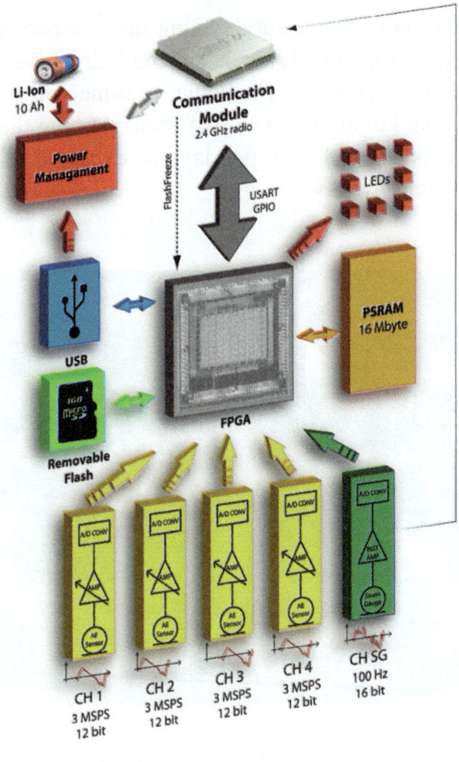

Fig. 2 AEPod Architecture

signal is also connected to one of the input channels of the microcontroller on the wireless communication module. The excitation voltage level is tunable to decrease the necessary power in sleep mode.

The on-board SD card and the provided USB connectivity increase the flexibility of the node tremendously. The SD card can store the measurements for a long deployment; it can be swapped out without having to download potentially large amounts of data. The USB provides fast data downloads and is also used to charge the battery. It is connected through the FPGA and not the microcontroller to support the highest data rates. The on-board SRAM memory can be utilized for short-term waveform storage, for example. Low power and high intensity LEDs are used to display basic status information. A real time clock is included to correlate measurements with train schedule.

The battery selected is a 10 Ah lithium ion with a small form factor. A switching regulator with high efficiency is utilized. Remaining battery capacity is monitored with a coulomb counter.

Figure 3 shows the prototype board. Table 1 summarizes the current draw of the AEPod at 3 V in active mode. Considering the utilized 10 Ah battery, the board supports approximately 80 hours of active mode. Note that these numbers do not include any wireless data download.

The data for sleep mode (with duty cycling the microcontroller to monitor the strain channel) is summarized in Table 2. The 5mA draw means that the board can sustain 2000 hours of sleep mode. The actual lifetime will depend on the ratio of active to passive mode, i.e. the frequency of trains passing through the bridge. For example, if the node is active 1 hour per day, the expected lifetime of the node on a single charge is about 6 weeks.

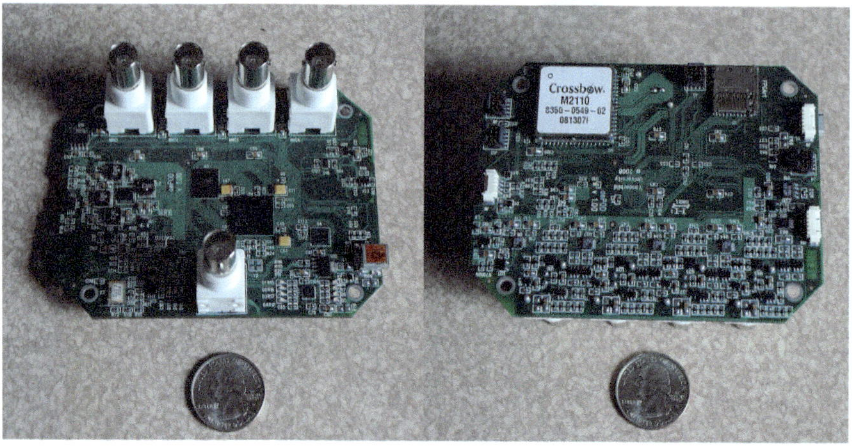

Fig. 3 First Generation Prototype

Table 1 Current draw in active mode

Component	mA
4x AE channel	48
FPGA	35
Communication module with radio off	6
Communication module with radio on	25
Strain Gage channel	3
Other components/loss	3
Power conversion efficiency	80%
Total (no radio):	~125
Total (with radio):	~150

Table 2 Current draw in sleep mode

Component	mA
4x AE channel	0
FPGA	0
Comm module (with duty cycling)	1
Strain Gage channel (lower voltage)	1
Other components/loss	2
Power conversion efficiency	80%
Total:	5

Sensor Node Revision

The prototype system proved that the flash-based FPGA technology enables high sampling rate with multiple signal streams and powerful node level data processing without significant impact on the power budget. It also demonstrated that duty cycling with smart wake-up triggers are essential for taking advantage of the benefits of the new platform (extremely fast wake-up and low static power consumption).

Based on our experience with the prototype hardware platform and taking into account additional requirements and opportunities, we have redesigned the platform. The changes add new sensor modalities to enable this platform to be used in a much wider range of applications and to provide the necessary foundation for advanced duty cycling and triggering mechanisms to be developed. Figure 4 shows the architecture of the revised sensor node.

We opted for a slightly different integrated module (Meshnetics ZigBit Amp [9]), which is code compatible with the originally used Crosbow IRIS module, but has an integrated 20dB RF amplifier providing significantly higher communication ranges eliminating many deployment constraints.

The prototype system was designed to be deployed and operational for several weeks autonomously. Now we are aiming at much longer periods between service events or any human interactions with the nodes. For this, we extended the power management subsystem with energy harvesting options. The sensor platform will support renewable energy sources with special emphasis on vibration-based energy harvesting.

Other related projects [10][11] were built around MEMS accelerometers as the single sensing source. These sensors are widely available, inexpensive and the power requirements of the sensor itself and that of the signal processing tasks are low, making this approach feasible for wireless sensor networks. We incorporated 3D MEMS accelerometers in the revised sensor platform. We also extended the prototype with additional low-frequency high-precision strain gauge channels, since these are excellent candidates for application specific wake-up triggers. Based on these sensor modalities, we will be able to use the same sensor platform in a wide range of applications where vibration, stress, ultrasonic elastic waves are good indicators of the health of the physical structure.

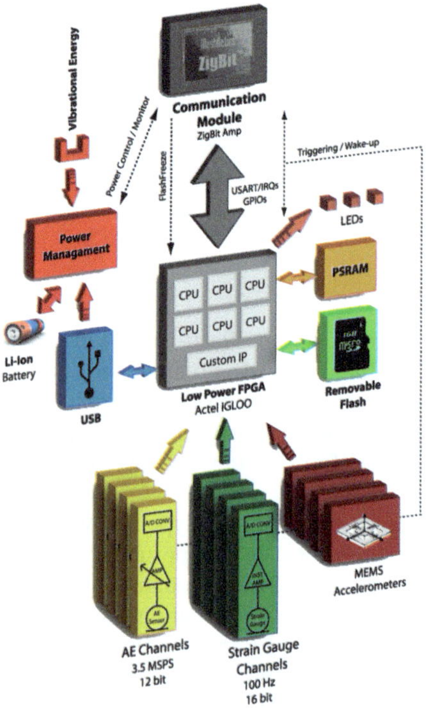

Fig. 4 Revised Sensor Node Design

Signal Processing

The objective of interpretation in acoustic emission bridge inspection is to assess the significance of sources of emission. The general approach begins with filtering out non-relevant emissions. A variety of acoustic signals occurs during the monitoring process, such as noise from loose fasteners and working members, mechanical noise transferred from the track and random electrical signals. These may mask the acoustic signals from a growing crack. Since an AE event from a growing crack has a typical, characteristic waveform, signal characteristics (features) are used to identify and filter crack-related acoustic events from noise.

AE data are evaluated in terms of activity and intensity. Activity is defined in terms of acoustic events that are detected inside the sensor array by all four sensors. Intensity is defined as the average signal strength of the acoustic events in dB:

- **Activity:** The number of events that occur within the sensing array. For an acoustic source to be classified as an event, it must be picked up by all four sensors and originate from inside the array. Activity may be classified as ***Critically Active*** if events are observed consistently at peak load, ***Active*** if randomly observed over the load spectrum, and ***Inactive***.
- **Intensity:** The average amplitude, in dB, of the events. Acoustic emission may be classified as ***Low Intensity*** (< 50 dB), ***Intense*** (50 - 75 dB), and ***Critically Intense*** (> 75 dB).

Based on AE activity and intensity, the AE source index is developed as shown in Figure 5. Activity and intensity metrics are derived from the features of the AE signals and their dependence on the load used to stimulate AE.

Feature extraction and source localization are carried out in the FPGA. The frequency response of the AE sensors themselves provides sufficient filtering [17] to enable a relatively simple time-domain based signal processing approach. This fits the problem well since the relevant AE signal features are all time-domain parameters. The configurable hardware implementation enables signal processing in a streaming manner at the sampling frequency; each sample is fully processed before the next one arrives. That is, there is no need to buffer the signals.

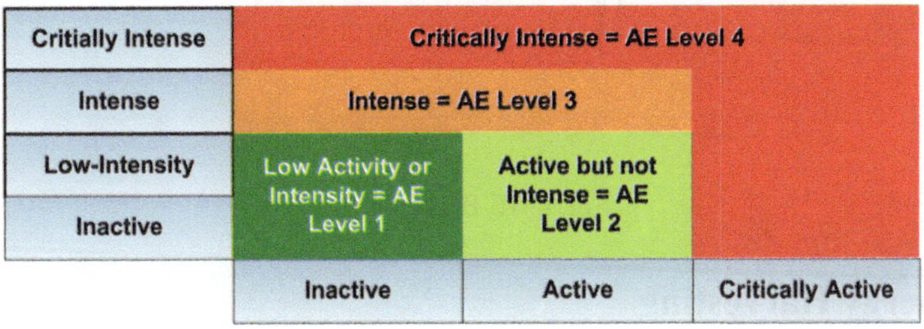

Fig. 5 AE Classification

The most important task of the processing core is to detect and measure the time of arrival of the acoustic events and to extract its characteristic features. Last but not least, the detection logic should work reliably with a few parameters to minimize the calibration requirements of the system. Figure 6 shows the time series of a typical acoustic event along with the current operational parameters (letters) and the extracted features (numbers).

The detection is triggered by a simple threshold (A) crossing condition. The start of the event (1) is the time instant of this threshold crossing. The end of the acoustic emission is identified if the signal does not cross the threshold level for longer than a timeout parameter (B). Between these two events the signal is monitored and the following features are calculated: the number of threshold crossings (using hysteresis to eliminate the effects of noise or riding waves) (5) – this is a good estimate of the fundamental frequency of the signal, maximum amplitude (4), rise time (3) – the elapsed time between the initial threshold crossing and the time when the signal reaches the maximum amplitude, the length of the event (2) – the time span between the initial and last threshold crossings and the energy of the signal (6) – sum of the squared sample values.

Events on multiple channels are then evaluated. If at least three channels detect AE, then the TDoA values are checked for consistency. If the difference between any two time stamps is larger than it takes for the sound to travel the distance between the corresponding sensors, the event could not have come from the same source. Such inconsistent observations are discarded. If the timestamps are consistent, then the source is localized using the standard TDoA equations. If the AE did not originate from within the sensor array, it is also discarded.

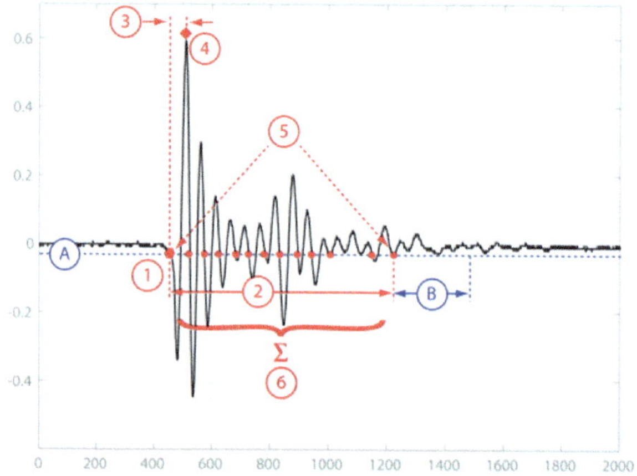

Fig. 6 AE Event Features

3 Energy Harvesting

The goal is to make the system self-sufficient from a power standpoint by harvesting kinetic energy from the structural vibrations of the bridge at, or very near, the location of each acoustic emission sensor node to provide power for its on-board sensing, processing and wireless communication functions. Given that the power harvesting for each node will be done locally and not in a centralized location, it is required to design an energy harvesting module that can accept and adapt to a broad range of excitation frequencies. The excitation frequency will vary by bridge, location of the sensor on the bridge, and traffic load on the bridge. The goal is to therefore design a modular energy harvester that will extract vibrational kinetic energy for a changing primary vibration mode by optimally changing its natural frequency.

Energy harvesters have been a growing topic of research interest and show their greatest potential for wireless sensor node applications. In particular, a survey of recent work on energy harvesters shows the greatest effectiveness for devices in the frequency range of 10-100 Hz [18]. Of the types that harvest energy from motion, three transduction methods are generally available: 1) electromagnetic, 2) electrostatic, and 3) piezoelectric. Electromagnetic transduction, in either a linear device or a rotary device, is generally not well suited for MEMS scale devices given the challenge of manufacturing coil windings and the integration of permanent magnets. Electromagnetic transduction is however practical at more macroscopic scales such as that under consideration here. Electrostatic transduction is impractical and inefficient at macroscopic scales, suitable only for the microscale [18]. Piezoelectric materials such as PZT (lead zirconate titanate) require a mechanical transmission system for scales larger than MEMS, require high voltage power electronics and are typically not well impedance matched for mechanical vibrations characterized by the amplitudes and frequencies found in a bridge structure.

Of the electromagnetic transducer variety of energy harvester, most utilize a proof mass suspended by a mechanical spring such that the mass-spring system's resonant frequency (damped natural frequency) is tuned to the largest frequency component of the excitation [19]. Commercial incarnations of this concept appear in such applications as self-winding watches and self-powered flashlights. One such shake-powered flashlight contains a 150 gram energy harvester and is able to produce 200 mW when excited at its resonant frequency of 3.3 Hz [19]. The down side of such devices is that they must be excited near their resonant frequency to generate an appreciable amount of power. A recent effort to design an energy harvester for a bridge monitoring system resulted in a device with a resonant frequency of 3.12 Hz and an energy extraction mechanism that behaved as a damper [20]. Such a system, where only the damping behavior is controlled, has relatively little ability to tune the resonant peak. Unfortunately this is typical of the research to date for such applications.

For bridge monitoring, the ability to alter the resonant frequency of the harvester to match that of the excitation frequency is imperative. Modern highway bridges posses a fundamental frequency typically in the range of 2-5 Hz, and very stiff bridges have fundamental frequencies in the range 10-15 Hz. [21]. This range is dependent on the design of the bridge, but it is also dependent on the traffic load on the bridge. The excitation frequency imparted to the harvester can therefore vary for a given bridge and even for a given time of day. For this primary reason, an energy harvester needs to be developed that has the novel ability of altering its damped natural frequency. A secondary reason to design for such an ability is to promote modularity in sensor node systems for bridges. In this way, one common sensor node system can be utilized for a wide variety of bridges. The energy harvester concept presented here offers a novel method for altering the resonant frequency by one or two orders of magnitude in real-time. To the authors' knowledge, such an approach does not currently exist.

Resonant Peak Shifting via Control

The novel harvester contains an inertial element vertically suspended in parallel by a spring and a linear generator. Alternate designs with a cantilevered mass and typical motor/generators are also possible. The extraction of vibrational kinetic energy can be accomplished through a combined design of mechanical and control elements within the harvester. The mechanical mass-spring portion of the harvester offers a device with a natural frequency designed to be in the center of the expected excitation frequency range of all bridges intended for monitoring. The control design and resulting control action results in a dynamic behavior of the linear generator that mimics a damper, a spring, and a mass. The damping behavior will be used for power extraction. The spring and inertial behaviors will require that the linear generator also act as a linear motor, and will require regenerative electronics. This spring behavior will add to, or subtract from, the influence of the mechanical spring to allow a broad range of frequency shifting of the system's overall damped natural frequency. Likewise, the mimicked inertial behavior can be used to alter the damped natural frequency. In this manner, the device will be able, in real-time, to adjust its resonant response so as to capture more energy than with a fixed resonant frequency harvester.

Referring to Figure 7, consider an energy harvester with a proof mass M and a mechanical spring with stiffness k. Declaring $y = 0$ at the static hung length of the spring with the proof mass attached under the influence of gravity, the following equation relates the absolute motion y of the proof mass to the excitation motion x as influenced by the spring force and the controllable force imparted by the voicecoil (linear generator/motor) u:

$$M\ddot{y} = u - k(y - x) . \tag{1}$$

Conventional approaches essentially dictate the voicecoil to behave as a damper acting on the relative motion of the base and the proof mass by utilizing a control law such as,

$$u = -b_c(\dot{y} - \dot{x}) . \tag{2}$$

Consider instead a control law that requires the voicecoil to behave as a damper, a spring and an inertia through the measurement and feedback of acceleration, relative velocity and relative position,

$$u = -M_c\ddot{y} - b_c(\dot{y} - \dot{x}) - k_c(y - x) . \tag{3}$$

The transfer function of the closed-loop system relating the proof mass motion to the excitation motion therefore appears as,

$$\frac{Y(s)}{X(s)}=\frac{\frac{b_c}{(M_c+M)}s+\frac{(k_c+k)}{(M_c+M)}}{s^2+\frac{b_c}{(M_c+M)}s+\frac{(k_c+k)}{(M_c+M)}}=\frac{2\xi\omega_n s+\omega_n^2}{s^2+2\xi\omega_n s+\omega_n^2}\ . \tag{4}$$

From Equation (4) it can be seen that the natural frequency of the harvester is $\omega_n=\sqrt{(k_c+k)/(M_c+M)}$. It can also be seen that for the conventional control law of Equation (2) lacking a spring-like or inertia-like behavior, the natural frequency of the harvester cannot be changed. The resulting damped natural frequency of the system can be changed only slightly. In contrast, by including a spring-like contribution and/or an inertial-like contribution to the system through the use of a non-zero value for k_c and M_c in Equation (3), it allows us to influence the natural frequency of the system and the resulting damped natural frequency by potentially orders of magnitude. The fact that both k_c and M_c can be altered in concert extends the range of adaptability of the natural frequency as limited by sensor noise in position or acceleration alone. The control approach also allows us to arbitrarily influence the amplified proof mass motion so as to magnify it as much as possible exceeding the mechanical limits of the device. Power extraction can then be optimized in real-time by optimizing the average power $\int_T b_c(\dot{y}-\dot{x})^2dt$ dependent on b_c and the height of the appropriately shifted resonant peak as influenced by all three specifiable parameters b_c, k_c and M_c.

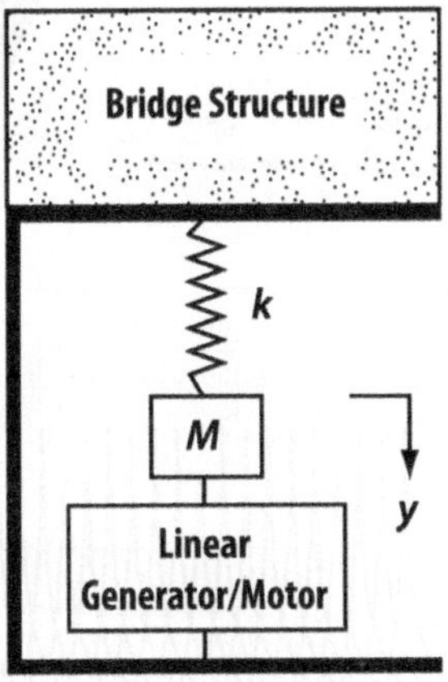

Fig. 7 Schematic of a vibrational energy harvester

Comparison of Conventional and the New Approach – a Case Study

Presented below is a case study comparing the conventional energy extractor control approach to the adaptive resonant peak shifting control approach. For this study, we will restrict our attention to varying the stiffness of the system. Similar conclusions hold for varying the inertial properties of the system. For the case presented, the proof mass M = 0.227 kg (0.5 lbs), and the mechanical spring stiffness k = 224 N/m (1.28 lbs/inch). Consider the following excitation,

$$x(t) = A\sin(\omega t) \qquad (5)$$

where the amplitude is set to unity and the frequency of excitation can take on any value between 0.1 and 20 Hz (corresponding to the expected fundamental frequencies of most bridges under most conditions).

For the conventional control approach utilizing the control law of Equation (2), Figure 8a shows a family of proof mass magnitude responses for a range of values for b_c. As can be seen, the frequency of the peak is not able to be shifted and results in low vibration amplitude when the excitation departs from the designed mechanical natural frequency of $\omega_n = \sqrt{k/M} = 5Hz$.

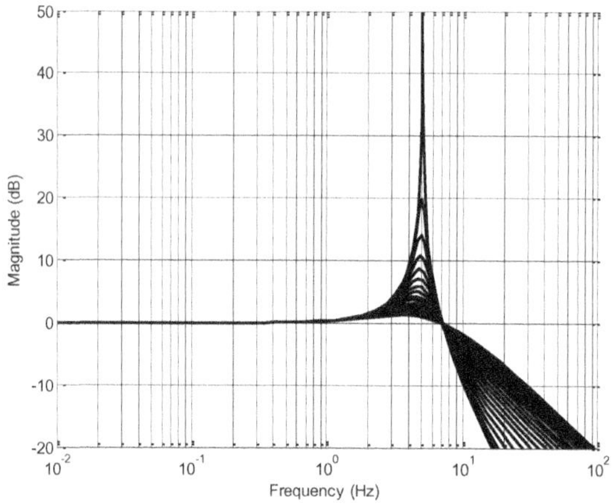

(a)

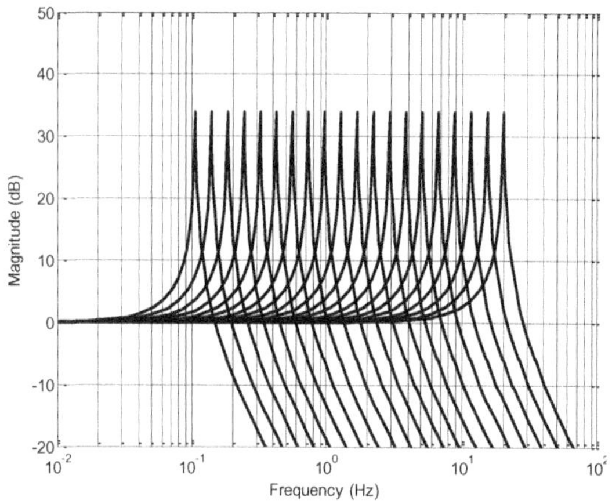

(b)

Fig. 8 Magnitude responses of the (a) proof mass for a range of controllable damping values and (b) proof mass for a range of spring and damping controller parameters

For the control approach utilizing the control law of Equation (3), Figure 8b shows a family of proof mass magnitude responses as both k_c and b_c are allowed to vary. As can be seen, the extra control degree of freedom offered by k_c in addition to b_c allows two orders of magnitude of resonant peak shifting. This allows a system capable of centering its resonance peak on excitation frequencies from 0.1 Hz to 20 Hz while maintaining a large amplitude of the proof mass for adequate power extraction. Additionally, the control law allows us to arbitrarily set the height of the peak. For the case shown below, a damping ratio of $\xi = 0.01$ was selected resulting in a magnitude of about 34 dB (an amplification in the proof mass amplitude of 50 times that of the excitation amplitude). The control parameters were set according to the frequency of excitation ω, which can be easily measured by the on-board accelerometer (ADXL330), and the desired damping ratio:

$$k_c = M\omega^2 - k\,, \tag{6}$$

$$b_c = 2M\xi\omega\,. \tag{7}$$

For the excitation frequency range of interest that would encompass nearly all bridges and bridge conditions (0.1 Hz to 20 Hz), the resulting range of controlled stiffness is -223.9 N/m to 3360.6 N/m and the resulting controlled damping coefficient range is 0.003 Ns/m to 0.57 ns/m, both well within achievable limits. It should be noted that negative stiffness values that subtract from the mechanical stiffness of the system are possible. It should also be noted that regenerative power electronics are needed to implement the control law; but these are available as off-the-shelf components.

For a common bridge frequency of 5 Hz [22], and an amplitude of 1mm (2mm peak-to-peak), the harvester will generate an average of 170 mW at 100% conversion efficiency. At a conservative estimate of 50% harvester conversion efficiency, this results in an average generated power of 85 mW. The maximum power draw from the sensor node is 300 mW. The harvester would therefore enable a 28% duty cycle. On the other hand, an excitation frequency of 10 Hz and a conversion efficiency of 50% result in 670 mW, or enough to power the sensor node all the time.

Initial Experimental Results for Resonant Peak Shifting via Control

Shown in Figure 9 is the experimental setup used to verify the notion of resonant peak shifting by controlling the overall stiffness of the harvester. The setup consists of two pinned beams. The lower beam represents the bridge motion by using a voice coil to actuate the beam at different frequencies and amplitudes. The upper beam represents the proof mass sprung to the base. The harvester voice coil serves the function of the linear generator/motor and of implementing Equation (3). The pinned beams isolate the motion to one dimension and also allow accurate measurement and scaling of the motions.

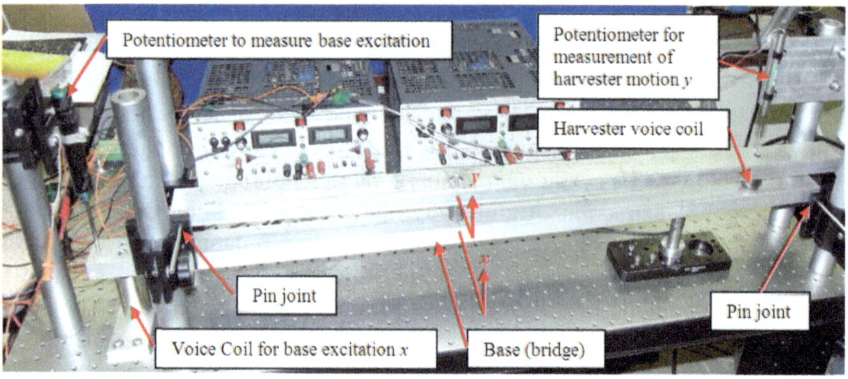

Fig. 9 Photograph of the experimental setup

Figure 10 shows amplitude data taken from the experimental setup. Two cases are shown: one where the harvester acts only as an energy extractor (solid line), and a second case where the harvester includes controlled spring behavior. As seen in the plot, the harvester has a natural frequency of about 3.4 Hz. By including spring behavior, the harvester is able to augment the physical spring in the system and subsequently shift the resonant peak to 6.4 Hz. This demonstrates that should the excitation frequency vary, the harvester will be able to alter the resonant frequency in order to achieve a large amplitude motion at the new excitation frequency and consequently generate power. The use of regenerative power electronics will be critical in realizing this concept.

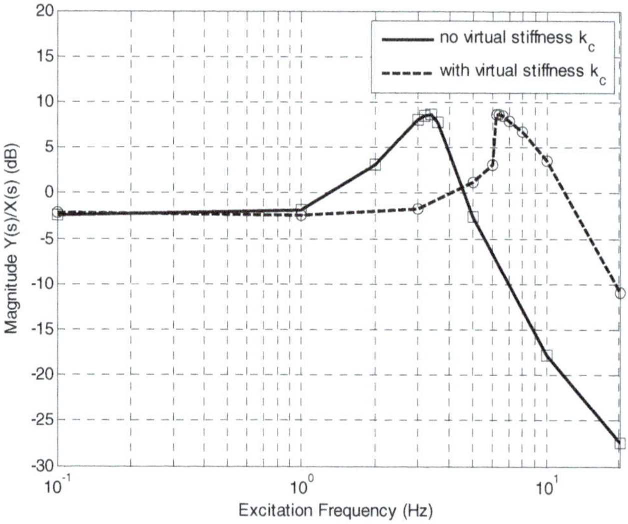

Fig. 10 Experimental resonant peak shifting

4 System Architecture and Operation

The architecture of overall system is shown in Figure 11. It consists of a number of sensor nodes and a base station. The sensor nodes have piezoelectric AE sensors (for accurate crack localization in 3D), MEMS accelerometers and strain gauges attached to them. Power to the sensor node is provided by the on-board battery and depending on the location of the sensor node and its environment, by a vibration energy harvesting unit that is connected and mounted at a carefully selected nearby position that offers the most vibration.

Upon installation, the sensor nodes form an ad-hoc wireless network, monitor the AE, MEMS accelerometer and strain gauge channels and execute local signal processing and sensor fusion tasks and exchange radio messages with other nodes and the base station.

The node level signal processing algorithms detect transient events (e.g.: acoustic emissions) and extract their salient features, such as maximum amplitude, duration, total energy, are extracted and the arrival times on the different channels are recorded. Local data fusion tasks filter out inconsistent data and execute preliminary localization and classification steps based on the extracted features. Insignificant events are discarded. Events and their features can be stored on-board and optionally sent to the base station or neighboring nodes. The decision, whether and if so, when to report events and/or involve other nodes in the data fusion, depends on the extracted features and the energy available to the node. We leave the algorithm that will schedule event reporting and distributed data fusion based on the severity of the event and the energy level of the nodes in the network for future work. Note, however, that unlike in delay-tolerant networks [23] critical events will need to be sent to the base station immediately using guaranteed delivery irrespective of the energy levels. These are events that may demand urgent action, such as potentially evacuating the immediate area.

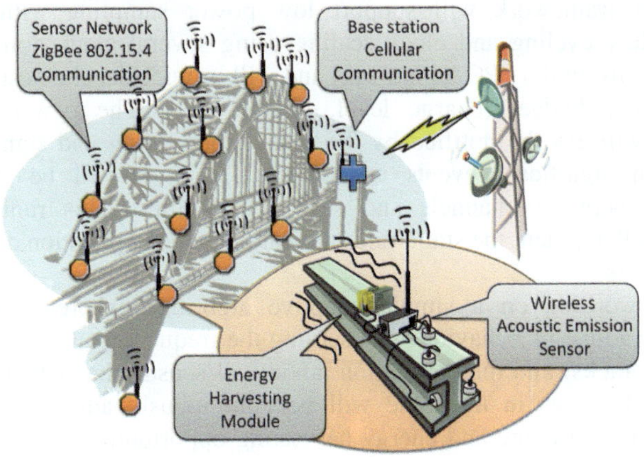

Fig. 11 System Architecture

The base station, an embedded PC class device, has a dual purpose in the system. First, it runs high-level structural health assessment algorithms based on the model of the given structure. Note that this aspect of the system is beyond the scope of this paper. Second, it is equipped with a GSM modem to report to a central monitoring station.

Power management

Node-level power management is a key component of the system. The sensor nodes have relatively high power consumption due to multichannel signal processing, the required high sampling rates on some of these channels (AE transducers) and node level data fusion and (de)compression. The worst case power consumption of the revised board is estimated at 300mW with every component turned on. Given a 10 Ah battery (3.6V Li-Ion cell), that comes to 120 hours of operation at full power. Even with energy harvesting, we do not expect that the node will be able to sustain continuous operation indefinitely. Although, low-power FPGAs – due to their several clock networks, clock scaling options, deep sleep modes and fast wakeup times – provide an excellent research platform for experimenting with various power-saving schemes, the triggering mechanism driving these modes is a cornerstone issue in any application. Our first generation system solved this problem specifically for railway bridges.

There, AE events are only expected when a train passes over the bridge. As the train enters the bridge, stresses are applied to the structure. The strain gage channel is slowly sampled by the duty-cycled microcontroller and if elevated values are observed, it wakes up the rest of the board. The prototype has an estimated lifetime of 6 weeks on a single charge on a typical railway bridge. Clearly, the same strategy is not applicable to highway bridges which have more or less continuous traffic.

The revised platform provides a more general framework for various triggering schemes. These triggering mechanisms need to minimize the chance of missing significant sensor events at the lowest possible consumed energy. The power management framework will support low power sampling with periodic or stochastic duty cycling and clock scaling using several clock domains (a clear advantage of using the FPGA platform) and will provide accurate estimates on the current energy budget (charge level, charge rate). The power management framework will also be notified by the sensor monitoring and signal processing layers when significant events are detected, thus it will be able to learn correlations between channels and sensor modalities. This runtime learning capability will augment the static ruleset created by the application developers and domain experts.

We are working on a simple adaptive algorithm whereas the node will dynamically adjust its behavior by observing the frequency and severity of sensor events (i.e. cracks) and the correlation among all sensor channels. Consequently, the threshold values in the table will be continuously adjusted based on the behavior of the structure and energy harvesting opportunities. This is well suited for the envisioned very long term deployments, since the behavior of the components is expected to slowly change as the structure ages. The algorithm will follow this trend. Note, however, that the algorithm needs to remain relatively simple, as it will run on a low-power, resource constrained microcontroller.

Low power listening

When the radio transceiver is turned on, it draws approximately 15mA operating at 3V, which can deplete the batteries quickly. Therefore, in order to extend battery life, radios must duty-cycle, i.e. wake up for short periods while staying turned off the majority of time.

The low-power radio stack we implemented for the transceiver works as follows. In receive mode, the transceiver is configured to duty-cycle, waking up periodically to check if a transmission is on the way. If no signal is detected, the transceiver goes back to sleep mode. If there is a transmission in progress, the transceiver stays awake to receive (and optionally acknowledge) the packet. Since packets are often received in bursts, the receiver stays on for a short period of time after a reception to wait for successive packets. When no more packet transmissions are detected, the receiver goes to sleep mode and continues duty cycling.

While the power consumption of the receiver can be drastically decreased this way, the transmitter must ensure that the radio channel is modulated long enough for the receiver to detect an incoming message. Therefore, the transmitter must keep the radio channel modulated longer than the sleep interval of the recipient.

The longer the receiver's sleep interval is, the less power is consumed. However, long sleep interval at the receiver mandates that the sender must modulate the channel long enough for the receiver to detect the transmission – which, results in higher power consumption of the transmitter.

Since such tradeoffs are application specific, we implemented the low power radio stack such that the receiver's sleep intervals, as well as the modulation durations are configurable during run-time. This implementation is suitable for a wide range of applications and allows for reconfiguration to adapt to operating conditions (e.g. available battery power) in a flexible way.

Other network services

The most important distributed service necessary in the system is multi-hop message routing. We utilize the Directed Flood Routing Framework [15] developed previously for our acoustic countersniper system [6]. For source localization we use the four AE sensors attached to the same AEPod sharing the same clock. In the future, we may want to correlate AE events across sensor nodes requiring precision time synchronization. The Routing Integrated Time Synchronization (RITS) protocol [14], also developed for the countersniper system, can provide 1-2 microsecond accuracy per hop.

Reliability

The FPGA-based architecture also promotes a more robust approach for implementing deeply embedded but still software driven system. It is a well-known problem that traditional (microcontroller-based) embedded systems are extremely sensitive to firmware/software errors. While many of these errors are similar to those in normal desktop applications, cyber-physical systems also experience more hidden problems due to their long-term deployment [24]. The typical answer for these problems is the use of watchdogs, grenade timers [25]. These "solutions" have their own negative side effects (application state is completely lost, non-trivial transient management on the cyber-physical boundary during reset). Instead of a purely software driven architecture we are using a layered approach, where lower level sensing, basic signal processing and communication tasks are implemented in the FPGA fabric. These hardware-driven tasks can execute autonomously and need software interaction for configuration and higher level services only. By decoupling the more complex and error prone software layer (running on a CPU softcores) from the physical interfaces, a potential failure and/or reset is less visible to the outside world.

As an added benefit of this flexible hardware/software boundary, the standard and rudimentary watchdog approach can be enhanced by additional application specific checks enforced by the deterministic hardware layer (sophisticated memory/IO protection, which typically not present in MCUs, temporal rules, duty cycle enforcement). The development of such smart hardware (IP core)-based supervisors results in a rich set of general schemes potentially applicable in other domains as well.

Offline Evaluation

It has been shown that the AE event rate per cycle is proportional to the crack propagation rate per cycle [24]. In experiments and from the proportionality between events rate per cycle and crack propagation rate per cycle, this study suggested a relation between the observed event count over any cyclic interval, and the crack area created in this interval. These findings are mostly empirical and are obtained experimentally. They allow the determination of the fatigue life curves based on AE test data. Such curves can be derived for a material or structure and provide an assessment of fatigue damage to material containing a crack. At higher stress intensity levels, the yield of emission per unit of crack extension is higher, a consequence of the larger amounts of stored energy available at higher stress intensities. This provides a basis to link acoustic emission with the fracture mechanism and to establish the relationship between emission and stress intensity factor.

A Fatigue Assessment Index (FAI) is then defined based on the AE source activity, intensity and the related fatigue crack. The corresponding recommended actions can be applied to each zone ranging from no action required, through various levels of follow up NDE or analysis, up to taking the structure out of service. These recommendations provide bridge engineers with information to plan, schedule and prioritize maintenance or replacement operations.

5 Initial Field Testing

The objective of the field test was to benchmark the wireless system against the wired system. The tested component is shown in Figure 12. The sensors connected to the AEPod are marked by the circles in the figure. The four sensors connected to the traditional wired system are shown inside the wireless sensors.

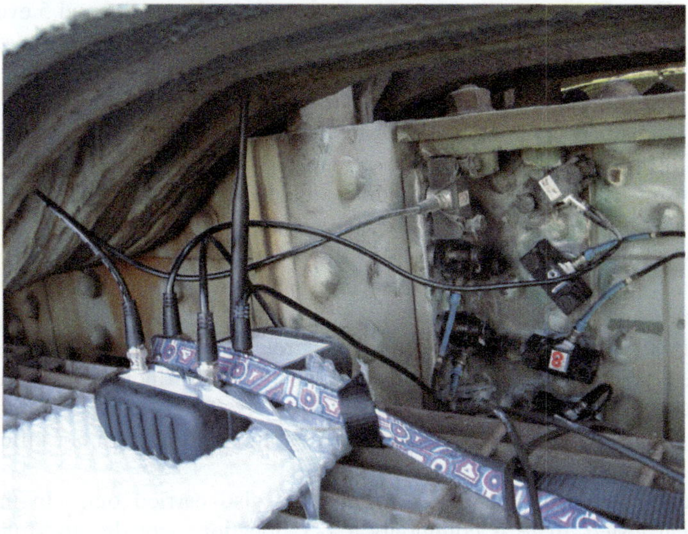

Fig. 12 Field Experiment

The events recorded by the wireless system are shown in Figure 13. In this figure, five different train passes are observed. The events recorded inside the array are superimposed upon the Train 1, 2-3, and 5 strain curves. Note that there was some overlapping of trains 2 and 3 as they passed over opposite tracks. For this analysis, they were treated as a single train. No events were recorded for train 4 by either the wired or wireless systems.

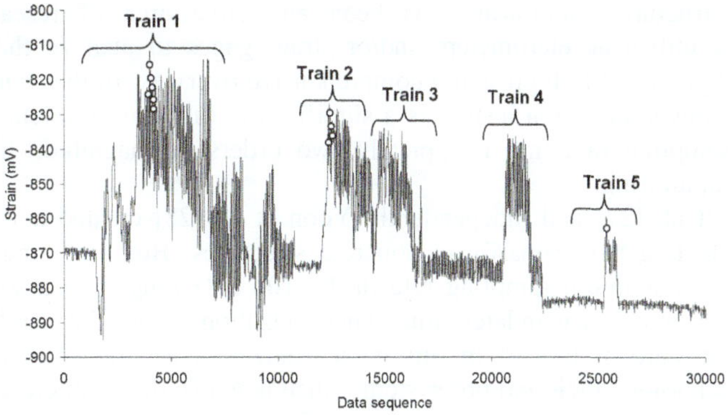

Fig. 13 Detected AE events (circles) superimposed on the strain signal

The events were further analyzed for intensity levels. The wireless system detected a total of 11 events over 5 train passes at an average intensity of 52 dB. For the same 5 trains, the wired system detected 9 events at an average intensity of 54 dB. For train 1, the wireless and wired systems detected 6 and 5 events from within the array. These numbers are close enough to suggest that the two systems are performing comparably since a missed event may be attributed to sensor location, surface preparation, and sensor coupling to the structure. Similarly, the average intensities are comparable. The 4 dB difference, again, is well within the realm of the considerations cited above.

The results from trains 2-3 also indicate that the wireless system is detecting the same events the wired system is detecting. Both systems detected 4 events inside the array at comparable intensities ~ 51 dB (wireless) and 58 dB (wired). Train 4 data results suggests further that the wired and wireless systems are performing comparably since neither array detected any events.

Finally, the train 5 result shows that the wireless system detected one event that the wired system did not pick up. The result is not indicative of sensitivity differences between the two instruments. It is again suggestive that sensor location, surface preparation, and acoustic coupling will have minor influences on activity and intensity.

A location comparison of the events was also carried out. In the bridge component tested, there is commonly a 1-3" location error due its structure and multiple fasteners in the joint. These features affect line-of-sight between the sensor and the source as well as the sound wave velocity, both of which influence accurate source localization. In this test, all events were clustered in an approximate 3" x 2" area. They were located in the vicinity of the crack tip (leading edge of crack) and are within the margin of location error associated with such bridge components.

6 Related Work

Wireless structural monitoring has been an active area of research. Most approaches utilize accelerometers and/or strain gages to analyze the vibrating structure. Lynch and Loh present a comprehensive overview of the state of the art in [26]. Acoustic emission testing is a significantly different problem due to the required sampling rate that is typically two orders of magnitude higher than vibration monitoring.

Grosse et al. [27] and independently Yoon et al. [28] created a wireless AE sensor node targeted primarily at concrete structures. Both are single channel sensors with maximum sampling rate in the 100 kHz range. Localization using separate sensor nodes mandates time synchronization across the wireless nodes. The current state of the art in time synchronization accuracy on the kind of wireless technology their and our system utilize is worse than a microsecond [14]. This translates to localization error of over 30 cm in steel. The 4 channels on our board share the same physical clock completely eliminating this source of error. Also, the order of magnitude higher sampling rate of our node makes TDoA measurements and hence, source localization much more accurate.

7 Conclusions

The paper presented a prototype wireless 4-channel acoustic emission sensor node that supports high sampling rates and hence, enables the detection and accurate localization of fatigue cracks. Having a wireless bridge monitoring system has many advantages. First of all, current wired systems were designed for short-term inspection and are not cost-effective or practical for long-term monitoring. Hence, our system enables a revolutionary paradigm shift in infrastructure maintenance. As such, the change will not happen overnight. We expect that our system will be initially used for inspection before it will be widely adopted for the permanent instrumentation of bridges. Even then it will demonstrate significant savings in time, effort and cost not having to deploy long cables in sometimes hard to access areas.

Being a first generation prototype, the current system does have some shortcomings. The lifetime of the nodes on a single charge under real life conditions will be probably be two to four weeks depending on the traffic on the bridge. Wireless data download is also limited primarily due to power constraints also. In our latest generation design, we are addressing these problems and extending the capabilities of the node to be able to support monitoring of highways bridges as well.

To this end, we presented a novel energy harvester design that utilizes the vibrations of the bridge itself due to wind and traffic. Laboratory experiments show that the amount of energy that can be gathered with it is an order of magnitude higher than what is provided by current piezoelectric designs.

Acknowledgement. This research was supported in part by the National Science Foundation awards CNS 0964592 and CNS 1035627 and the U.S. Transportation Research Board.

References

1. Deficient Bridges by State and Highway System, FHWA, `http://www.fhwa.dot.gov/bridge/deficient.htm`
2. Reliability of Visual Bridge Inspection, Turner-Fairbank Highway Research Center, Federal Highway Administration (March 2001)
3. TechBrief: Reliability of Visual Inspection for Highway Bridges, Turner-Fairbank Highway Research Center, FHWA (September 2001), `http://www.tfhrc.gov/hnr20/nde/01105.pdf`
4. Bridge Structural Monitoring System, `http://www.dataq.com/applicat/articles/bridge-structural-monitoring.html`
5. Issues and Options in Infrastructure Investment, Congressional Budget Office (May 2008)
6. Ledeczi, A., et al.: Countersniper System for Urban Warfare. ACM Transactions on Sensor Networks 1(2), 153–177 (2005)

7. Selavo, L., et al.: LUSTER: wireless sensor network for environmental research. In: Proc. of the 5th International Conference on Embedded Networked Sensor Systems (SenSys), Sydney, Australia (November 2007)
8. Crossbow Inc. eKo System, `http://www.xbow.com/eko/index.aspx`
9. Meshnetics Zigbit Amp module (2009), `http://www.meshnetics.com/zigbee-modules/amp/`
10. Xu, N., Rangwala, S., Chintalapudi, K., Ganesan, D., Broad, A., Govindan, G., Estrin, D.: A Wireless Sensor Network For Structural Monitoring. In: Proceedings of the 2nd ACM Conference on Embedded Network Sensor Systems (SenSys 2004), Baltimore, MD (November 2004)
11. Kim, S., Pakzad, S., Culler, D., Demmel, J., Fenves, G., Glaser, S., Turon, M.: Health Monitoring of Civil Infrastructures Using Wireless Sensor Networks. In: 6th International Symposium on Information Processing in Sensor Networks, IPSN 2007, April 25-27, pp. 254–263 (2007)
12. Hay, T., Jayaraman, S., Ledeczi, A., Volgyesi, P., Al Sammane, G.: Wireless Technology for Steel Bridges.In: Proceedings of the American Society for Non-destructive Testing Conference on Structural Materials and Technology, Oakland, CA (September 2008)
13. Miller, R.K.: Acoustic Emission Testing. In: Nondestructive Testing Handbook, 3rd edn., vol. 6. American Society for Non-destructive Testing, Columbus (2006)
14. Kusy, B., Dutta, P., Levis, P., Maroti, M., Ledeczi, A., Culler, D.: Elapsed Time on Arrival: A simple, versatile, and scalable primitive for canonical time synchronization services. Int. Journal of Ad Hoc and Ubiquitous Computing (2006)
15. Maroti, M.: The Directed Flood Routing Framework. In: Proc. of Fifth ACM/IFIP/USENIX International Conference on Middleware, Toronto, Canada (October 2004)
16. Sinclair, A.C.E., Connors, D.C., Formby, C.L.: Acoustic Emission Analysis during Fatigue Crack Growth in Steel. Journal of Material Science Engineering 28 (1977)
17. Huang, M., Jiang, L., Liaw, P.K., Brooks, C.R., Seelev, R., Klarstrom, D.L.: Using acoustic emission in fatigue and fracture materials research. JOM 50(11), 1–14 (1998)
18. Mitcheson, P.D., Yeatman, E.M., Rao, G.K., Holmes, A.S., Green, T.C.: Energy Harvesting From Human and Machine Motion for Wireless Electronic Devices. Proceedings of the IEEE 96(9), 1457–1486 (2008)
19. Paradiso, J.A., Starner, T.: Energy scavenging for mobile and wireless electronics. IEEE Pervasive Computing 4(1), 18–27 (2005)
20. Li, H., Pillay, P.: A Methodology to Design Linear Generators for Energy Conversion of Ambient Vibrations. In: IEEE Industry Applications Society Annual Meeting, IAS 2008, pp. 1–8 (October 2008)
21. Paultre, P., Chaallal, O., Proulx, J.: Bridge Dynamics and Dynamic Amplification Factors – A Review of Analytical and Experimental Findings. Canadian Journal of Civil Engineering 19, 260–278 (1992)
22. Jozef, M.: Vibration Measurement of Highway Bridges. In: Proceedings of the 40th International Conference Experimental Stress Analysis, Prague, Czech Republic, pp. 169–174 (2002)
23. Juang, P., Oki, H., Wang, Y., Martonosi, M., Peh, L., Rubenstein, D.: Energy-Efficient Computing for Wildlife Tracking: Design Tradeoffs and Early Experiences with ZebraNet. In: Tenth International Conference on Architectural Support for Programming Languages and Operating Systems, ASPLOS-X (October 2002)

24. Huang, Y., Kintala, C., Kolettis, N., Fulton, N.D.: Software rejuvenation: analysis, module and applications. In: Twenty-Fifth International Symposium on Fault-Tolerant Computing, FTCS-25. Digest of Papers, Pasadena, CA, USA, pp. 381–390 (June 1995)
25. Dutta, P., Hui, J., Jeong, J., Kim, S., Sharp, C., Taneja, J., Tolle, G., Whitehouse, K., Culler, D.: Trio: enabling sustainable and scalable outdoor wireless sensor network deployments. In: Proc. 5th International Conference Information Processing Sensor Networks (IPSN 2006), pp. 407–415 (2006)
26. Lynch, J.P., Loh, K.J.: A Summary Review of Wireless Sensors and Sensor Networks for Structural Health Monitoring. The Shock and Vibration Digest 38(2), 91–128 (2006)
27. Grosse, C., McLaskey, G., Bachmaier, S., Glaser, S.D., Krügera, M.: A hybrid wireless sensor network for acoustic emission testing in SHM. In: Proc. of SPIE Sensors and Smart Structures Technologies for Civil, Mechanical, and Aerospace Systems 2008, vol. 6932 (2008)
28. Yoon, D., Lee, S., Kim, C., Seo, D.: Acoustic Emission Diagnosis System and Wireless Monitoring for Damage Assessment of Concrete Structures. In: NDT for Safety, Prague, Czech Republic (November 2007)

Deformation Detection in Structural Health Monitoring

Pierantonio Merlino[1] and Antonio Abramo[2]

[1] PTLab - Agemont SpA, via J.Linussio 1, 33020 Amaro, Italy
pierantonio.merlino@agemont.it
[2] DIEGM - Università degli Studi di Udine, via delle Scienze 208 - 33100 Udine, Italy abramo@uniud.it
and
ETH Lab - Eurotech Group, via Fratelli Solari 3/a - 33020 Amaro (UD), Italy
a.abramo@ethlab.com

Summary. In this contribution the issue of the embedded monitoring and detection of structural unhealthy conditions is addressed. The recent work on the design of a self-organizing architecture of sensing/communication nodes able to monitor the topological modification of structural surfaces is reviewed. The node design, purposely carried out to attain both contactless communication and sensing abilities, makes use of near-field coupling among nodes to implement both features, i.e. to monitor structure displacements and deploy a local communication network for the transfer of information. This technology shows low realization costs and lower power consumption compared to traditional wireless communication. A simple experimental setup is presented, demonstrating the architectural ability to trace the evolution of single structural fractures as well as of topological in-plane deformations, thus crediting the design as viable for the embedded surveillance of civil infrastructures.

1 Introduction

Complex civil infrastructures, such as bridges, buildings and dams, are often subject to severe environmental conditions and abnormal loads, e.g. strong winds, heavy rains, high humidity and huge temperature variations, that cannot be easily anticipated during their design [1]. This results into long-term structural deterioration that often is not detected by conventional visual inspection [2]. Moreover, catastrophic events, such as earthquakes, hurricanes or floods can severely affect the health of the structure and induce potential life-threatening conditions [3]. For this reasons, in recent years so called *Structural Health Monitoring* (SHM) technologies have emerged, opening interesting research fields inside the different branches of the engineering disciplines [1]. SHM systems involve large arrays of nodes that continuously monitor the quantities of interest by means of proper transducers, thus tracking the health of the particular structure. SHM systems are able to estimate the state of structural health and to evaluate the changes of the geometric properties [4, 5],

S.C. Mukhopadhyay (Ed.): New Developments in Sensing Technology for SHM, LNEE 96, pp. 41–62.
springerlink.com

both in amplitude and on a time basis, that effect the performance of the monitored structure. Usual employment of SHM systems, indeed, are that of damage[1] detection, damage localization and severity damage estimation [7].

Traditionally, SHM systems ground on wired-based technologies, but recently, the use of *Wireless Sensor Networks* (WSN) has emerged [7]. The reason stems from the large cost connected with the deployment of complex wired sensor arrays, which can be significantly reduced switching to their relatively cheaper wireless counterparts [1]. Moreover, wireless technologies are not subjected to wires wear and tear or damage caused by harsh weather conditions or other extreme events [3]. WSNs, in fact, do not require wire connections among sensors, and from them to the base-station, allowing the deployment of wide sensor networks even in almost inaccessible places. In addition, WSN can process the data collected by the sensors locally, and communicate summary information only [7].

These features — namely lower costs, cable-less installation and local computation capabilities — enable the deployment of hundreds of sensor nodes on a single structural element, thus enabling *local-based* damage-detection strategies [1].

A typical wireless sensor node architecture for SHM consists of a radio/computing system to which specific transducers are attached, such as strain-gauges, accelerometers or others. As a consequence, the research on WSNs for SHM systems has mainly focused on new hardware architectures [8, 7], power consumption and node size reduction [8], or network organization [9] and implementation of distributed sensing and computation architectures and strategies [10]. Moreover, the recent development of very low power architectures for wireless sensor nodes has enabled the implementation of energy harvesting technologies [11] on SHMs systems.

2 Structural Deformation Detection Using Wireless Sensor Networks

A different approach for the solution of SHM problems was proposed in [12]. In this work a novel concept for the architecture of SHM nodes and network that exploits the near-field coupling between adjacent nodes for both the communication and the distance measurement was developed. The system is based on the idea that the deployment of a multitude of nodes on a structural element can enable the autonomous setup of a connected network of nodes that can, at the same time, monitor the local node-to-node displacements, hence acting as fracture monitor, and as a network on the whole, mapping the surface of the structural element under control on which the nodes have been laid, thus monitoring its surface deformations through the corresponding network topology modifications.

[1] The term *damage* can be defined as changes introduced in the system that adversely affect its current or future performance. Its definition is commonly limited to changes to the material or geometric properties of the system [6].

The single fractures can be detected and monitored locally through the measurement of the mutual distance between two adjacent nodes. Conversely, the monitoring of structural deformations requires the mapping of the structure geometry, hence the determination of all nodes relative positions.

Consequently, as far as the structural deformation software procedure, the core of the system is the distributed localization algorithm described in [13]. Each monitoring node determines its position by means of the sole knowledge of the distance measured from its connected nodes, and based on the estimated positions those have made about their own positions. In this way each node can determine its positions in a *relative coordinate system*, from which the structure deformation can be monitored. A sketch of the described monitoring setup is shown in Fig. 1. The only requirement for the correct operation of the algorithm is the attribution to at least three of the nodes of the status of *anchors*, namely those nodes who know their exact (relative) position (e.g. the three unitary versors $[1,0,0]^T$, $[0,1,0]^T$, $[0,0,1]^T$ of what we called the *relative coordinate system*).

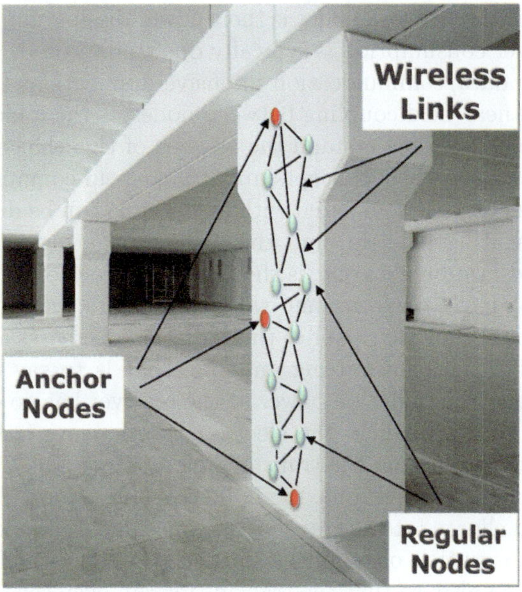

Fig. 1 A sketch of a near-field monitoring communication network

The algorithm of [13] assumes that each node collects the positions of the neighboring ones, temporarily acting as *local anchors*, and updates its own position through an asynchronous, decentralized optimization procedure. The localization algorithm guarantees the complete decentralization of the computation and implements a localization strategy largely insensitive to the peculiarities of the network topology.

As far as the hardware design is concerned, instead, the keystones of the proposed monitoring system are the near-field transmission technology adopted for the network communication, and the displacement measurement technique used for the estimation of the nodes relative distances.

After the brief review of Sect. 3 on the near-field communication, clarifying some basic concepts about this technology, the problem of the antenna design and its design procedure are illustrated in Sect. 4. The distance measurement problem is analyzed in Sect. 5, where the adopted distance measurement technique based on Received Signal Strength (RSS) is also presented. The node architecture and its performance are presented in Sect. 6, which also describes the implementation of the network of monitoring nodes. Some recent improvements made on the measurement part of the analog circuitry are illustrated in Sect.7, before drawing the conclusions of the work in Sect. 8.

3 Near-Field Magnetic Communication

Since in SHM applications WSNs must guarantee operational lifetimes of several months, an important aspect to be carefully considered in designing the hardware architecture of the network nodes is their power dissipation. In WSNs, the largest part of power consumption is typically due to inter-node communication, especially for data/communication intensive applications [14]. For this reason we adopted near-field coupling between nodes as the underlying communication technology. To understand the reasons of this choice, it is worth to briefly introduce some basic concepts about near-field communication.

The electromagnetic field associated with an antenna can be divided in two regions: the propagating far-field, and the non-propagating near-field [15]. The far-field, called Fraunhofer zone, is the region where the electromagnetic wave possesses a planar wave front, and where its electric and magnetic field are in phase. In this region the power of the radiation decreases as the square of the distance from the transmitting antenna, that is to say $-20\,\mathtt{dB/dec}$, and the absorption of the radiation power at the receiver has no effect on the transmitter itself. In the far-field the electromagnetic wave is fully formed and completely independent on the transmitting antenna [16]. Conversely in the near-field region, or Fresnel zone, the inductive and capacitive effects due to the currents and charges at the transmitting antenna are predominant[15]. In this case, the absorption of power at the receiver side has effects on the transmitting antenna also, so that the transmitter can even sense that power is absorbed from its emission. In near-field conditions the field strength decreases as $1/\mathtt{r}^3$, or $-60\,\mathtt{dB/dec}$, where $\mathtt{r}$ is the distance from the antenna. (See, e.g., Fig. 4.57 in [16]) Such a rapid roll-off of the field strength implies that inductive coupling effects are limited to a region relatively close to the antenna. As a consequence, wireless technologies based on near-field communication have a short range character, and typically do not interfere with other RF systems.

The boundary between the near- and far-fields, that is to say the range of a near-field transmission, is determined by the kind and size of the antenna, and by the frequency of the electromagnetic radiation. As a rule of thumb, for a coil antenna this boundary is set to be $\lambda/2\pi$, where λ is the wavelength of the electromagnetic field [16].

The *short-range* character of the near-field communication allows to attain significant reductions in the energy budget required for the communication among nodes, especially if non-radiative, resonant conditions are attained, thus increasing the operation lifetime that a WSN can feature [12].

4 Inductive Antenna Design

As presented in [12], we implemented a near-field transmission system using a PCB-based inductor antenna. A baseband communication is obtained between adjacent nodes by electrically modulating the magnetic flux of their coils with the transmitting data signal. Since the performance of the wireless communication, i.e. its communication range and datarate, depends mainly on the shape of the antenna and on its geometric dimensions, such as the track width and thickness, number and diameters of its turns, the accurate characterization and design are necessary in order to achieve the required figures.

4.1 Equivalent Circuit Analysis

The first activity of the whole design process was the modeling of the physical phenomena involved with near-field communication, and the first step of such a modeling activity was the identification of an equivalent circuit able to properly reproduce the inductive coupling between transmitting and receiving antennas. We adopted the circuit presented in [17, 18], which is depicted in Fig. 2. As can be seen, both the transmitting and receiving parts of the circuit are modeled as ideal inductors. However, the circuit is completed with series resistors representing the coils' ohmic losses, and with a parallel capacitor that model the high-frequency shunt of the circuit. The

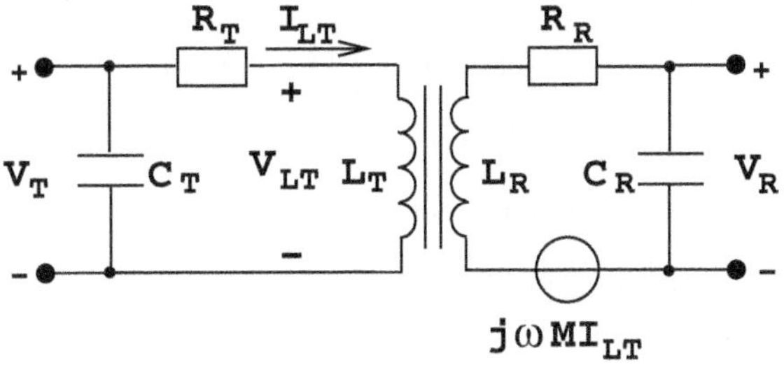

Fig. 2 The equivalent circuit used for the modeling of the inductive coupling between adjacent coils

received voltage, V_R, emerges from the presence of the current-controlled voltage generator, $j\omega M I_{LT}$, where $M = k\sqrt{L_R L_T}$ is the mutual inductance between transmitting and receiving inductors, k is the coil coupling coefficient, and I_{LT} is the current flowing through the transmitting coil. More complex circuits can be found in literature [19]. Nevertheless the adopted one, despite its simple structure, is able to describe the behavior of the near-field coupling with sufficient accuracy, and it can be effectively used to characterize the communication between adjacent nodes [12].

The analysis of the equivalent circuit, in particular of its step response, was performed to understand what the performance of the designed coil in terms of maximum datarate, power consumption, and communication range could be. Following [12], it can be found that[2]:

$$\begin{aligned} DR_{10\%} &= R_T / (2.3\, L_T) \\ P_{TXmax} &= V_O^2 / R_T \\ V_{RXmax} &= M\, V_{TXmax} = k\, V_O \sqrt{L_R / L_T}, \end{aligned} \quad (1)$$

where $DR_{10\%}$ is the maximum datarate[3], P_{TXmax} is the peak transmitted power, V_{RXmax} is the peak received voltage and V_O is the maximum input voltage level.

The pulse duration can be reduced, hence the transmission datarate increased, using coils characterized by low inductance and high resistance values. Moreover, the maximum datarate can be finely tuned adding a resistor R_S of proper value in series with the coil. Since C_T and C_R are low enough to be neglected, the resistance R_S results in series with the equivalent resistance of the coil, R_T, allowing the trimming of the datarate. Unfortunately, high values of the tuning resistor R_S tend to reduce the inductor peak voltage, V_{TXmax}, thus decreasing the effective communication range. In fact, if a voltage step with a rising time of t_r is applied to the input, that is to say:

$$v_T(t) = \frac{V_O}{t_r} t \times (\mathbf{1}(t) - \mathbf{1}(t - t_r)) + V_O \mathbf{1}(t - t_r), \quad (2)$$

where $\mathbf{1}(t)$ is the step function, then the voltage emerging at the inductor, V_{LT}, is going to be:

$$\begin{aligned} v_{LT} = & \frac{V_O}{t_r} \frac{L_T}{R_T + R_S} (1 - e^{-t/\tau}) \mathbf{1}(t) - \\ & - \frac{V_O}{t_r} \frac{L_T}{R_T + S_S} (1 - e^{-(t-t_r)/\tau}) \mathbf{1}(t - t_r) + \\ & + V_O e^{-(t-t_r)/\tau} \mathbf{1}(t - t_r) \end{aligned} \quad (3)$$

[2] The formulas of [12] are computed under the assumption of low C_T and C_R values ($\leq 10\,\mathrm{pF}$).

[3] Since the voltage V_T at the coil terminals is a train of bipolar pulse signals [12] whose positive parts correspond to the rising edges of the input and whose negative ones correspond to its falling edges, the datarate is computed as the inverse of the pulse time length at 10% of the pulse peak voltage, $DR_{10\%} = 1/t_{10\%}$. Assuming that $v_{LT}(t_{10\%}) = v_{TO}\, e^{-t_{10\%} R_T / L_T} = 0.1\, V_O$, it can be found that the pulse time length is $t_{10\%} = 2.3\, L_T / R_T$.

where $\tau = L_T/(R_T + R_S)$. As can be noticed, the maximum V_{LT} of the transmitting antenna is obtained when $t = t_r$ and $V_{LTmax} = \frac{V_0}{t_r}\frac{L_T}{R_T+R_S}(1 - e^{-t/\tau})$. Consequently, from Eqs. (1)-(3) it can be observed that if high R_S values are chosen, the datarate increases but the communication range decreases due to the reduced received voltage $V_{RXmax} = M\, V_{TXmax} < k\, V_0\, \sqrt{L_R / L_T}$.

4.2 Antenna Modeling and Design Strategy

Having analyzed the equivalent circuit of the near-field coupling, the design of the transmitting and receiving antenna can be performed so as to obtain the required performances in terms of datarate, power consumption and communication range. Using the simulator presented in [12], we are able to extract the electrical parameters of planar, multi-turns, rectangular and circular coil configurations. For the sake of clarity, we briefly review here some results about coil dimensioning.

For a coil of arbitrary shape realized with the PCB technology, the geometrical parameters used for the design are the trace width, w, and thickness, h, of the deposited metal, the number of turns of the inductor, n, and the diameter(side) of the circular(square) coil, d.

Fig. 3 shows how the datarate depends on the geometrical parameters of the coil. As expected, the datarate increases at decreasing values of both w and h, since this corresponds to high values of the series resistance R_T. However, this condition results into the reduction of the magnetic coupling of the coils. (See Fig. 4-(c),(d)).

It must be also noticed that the coupling coefficient k, hence the received voltage V_R, depends additionally on the coil diameter, d, and on the number of turns, n. (See Fig. 4-(a),(b)) Since high values of k are desirable, wide diameters and high number of turns should also be designed. As a consequence, a trade off between the geometric parameters of the inductor is necessary.

Based on the considerations above, we implemented a simple procedure that, accounting of the performance requirements and the geometrical limits

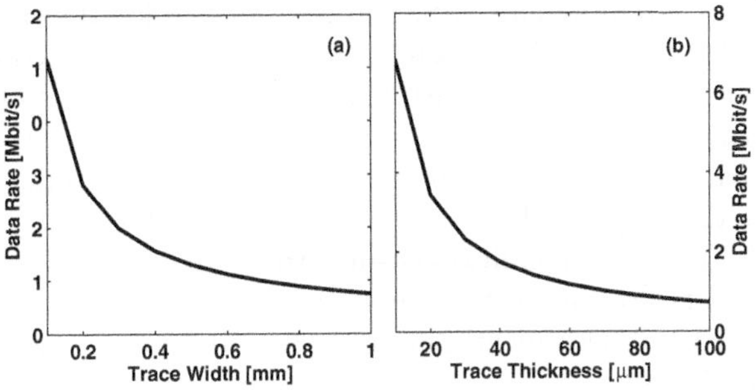

Fig. 3 The communication datarate plotted as a function of the coil geometrical parameters.

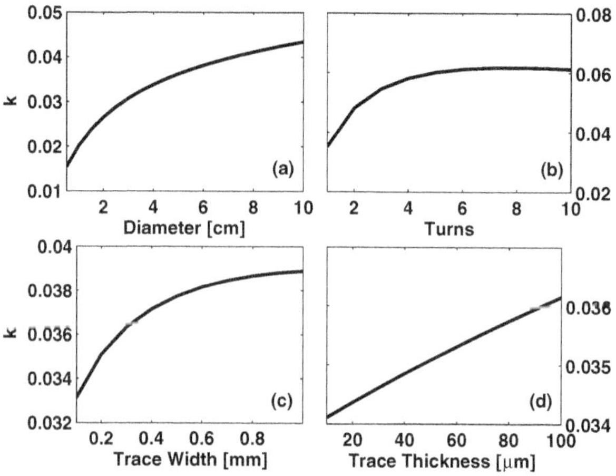

Fig. 4 Coupling coefficient, M, between two identical coils, plotted at varying coil diameter and number of turns.

of the PCB technology, searches the optimal values of the inductor geometrical parameters. The strategy, depicted in Fig. 5, can be described as follows:

Step 1: Given a specific application, the minimum datarate, DR_{min}, the minimum received voltage[4], V_{RXmin}, and the maximum power consumption, P_{TXmax}, are determined. The technology chosen for the antenna realization determines the span of feasible values of the geometrical parameters. In our application we chose the PCB technology and set feasible values for the diameter, I_d, trace width, I_w, thickness, I_h, and number of turns, I_n.

Step 2: The actual peak received voltage, V_{RX}, is computed setting the geometrical parameter at their minimum values. It must be noticed that we decided to implement circular inductors for both the transmitting and receiving coils in order to obtain isotropic field conditions around the circuits. This situation is favorable for the nodes reciprocal distance, as will be seen in Sect. 6. Finally, to reduce power consumption, the tuning resistor, R_S, is initially set to its maximum value, R_{Smax}.

Step 3: If the peak received voltage is larger than its allowed minimum, that is to say $V_{RX} \geq V_{RXmin}$, the procedure proceeds with the next step; as a matter of fact, this condition ensures that the communication range requirements are satisfied. Otherwise, the tuning resistor is reduced by a fixed small decrement, ΔR_S, and the procedure iterates until the condition is met.

[4] The minimum received voltage is computed given a desired signal-to-noise-ratio and communication range, as will be explained in the next Subsection.

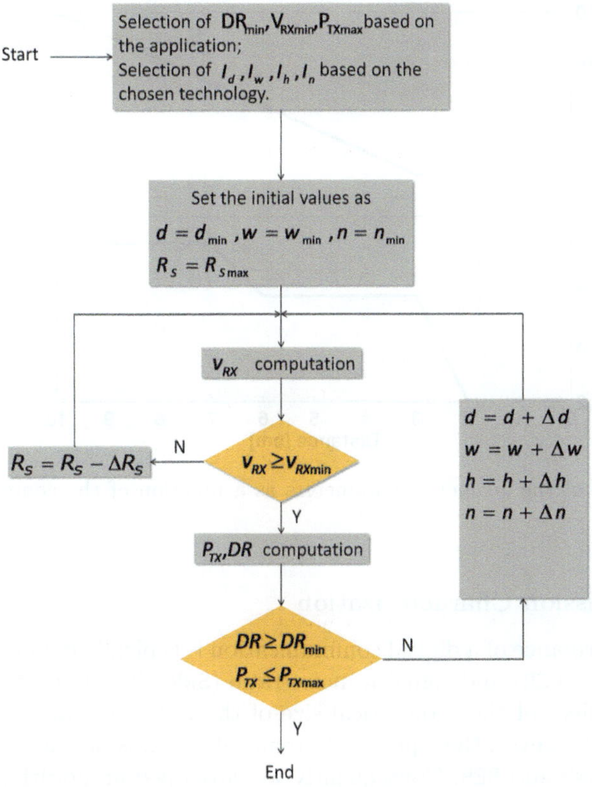

Fig. 5 Flowchart of the antenna design procedure.

Step 4: The actual datarate and power consumption are computed. If their values meet the requirements, that is to say $\mathtt{DR} \geq \mathtt{DR_{min}}$ and $\mathtt{P_{TX}} \leq \mathtt{P_{TXmax}}$, then the antenna geometric parameters are identified and the procedure stops. Otherwise, Step 2 is resumed with incremented values of the geometric parameters.

Since compact antennas are desirable, the procedure was set to privilege small antenna designs first. Fig. 6 shows the results obtained with the procedure in our case, i.e. the dependence of the geometrical parameters of the circular coils on the communication range. As expected, both diameter and turns must increase at increasing communication range, since the mutual inductance must be increased with distance.

In our case the design strategy found the optimal geometric parameters as $\mathtt{d} = 50\,\mathtt{mm}$, $\mathtt{n} = 8$, $\mathtt{w} = 0.2\,mm$, $\mathtt{h} = 50\,\mu\mathtt{m}$. The circular inductors overlapped on 4 PCB layers. The tuning resistance was set at $3k\Omega$, yielding a maximum datarate of 20 Mbit/s. The maximum communication range was found to be 10 cm, while the peak power consumption for the transmission was estimated in 8 mW.

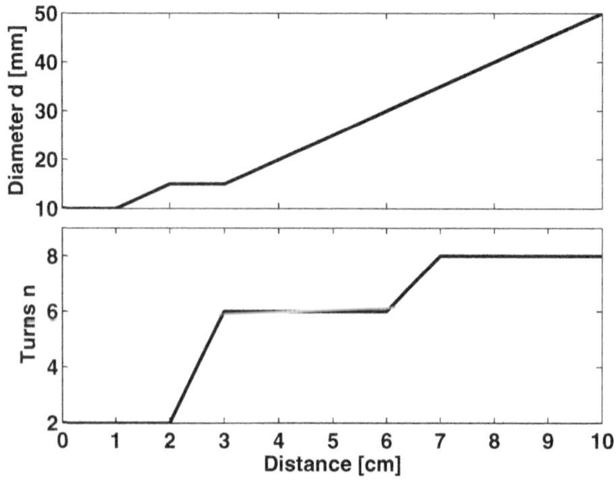

Fig. 6 Behavior of the geometric parameters as a function of the communication range.

4.3 Transmission Characterization

Since the performance of a digital communication is typically defined in terms of bit-error-rate (BER) and signal-to-noise-ratio (SNR), it is important to understand the effect of the geometrical size of the inductors on these performance figures. However, the equivalent circuit of Fig. 2 is not devised for the estimation of SNR and BER. Consequently we developed an additional model for the simulation of the whole transmission system [12].

The model was implemented in MATLAB^{TM}, and was describing the communication chain as the cascade of the filter elements shown in Fig. 7.

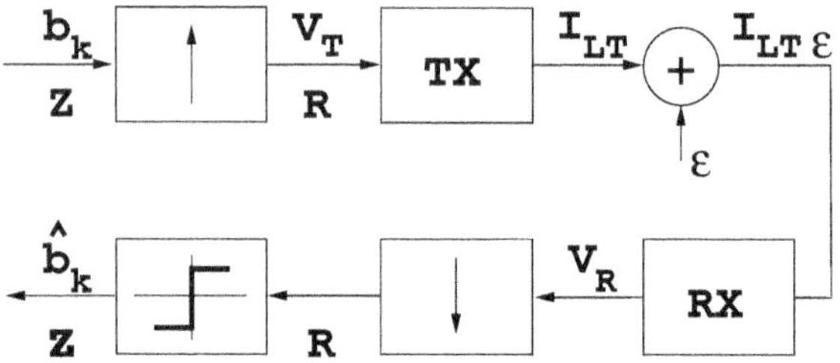

Fig. 7 Schematic view of the near-field communication system as modeled in software.

The first stage is an interpolation filter, generating the transmitted voltage, V_T, from the input bit stream, b_k. V_T is then elaborated by the transmitting block, TX, whose transfer function:

$$\frac{I_{LT}}{V_T} = \frac{1}{R_T + j\omega L_T} \tag{4}$$

provides the transmission inductor current, I_{LT}. Due to the short range of the transmission we decided to model the channel simply as an additive white Gaussian noise, ε.

Proceeding along the communication chain, the receiving stage, RX, is responsible for the conversion between the received current, $I_{LT\varepsilon}$, and the corresponding received voltage, V_R, which is obtained through the following transfer function:

$$\frac{V_R}{I_{LT\varepsilon}} = \frac{j\omega M}{-\omega^2 L_R C_R + j\omega R_R C_R + 1}. \tag{5}$$

Finally, the received voltage V_R is sampled and the received bits are decided using a threshold transfer function.

Fig. 8 shows the simulation results obtained in case of circular coils of different diameters. As can be seen, the SNR (thus BER) values vary accordingly with coil diameters: wider coils guarantee higher SNR values thanks to stronger coil coupling.

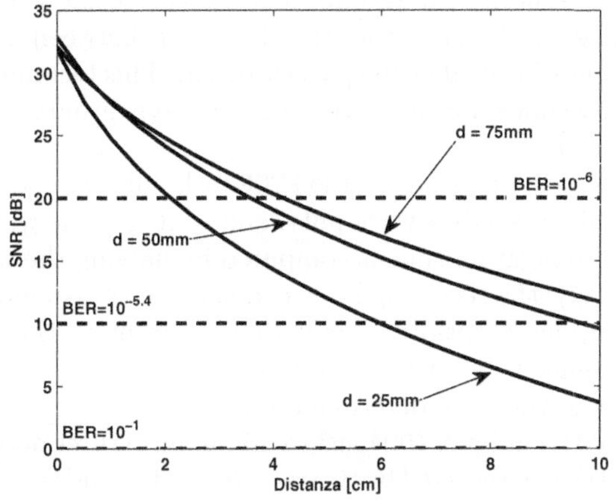

Fig. 8 SNR vs. communication distance for circular coils of different diameters, d

The BER values can be used to define the maximum communication range. For example, targeting a desired BER of 10^{-1}, the communication range exceeds 10 cm for a 50 mm circular inductor if a SNR = 0 dB is targeted.

5 Distance Measurement

In our application, the main ingredient for attain the desired network structural monitoring is the measurement of nodes relative distances. To this purpose, it is worth summarizing some of the most common ranging techniques that are used in WSNs before presenting the implementation of the one we chose for our case-study.

5.1 Distance Ranging Techniques in WSNs

Ranging techniques can be divided into several classes, depending on the physical principles exploited to measure the distance between nodes [20]. The more used techniques are based on the propagation time of the electromagnetic wave, or on the received power. The first class includes *Time Of Arrival* (TOA), *Time Difference Of Arrival* (TDOA) and *Round-Trip time Of Arrival* (RTOF), while the RSS is included in the second class.

Time-based Techniques

Time based techniques exploit the propagation time of the radio signal from the transmitter to the receiver nodes. Since the propagation speed of an electromagnetic wave in the medium is c, the distance can be simply computed as $d = c \times t$, where d is the distance and t is the time of propagation. Therefore, the measure of distance between nodes can be obtained by measuring the propagation time of the transmitted signal.

The simplest way to measure distance in WSNs is the TOA technique. The measurement setup is made of a transmitter node, sending a data packet that incorporates the sending timestamp, and a receiver one that computes the propagation time of the signal as the difference between the received timestamp and the one obtained at the packet arrival. This technique provides an accuracy of microseconds, but it requires the time synchronization between the sender and receiver.

In order to bypass this requirement, the RTOF technique can be adopted. In this case, the transmitter sends a wave pulse and waits for the wave reflected by the target. The propagation time is computed by halving the wave round-trip time. Alternatively, the receiving node can act as a transponder, sending back a reply wave upon reception. This variant guarantees the presence of stronger returning signals, but the delay inherent to the resending process can introduce errors in the time determination.

The last time-based technique, TDOA, uses a minimum of three nodes. A transmitter sends a signal that is received by two receiver nodes, and the propagation time is computed using the time arrival differences. The TDOA algorithm assumes that the nodes are time synchronized and that they know their locations.

Received Signal Strength Technique

The RSS measurement method is based on the dependence of the field strength on the distance from the transmitting antenna. The measure of the distance is performed relating the signal strength at the receiver with a model of the decay over distance of the field strength. A commonly adopted evaluation of the decay is based on the *path loss* model (PL) [21]:

$$PL(d) = 10\,\log_{10}\frac{P_t}{P_r} = 10\,N\,\log_{10}\frac{d}{d_0} + 20\,\log_{10}\frac{4\pi d_0}{\lambda} + \chi_\sigma \tag{6}$$

where P_t and P_r are the transmitted and received power, respectively, d is the distance, d_0 is a reference distance (usually $d_0 = 1\,m$) and λ is the wavelength of the field, N is the path-loss coefficient that takes into account the specific propagation environment and others effects such as fading or multipath, and finally χ_σ is a zero-mean Gaussian process with standard deviation σ, modeling measurement noise. Since this technique does not require any synchronization between nodes, its implementation is simple and it is widely adopted in WSNs. However, the RSS technique suffers from multipath inaccuracy especially in indoor environments, and the PL coefficient can greatly vary making this range technique very inaccurate.

Nevertheless, we judged that in our case the short-range character of the envisioned application could strongly mitigate both the multipath and distortion effects, and that the measurement accuracy could be more than satisfactory for our application. For this reason, we decided to choose the RSS in consideration of its simpler structure.

As a final remark, it can be noticed that Eq. (6) is valid only in far-field conditions and cannot be used in the present near-field case. For this reason in the next Section we will make use of the Eqs. (1) and of the simulation framework previously described for the characterization of the measurement technique.

5.2 RSS Ranging Technique Implementation

As previously mentioned, Eqs. (1) show that the received voltage, V_R, is proportional to the mutual inductance, M, and how the latter strongly depends on the distance between transmitting and receiving coils. Consequently, distance information can be extracted from the transduction of M values, i.e. from the measurement of the received signal level.

To this purpose, we used the simulation framework previously described to quantify the dependence of the mutual inductance of nodes on their mutual distance.

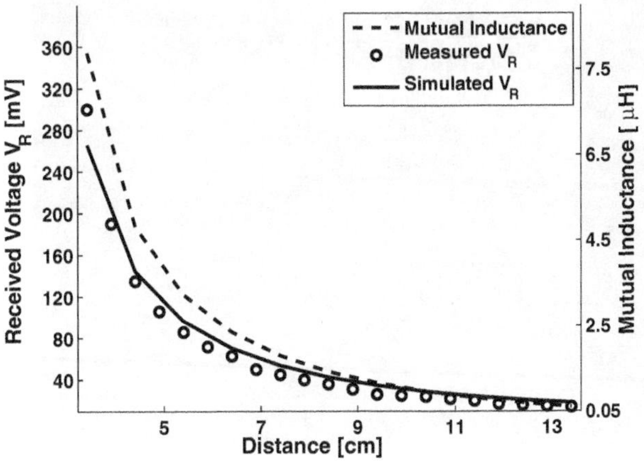

Fig. 9 Measured (circles) and simulated (line) received voltage as a function of the distance between circular coils. The coil parameters are: d = 50 mm, n = 8, w = 0.2 mm, h = 50 μm. The plot of the mutual inductance is also included.

As a first step we tabulated the V_R vs. r (i.e. M vs. r) relationship, as experimentally extracted using two template inductors. A look-up table was then stored on the node, and used to convert M variations, measured at run-time, into the correspondent distance measure. (See Fig. 9 for the case of a circular coil).

Since the mutual inductance of adjacent coils, and consequently the received voltage level, do not vary linearly with distance, but rather as $1 / r^3$ (see Fig. 9), the voltage variations ΔV_R corresponding to equal distance variation Δr is larger at small r, that is to say when the coils are closer. This evidence sets the limits to the precision of the measurement, since the system is able to resolve small distance variations only at close distance, where the mutual inductance is high. The interested reader can found a more detailed explanation of this point in [12].

6 Node Design and Network Implementation

In order to validate the proposed near-field sensing/communication strategy, a few versions of the node were realized [12]. (See Fig. 10 showing the second circular prototype. For simplicity, a first version had been realized in square shape, but it was soon abandoned because of the limited communication range and the anisotropic character of the electromagnetic field distribution.) The

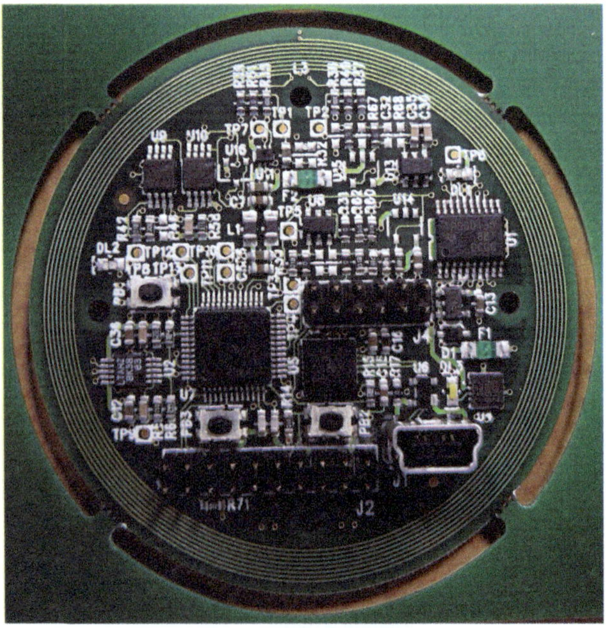

Fig. 10 Circular prototyping board for the evaluation of the sensing/communication monitoring system: 8-turns external, concentric coils; $w = 0.2\,mm$; $h = 50\,\mu m$; $d = 5\,cm$

system showed encouraging results both in terms of power consumption and datarate, as well in terms of accuracy of the distance measurement.

The node was designed following the indications of the simulation framework described above, on whose prediction ability we gained high confidence thanks to the very good comparison between simulations and experimental verification.

The digital part of the design is based on the use of a NXP™ LPC2106 microcontroller, where the main functions of the systems, such as distance computation, positioning algorithms and communication through nodes and to a host PC, are implemented in software. The choice of the specific microcontroller was made considering its computational capability, the availability of several on-chip peripherals (such as counters, UART and SPI ports, which were found very useful for PC and ADC interfacing, actually allowing radical simplifications on the PCB layout), and its limited power consumption, obtained thanks to the presence of an efficient power management unit.

As far as the analog part of the circuit[5], the near-field transmitter is based on a simple power-CMOS inverter directly driving the transmission coil, whose impedance was adapted by means of a tuning resistor, R_S. (See Fig. 11) The receiver, instead, was set up in a two-stage topology. (See Fig. 12).

The first stage acts as a differential amplifier, boosting the received differential voltage, V_{RX}, while the second one is a Schmitt-trigger, where the positive/negative received pulses cause the positive/negative saturation of the amplifier and reshape the received signal into a square pulse train. As a result, the output of the second stage is a NRZ signal identical to the transmitted data, but with a voltage level that relates, as said, to nodes mutual distance.

The characteristics of the near-field communication were experimentally tested, yielding[6] a datarate of 20 Mbit/s. In very good agreement with the performed simulations, we found that the coupling coefficient started from a value of 0.13 for nodes that were positioned so as to touch, and decreased down to 0.01 for a node distance of 10 cm. Consequently, a maximum communication range of 10 cm was set. (See Fig. 8).

In order to convert RSS measurements into distance, the peak voltage of the received digital signal, i.e. of the output of the Schmitt-trigger, is extracted by the simple diode-capacitor peak detector. (See again Fig. 12) This maximum value is then converted by the microcontroller using its internal ADC, and from this value the voltage-to-distance correspondence is extracted using the look-up table that, as said, was initialized with the mapping of the V_R vs. distance characterization. In terms of resolution, the measurement circuit was able to

[5] All transceiver circuits were simulated in SPICE to evaluate their functionality and performances. The magnetic coupling was modeled using a conventional transformer, whose leakage inductance was set to a value greater than the magnetizing one to account for the rather low values of the coupling coefficient and of the mutual inductance that are obtained in the actual inductors.

[6] This result was obtained with a tuning resistor $R_S = 3k\Omega$.

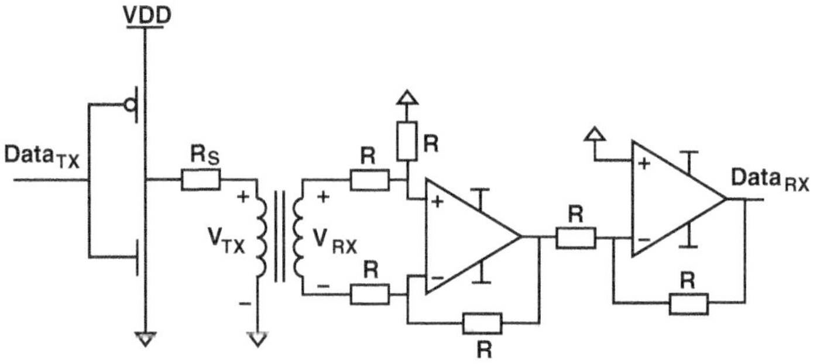

Fig. 11 Schematic view of the transmitting part of the transceiver circuit

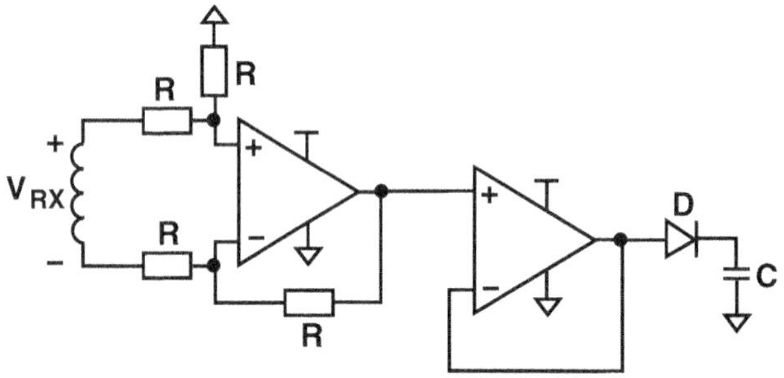

Fig. 12 The distance measurement circuit based on a peak detector

discriminate distance variations with an accuracy that, being dependent on node distance, was found to range between 48 μm at zero distance and 480 μm at 10 cm.

Since communication among nodes is necessary in the case of the monitoring of isolated fractures as well as in that of surface mapping, a protocol able to resolve the contention originating from the possible simultaneous node access to the communication channel was included, so as to properly treat the second case [16]. The simultaneous access to the channel, indeed, can hamper the nodes communication and irreparably corrupt the distance measurement.

Since the real-time requirements of the considered applications are rather limited, we decided to favor the simplicity of the software implementation at the expenses of the execution performance. Consequently, we chose to implement a simple *token-based* communication protocol to resolve the medium access contentions: only the node who owns he token can start broadcasting the data to the adjacent ones, who can only reply to an external request. Once the communication is completed, the token is passed to one of the adjacent node. If the token is repeatedly exchanged in a proper sequence, all nodes of the network will eventually receive it, and will accomplish to their software tasks. To guarantee a *democratic* periodicity it is sufficient to annotate each node with a unique network identifier. To this purpose we developed a fully decentralized identifier assignment procedure, specifically derived for the case

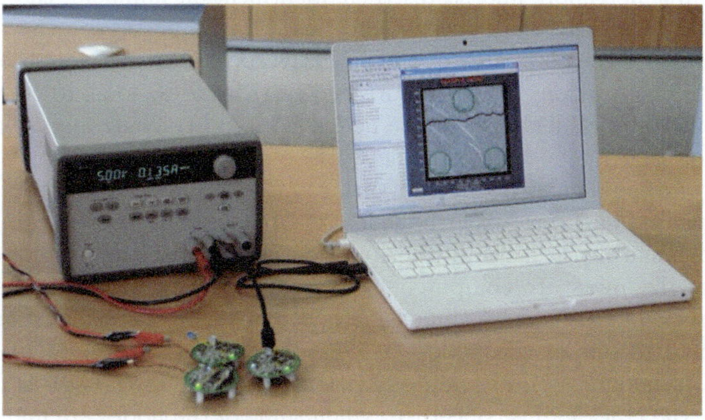

(a)

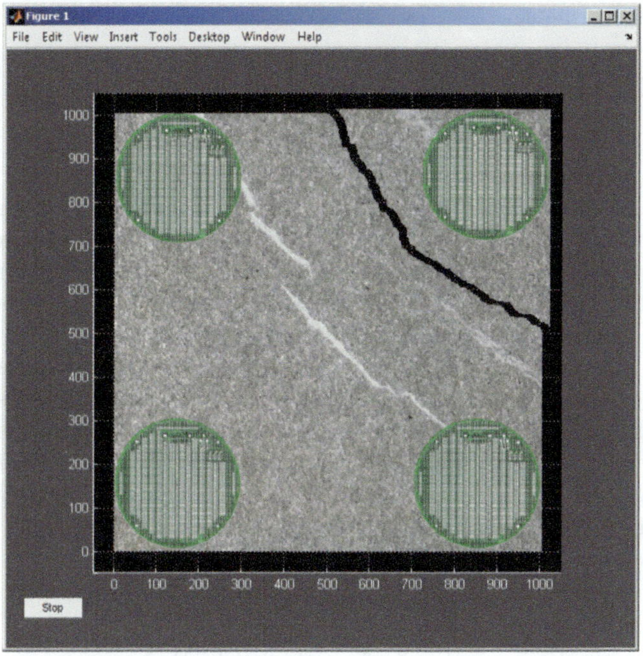

(b)

Fig. 13 (a): Demonstrator of the SHM system. (b): Close-up of the graphical sketch on the PC: the crack at the up-right corner of the marble tile widens proportionally as nodes are manually displaced in reality.

of token-based communication protocols (see [12] for more details): at reset the network proceeds to the unique node identification; then each nodes discovers its first neighbors and stores their identification numbers; the token is then introduced into the network, and based on its possession the nodes start exchanging the estimates of their relative positions, measured locally through RSS conversion; the procedure endlessly iterates, so as to converge to the actual mutual distances of the nodes [13], and tracking any topology modification that may occur to the network.

As a prototype demonstrator of a surface mapping application, the basic set up shown in Fig. 13(a) was arranged: a set of three nodes is mimicking the mapping of a marble tile surface, where an existing crack has to be monitored; the mutual distances are computed by the nodes following the procedure sketched above, and the crack dimension is displayed on the GUI of a laptop PC connected to one of the node via USB connection (see Fig. 13(b)); the network continuously updates nodes positions, and so does the GUI as far as the plot of the crack gap is concerned; when some of the nodes are manually displaced, the GUI enlarges or reduces the crack dimension according to the real node displacement.

7 RSS Circuit Improvements

After several test session, it was found that the design of the analog part of the circuit was hampered by severe limitations, mainly originating from the simple peak detector implementation. In fact, the pinning of V_R to its maximum value, that in [12] was obtained through the use of a simple diode-based peak detector, was shown to limit the dynamic range of the measurement, besides introducing a severe sensitivity of the very same measurement on temperature, attributed to the drift of the diode parameters.

Although alternative circuit topology exist that can limit this detrimental effect [22], we decided to switch to the design of a RF detector, due to its higher dynamic range ($> 40dB$) and good temperature stability. Consequently, to improve the performance of the measurement circuit we implemented the circuit of Fig. 14 that, as can be seen, makes use of the cascade of a Variable Gain Amplifier (VGA) and of a RF power detector.

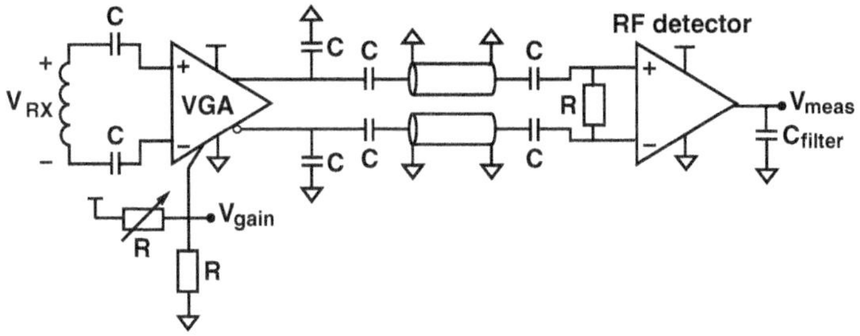

Fig. 14 The distance measurement circuit

In a VGA the gain is set by an external control voltage. In Fig. 14, a simple resistive trimmer is introduced to this purpose, but in reality we made use of the ADC available on the microcontroller to set the control voltage of the VGA. In this way, we were able to properly adjust the received voltage levels to the input requirements of the RF detector, and to compensate the errors introduced by PCB manufacturing mismatches.

The core of the RSS circuit is the RF power detector, extracting the power of its RF input. Its output, indeed, returns a voltage that is proportional to the power of the incoming signal that, in our case, corresponds to the RSS, which can be directly used to extract distance measures. As can be seen in Fig. 14, a filter capacitor was placed at the output of the RF detector, so as to limit the output voltage ripple to provide a more stable signal to the ADC, and to filter the high frequency noise that can be spuriously collected at the receiving antenna and amplified by the VGA.

To demonstrate the validity of the design we implemented it using commercial parts, assembled in the discrete test setup shown in Fig. 15. Here, the circular nodes previously developed were used only as antennas, that is to say completely bypassing their circuitry. As can be seen, the transmitting antenna is driven by a square wave, provided by an arbitrary signal generator (not shown), simulating the data transmission. The receiver coil is connected to a VGA board, and this, in turn, to the RF detector by means of coax connection. An impedance matching circuit was also implemented on the RF detector in order to avoid wave reflections. Finally the output voltage, i.e. the RSS, is extracted and displayed at the oscilloscope (not shown).

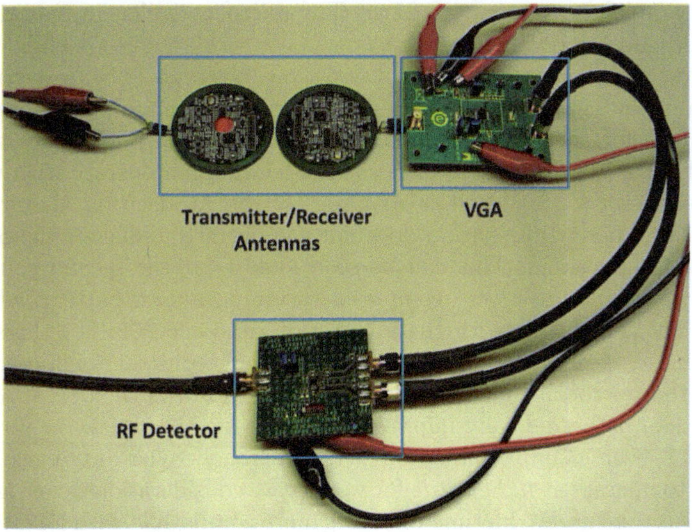

Fig. 15 RSS system setup used for evaluation and testing purposes

Table 1 Power dissipation figures of the prototyping system. On the left: Lifetimes of the different system components at the estimated operation duty=cycles. A battery featuring 1 Ah was assumed. On the right: instantaneous power dissipation of the different system components.

Duty Cycle	Lifetime [h]	Node functionality	Power Consumption [mW]
100%	48.3	CPU	18
50%	96.6	Transmission	8
4%	1207.5	Reception	27
1%	4830	Measurement	86.7

As far as the VGA component is concerned, we chose the Analog Devices^{TM} AD8330 because of its wide input dynamic range, low power and low noise characteristics. The chosen RF power detector, instead, was the Analog Devices^{TM} AD8310, featuring high dynamic and frequency ranges, and large temperature stability. The measurement circuit of Fig. 15 was then cascaded to a TI^{TM} ADS7884, that is a 10-bit, 3 MSamples/s ADC that we introduced for analog-to-digital conversion, and whose data samples are sent to the microcontroller for RSS vs. distance conversion.

The whole monitoring system was designed taking power dissipation in particular consideration. (See Tab. 1) The near-field transmission part of the analog circuitry can be considered rather parsimonious, requiring just 8 mW (1.6 mA@5 V) to operate, sensibly less than what required by typical ZigBee^{TM} transmitters. The receiver circuit power dissipation, mainly due to the two operational amplifiers, amounts to 27 mW. The microcontroller, instead dissipates a peak value of 18 mW (10 mA@1.8 V).

The largest contribution to power dissipation, however, is to be ascribed to the distance measurement circuit, and amounts to 86.7 mW, partitioned as follows: 52.8 mW for the VGA operation, 26.4 mW for the RF power detection, and 7.5 mW for the ADC. However, since the RSS circuit can operate with very small duty-cycles ($< 1\%$), as it is required by the localization algorithm, this rather large power dissipation does not significantly influence the overall lifetime of the system. This can be seen looking at the second column of Tab. 1, where lifetimes were computed assuming a 1 Ah battery, whose dimensions are compatible with the integration onto the PCB. For the sake of completeness, it must be noticed that the severe constraint imposed to lifetime by the microcontroller, limiting to about two days the operation of the system, can be be radically improved by aggressive power saving strategies. However, even a simple reduction of the microcontroller duty-cycle, assumed here to operate at *full throttle* for worst-case considerations, can significantly increase the nodes' lifetime to values more compatible with long-term applications.

8 Conclusions

To summarize, this contribution demonstrates that embedded monitoring of structural elements can be performed using low-complexity, low-cost, and low-dissipation systems. In other words, that SHM requirements are compatible with WSN specifications. Although applied to a laboratory case-study, the results obtained envision the deployment of large networks of monitoring nodes that, self-assembling as a network on the whole, can constantly trace the displacements of structural parts, or even map their topological deformations.

Acknowledgments. The work was partially funded by ETH Lab, Eurotech Group, Amaro (UD), Italy.

References

[1] Lynch, J., Loh, K.: A summary review of wireless sensors and sensor networks for structural health monitoring. In: Shock and Vibration Digest, vol. 91, Sage Publications, Thousand Oaks (2007)

[2] Sazonov, E., Janoyan, K., Jha, R.: Wireless intelligent sensor network for autonomous structural health monitoring. In: Smart Structures and Materials 2004: Smart Sensor Technology and Measurement Systems, vol. 5384, p. 305 (2004)

[3] Bocca, M., Cosar, E., Salminen, J., Eriksson, L.: A reconfigurable wireless sensor network for structural health monitoring. In: Meier, U., Havranek, B., Motavalli, M. (eds.) Proceedings of the 4th International Conference on Structural Health Monitoring of Intelligent Infrastructure, Zurich, Switzerland. International Society for Structural Health Monitoring of Intelligent Infrastructure (2009)

[4] Kim, S., Pakzad, S., Culler, D., Demmel, J., Fenves, G., Glaser, S., Turon, M.: Health monitoring of civil infrastructures using wireless sensor networks. In: IPSN 2007: Proceedings of the 6th International Conference on Information Processing in Sensor Networks, pp. 254–263. ACM Press, New York (2007)

[5] Rizzoli, V., Costanzo, A., Montanari, E., Benedetti, A.: A new wireless displacement sensor based on reverse design of microwave and millimeter-wave antenna array. IEEE Sensors Journal 9, 1557–1566 (2009)

[6] Farrar, C., Worden, K.: An introduction to structural health monitoring. Phil. Trans. R. Soc. A 365, 303 (2007)

[7] Wu, J., Yuan, S., Zhao, X., Yin, Y., Ye, W.: A wireless sensor network node designed for exploring a structural health monitoring application. Smart Material and Structures 18, 1898 (2007)

[8] Liu, L., Yuan, F.: Wireless sensors with dual-controller architecture for active diagnosis in structural health monitoring. Smart Material and Structures 17, 25016 (2008)

[9] Kottapalli, V., Kiremidjian, A., Lynch, J., Carryer, E., Kenny, T., Law, K., Lei, Y.: Two-tiered wireless sensor network architecture for structural health monitoring. In: Proceedings SPIE, vol. 5057, p. 8 (2003)

[10] Mitchell, K., Sana, S., Liu, P., Cingirikonda, K., Rao, V., Pottinger, H.: Distributed computing and sensing for structural health monitoring systems. In: Proceedings SPIE, vol. 3990, p. 156 (2000)
[11] Park, G., Rosing, T., Todd, M., Farrar, C., Hodgkiss, W.: Energy harvesting for structural health monitoring sensor networks. Journal of Infrastructure Systems 14, 64–79 (2008)
[12] Merlino, P., Abramo, A.: An integrated sensing/communication architecture for structural health monitoring. IEEE Sensors Journal 9, 1397–1404 (2009)
[13] Abramo, A., Blanchini, F., Geretti, L., Savorgnan, C.: A mixed convex/non-convex distributed localization approach for the deployment of indoor positioning services. IEEE Transaction on Mobile Computing 7, 1325–1337 (2008)
[14] Enx, C., Scolari, N., Yodprasit, U.: Ultra low-power radio design for wireless sensor networks. In: Proceedings RFIT, vol. 1 (2005)
[15] Evans-Pughe, C.: Close encounters of the magnetic kind (near field communications). IEE Review 51, 38–42 (2005)
[16] Finkenzeller, K.: RFID handbook: fundamentals and applications in contactless smart cards and identification. Wiley, Chichester (2003)
[17] Miura, N., Mizoguchi, D., Sakurai, T., Kuroda, T.: Analysis and design of inductive coupling and transceiver circuit for inductive inter-chip wireless superconnect. IEEE Journal of Solid-State Circuits 40, 829 (2005)
[18] Miura, N., Mizoguchi, D., Inoue, M., Sakurai, T., Kuroda, T.: A 195-Gb/s 1.2-W inductive inter-chip wireless superconnect with transmit power control scheme for 3D-stacked system in a package. IEEE Journal of Solid-State Circuits 41, 23 (2006)
[19] Neagu, C., Jansen, H., Smith, A., Gardeniers, J., Elwenspoek, M.: Characterization of a planar microcoil for implantable microsystems. Sensors and Actuators A: Physical 62, 599 (1997)
[20] Diao, Y., Fu, M., Zhang, H.: An overview of range detection techniques for wireless sensor networks. In: 8th World Congress on Intelligent Control and Automation (WCICA), pp. 1150–1155 (2010)
[21] Rappaport, T.: Wireless communications: principles and practice, 2nd edn. Prentice-Hall, Englewood Cliffs (2001)
[22] Rixon, A., Waugh, R.: A suppressed harmonic power detector for dual band phones. Applied Microvawe and Wireless 11 (1999)

MEMS Strain Sensors for Intelligent Structural Systems

Debbie G. Senesky and Babak Jamshidi

University of California, Berkeley

Abstract. The use of microelectromechanical systems (MEMS) technology to develop strain sensors (resonant and capacitive) is the main topic of this paper. Sensing technology can advance the design and integrity of structural systems in various industries by enabling monitoring of strains and stress concentrations within a mechanical structure in real-time. MEMS-based strain sensors enable performance improvements through increased resolutions, increased operation bandwidths and reduced sensitivity to noise. Therefore, the application of these devices can significantly improve the design robustness and efficiency by predicting catastrophic failures and enabling lightweight designs. MEMS strain sensors can impact the oil and gas, automotive, aerospace and buildings industries through the real-time monitoring of critical components. In addition to device performance, packaging, temperature compensation and long-term drift are important design considerations.

Keywords: sensors, MEMS, strain sensing, stress, structural monitoring.

1 Introduction

Since the early 1990's, the use of semiconductor fabrication techniques to create microelectromechanical Systems (MEMS) has been explored to create robust devices with decreased footprints at reduced costs [1]. Recently, the use of MEMS sensing devices in wireless sensor networks (WSN) has been explored to collect data from structures and environments in real-time [2,3]. One vision of the future is to utilize sensing technology to improve the design and efficiency of mechanical structures through real-time, condition-based monitoring [4]. Delamination, mechanical fractures and corrosion can be identified with proper implementation of sensing systems. This paper will review the design and fabrication of MEMS strain sensors that can be utilized to create intelligent structures. MEMS-based designs are advantageous due to the ability to create devices with high resolution and low noise. In addition, the high-volume manufacturability of MEMS devices reduces the production costs to a fraction of existing monitoring systems. Strain sensors with resonant and capacitive sensing schemes are typically employed and will be described here. It is important for the designer to consider the entire system and to choose a sensing method which exhibits the least environmental

S.C. Mukhopadhyay (Ed.): New Developments in Sensing Technology for SHM,LNEE 96, pp. 63–74.
springerlink.com

biasing (e.g. temperature). Advancements in packaging and electronics are required to enable monitoring systems that are robust and calibrated for offset drifts.

It should be noted that metal-foil strain gauges are commercially available for structural monitoring. Metal-foil gauges utilize the piezoresistive effect to transduce or convert a mechanical strain to an electrical signal. These devices typically have a large footprint and low resolution. Also, piezoelectric devices (e.g. surface acoustic wave or bulk acoustic wave) can be used to monitor changes in the acoustic emission of a material to observe mechanical degradation. This paper focuses on MEMS strain gauges that utilize free-standing, released sensing elements for direct strain detection and strain rate monitoring.

2 Applications for MEMS Strain Sensors

MEMS sensors are advantageous due to the ability to obtain extremely small sensor footprints and batch fabricate complex structures. Strain sensors enable monitoring of strains and stress concentrations and can be utilized for condition-based monitoring of structures. More specifically, these devices can be used to predict and assess mechanical failures such as delamination, mechanical fatigue cracks and corrosion.

Strain sensors can be applied to improve the performance of systems used in various industries such as

- Automotive
- Aerospace
- Buildings and bridges
- Machining tool
- Wind turbine power.

The improvement of these systems can have a significant impact on society by improving safety, increasing operation lifetimes and enabling energy efficiency. For example, strain sensors can be embedded into composite materials to monitor degradation and prevent catastrophic failures [5-6]. In addition, strain monitoring can be used to develop efficient and cost effective designs with decreased safety factors due to more accurate and reliable assessment of structural health. However, it is critical to carefully integrate the strain sensor and circuitry into the system to prevent undesirable and unpredictable failures [7].

It should be noted that the packaging and positioning of strain sensors should be engineered to enable strain transfer to the sensing element without impact to the performance of the underlying structure. Stress concentrations and delamination of existing structures should be avoided. Therefore, loading conditions should be determined for accurate measurements. In Fig. 1 schematic images of positioning strain sensors onto mechanical structures to monitor axial and torsional loading are detailed. Clearly, alignment to the structure is critical and should be considered. In addition, in-plane behaviours should be studied to ensure appropriate strain transfer to the sensing element. Therefore, packaging and bonding technology should be developed to enable efficient integration with the overall system.

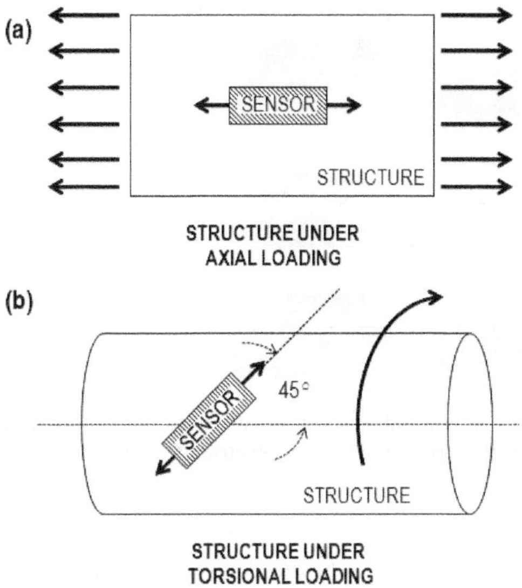

Fig. 1 Schematic images of configuring strain sensors on a mechanical structure to measure axial (a) and torsional loads (b)

3 Fabrication Technologies

The fabrication of MEMS sensors leverages processes developed by the semiconductor industry for integrated circuits (ICs). 2-dimentional patterns along with additive and subtractive processes are used to define 3-dimentional structures. Fig. 2 depicts a simplified fabrication sequence that can be used to design MEMS sensors. Typically, a silicon (Si) substrate is used as the base material for the device. It can also serve as electrical interconnect to the MEMS structures if the Si substrate is highly doped. A sacrificial material such as silicon dioxide (SiO_2) or a polymer thin film (e.g. photoresist or SU-8) is used as a temporary material to enable growth of the structural layer. To enable access of the structural material to the underlying substrate the sacrificial material is etched or patterned. The structural layer (polycrystalline Si in our example) is deposited and subsequently etched to define the top view geometry of the device and to enable access to the underlying sacrificial material. A dry release technique is preferred to avoid stiction effects. Therefore, vapour (dry) release with hydrofluoric (HF) vapour or XeF_2 is often utilized to etched the sacrificial material. To create electrical interconnect to the MEMS device, thin film metals are deposited (sputter deposition or evaporation) onto the structure. It should be noted that this fabrication sequence can be modified to implement new materials to enable alternative sense mechanisms. The packaging of the device can also use semiconductor fabrication techniques.

Designers that are interested in fabricating devices but do not have access to a clean room facility can utilize a multi-user fabrication processes such as MEMSCAP's polysilicon multi-user MEMS processes (polyMUMPS) [8].

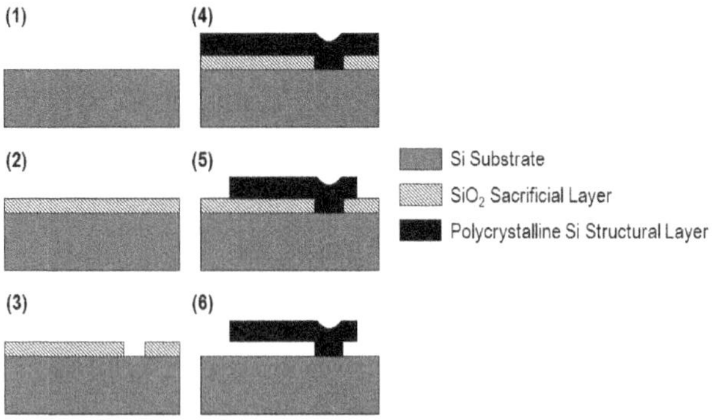

Fig. 2 Illustration of a simple fabrication process used to create released MEMS structures. It should be noted that packaging and electrical interconnect are not shown in this schematic

Furthermore, new materials can be implemented in the design of MEMS strain sensors to extend the performance of devices to extreme temperatures. For example, silicon carbide (SiC) is being utilized in the design of strain sensors [9-10]. In addition, advanced piezoelectric materials (e.g. PZT or AlN) have been extensively studied to design sensors that can monitor acoustic emissions [11].

4 Resonant MEMS Strain Sensors

MEMS strain sensors utilize free-standing mechanical elements to detect physical changes or deformations within interfacing structures. Observing shifts in the resonance frequency of a MEMS structure is one method for detecting strain and often leads to high sensitivity measurements with increased bandwidths and low-noise [12]. The shift in the resonance frequency with applied strain (sensitivity) can be measured and monitored with external electronics (e.g. oscillator circuits) [13-14].

A double-ended-tuning-fork (DETF) structure can be fabricated using MEMS processes and designed such that the resonant frequency of the DETF tines is highly sensitive to external forces. In such a design scenario, the DETF is used as the sensing element for strain detection. The DETF can be driven into resonance with electrostatic forces via interdigitated comb drives (Fig. 3) or parallel capacitive plates. A secondary set of electrostatic features are used for sensing changes in frequency. Fig. 3 details the design features of a MEMS strain sensor with interdigitated drive and sense electrodes and a DETF sensing element.

The DETF structure can be modelled as two clamped-clamped beams. The axial force applied to a single clamped-clamped beam is proportional to the strain (ε),

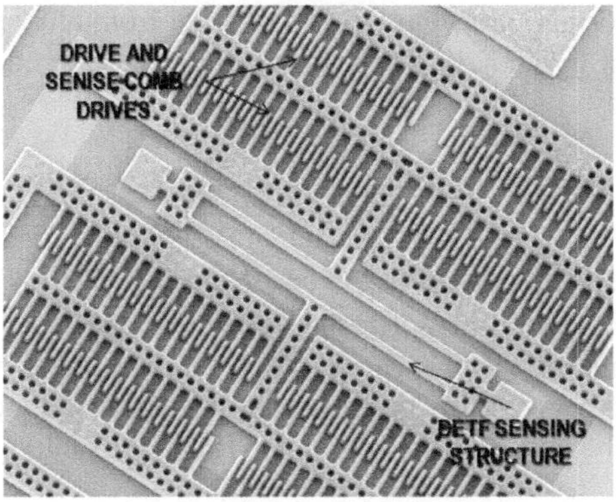

Fig. 3 SEM image of MEMS resonant strain sensor with a DETF sensing structure ad inter-digitated comb features used for drive and sense

$$F = 2wtE\varepsilon \tag{1}$$

where *w* is the beam width, *t* is the beam thickness and *E* is the Young's modulus of elasticity. Recalling from basic structural mechanics, ε is the ratio of the change in length and the original length,

$$\varepsilon = \frac{L - L_o}{L_o} = \frac{\Delta L}{L_o} \tag{2}$$

where L_o is original length of the beam and L is the final length of the beam (Fig. 4) [15]. Although changes in length are shown in Fig. 4, it should be noted that out-of-plane deformations contribute to the behaviour of the mechanical structure.

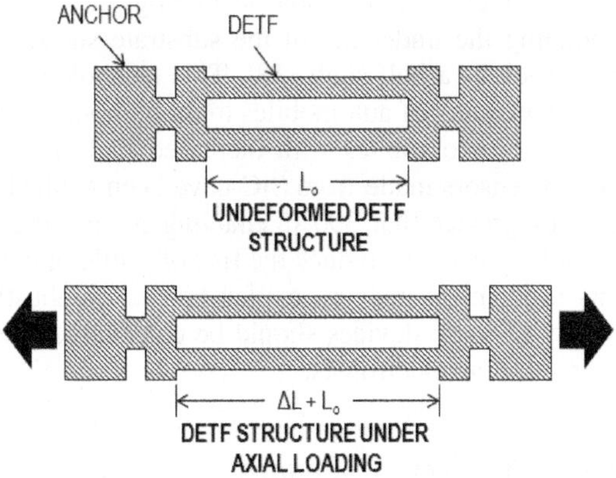

Fig. 4 Schematic image of undeformed DETF structure and DETF structure subjected to axial loading causing changes in the device dimensions

Ultimately, the deformation in the DETF structure from an applied force causes a shift in the resonant frequency. The resonant frequency, f_r, of a clamped-clamped beam is described by

$$f_r^2 = \frac{K_{eff}}{M_{eff}} \tag{3}$$

where M_{eff} is the effective mass of the beam and K_{eff} is the effective spring constant of the beam. It should be noted that the built-in strain (ε_{BI}) and the mass of the drive-sense actuators (M_{act}) which in this analysis are assumed to be lumped at the center of the beam. The change in the resonance frequency of a clamped-clamped beam can be approximated using the Rayleigh's energy method,

$$f_r^2 \approx \frac{EI\int_0^L\left(\frac{\partial^2\varphi(x)}{\partial x^2}\right)^2 dx + 2wtE\varepsilon\int_0^L\left(\frac{\partial\varphi(x)}{\partial x}\right)^2 dx + wt\varepsilon_{BI}\int_0^L\left(\frac{\partial\varphi(x)}{\partial x}\right)^2 dx}{\rho wt\int_0^L \varphi(x)^2\, dx + M_{act}} \tag{4}$$

where ρ is the density and $\varphi(x)$ is the trial function [16]. Using

$$\varphi(x) = \frac{16}{L^4}x^2(x-L)^2 \tag{5}$$

as the trial function and taking the derivative with respect to strain, the sensitivity can be approximated as

$$\frac{\partial f_r}{\partial \varepsilon} \approx \frac{1}{7}\sqrt{\frac{256ELt}{15w\left(\frac{128}{315}\rho tLw + M_{act}\right)\left(1+\frac{2L^2}{7w^2}\varepsilon_{bi}\right)}}\ [17]. \tag{6}$$

Resonant MEMS strain sensors using DETFs as sensing elements have been investigated by various groups [9,10,12,16,17]. These devices can readily be fabricated using the semiconductor processes described in Section 3. The devices have demonstrated high resolution (less than 0.1 με in a 10 kHz bandwidth) which is beyond the performance of commercially available technology. Such devices have been characterized by bonding the underside of the substrate surface to a macro-scale mechanical structure such as a half-shaft [18]. This technology can be further developed to monitor drive-shafts of automobiles to monitor signatures from combustion chambers leading to automobiles with increased fuel efficiency. In addition, resonant MEMS strain sensors made from SiC have been studied to extend the operation to temperatures greater that 300°C enabling monitoring in extreme environments. This technology can also reduce the risk of brittle or corrosion failures of critical components used in oil and gas exploration or combustion systems. The temperature sensitivity of these devices should be considered and can be compensated with signal conditioning electronics.

5 Capacitive MEMS Strain Sensors

Capacitive strain sensing is an alternative approach to resonant strain sensing, in which the strain is measured by monitoring the geometry [19] or permittivity [20]

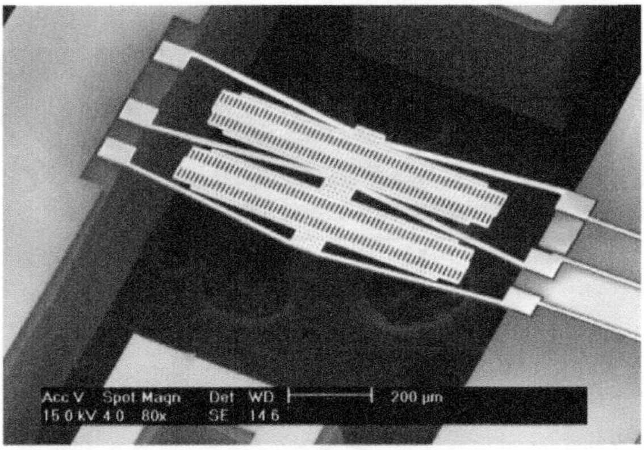

Fig. 5 Capacitive strain sensor using electrostatic comb drives [26]

change in parallel plate capacitors. The passive nature of the capacitive strain measurement requires low power and has nominal temperature dependency [21]. Consequently, it requires low voltage circuitry for continuous operation which makes it an attractive choice for industrial applications.

MEMS capacitive strain sensors generally consist of single or multiple capacitors [22] or a system of electrostatic comb drives [23]. The latter typically has a simple structure but requires amplification of the strain signals transferred from the medium by using sophisticated circuitry or customized mechanical designs to achieve acceptable rate of signal to noise ratio. In addition, a bulk micromachining fabrication technique on semiconductor grade wafers is typically used to manufacture the capacitive sensors and maximize the capacitive area. Therefore, these sensors are often fabricated on top of relatively thick substrate. However, the presence of a rigid substrate can dissipate up to half of the strain signal transferred from the medium [24]. Although a system of electrostatic comb drives (Figure 5) improves the capacitive area [25] and gauge sensitivity, it will introduce readout non-linearity, cross-axis strain sensitivity, lower mechanical bandwidth, and large parasitic and feed-through capacitance into output signal.

The capacitive sensing method is based on the detection of electrical flux variations between two electrically conductive electrodes when a differential voltage is applied across them. The amount of produced electrical flux (capacitance) depends on the geometry of the electrodes. For example, if we consider a parallel plate capacitor (Fig. 6) the capacitance, C depends on the area, A, the gap, g between the conductive plates and permittivity of the medium, $\varepsilon_o\varepsilon_r$ (Eq. 7).

$$C = \varepsilon_o \varepsilon_r \frac{A}{g} \qquad (A = bd) \tag{7}$$

Therefore, variation of the physical dimensions will have an impact on the voltage across the plates [27]. Furthermore, parametric mechanical design is a critical step in development of a capacitive sensor.

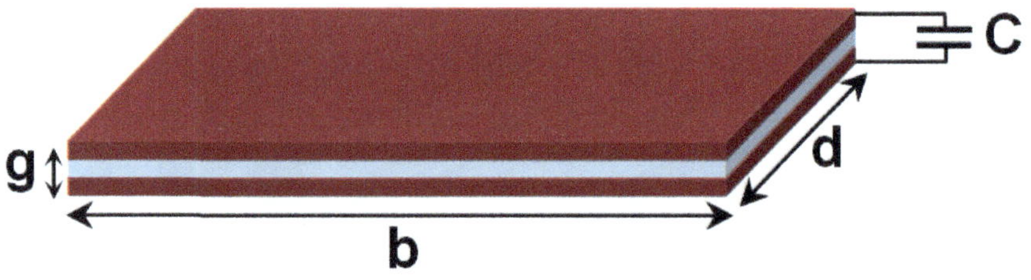

Fig. 6 Schematic image of a parallel plate capacitor

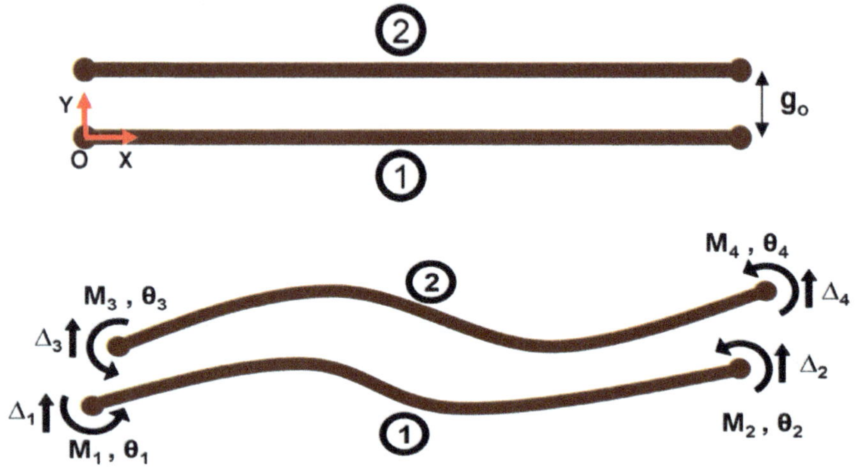

Fig. 7 Unstrained capacitive strain sensor (top), translated and deformed state of capacitive electrodes due to applied strain (bottom)

One of the major challenges of capacitive strain sensor design is to eliminate the effect of the undesired strain signals and achieve accurate and reliable measurements. The majority of strain sensors are bulk micro-machined so the state of active strain field can be presumed as plane strain. As described in Fig. 7, the transferred plane strain will deform and translate the capacitive electrodes which influences on both capacitive gap (g) and area (A).Therefore, the capacitance change due to the applied strain can be derived as:

$$\frac{dC}{dx} = -\varepsilon_o \varepsilon_r \frac{A}{g^2} \cdot \frac{\partial g}{\partial x} + \varepsilon_o \varepsilon_r \frac{1}{g} \cdot \frac{\partial A}{\partial x} \tag{8}$$

If we consider capacitive plates with the length, L, and unit heights, the deformation of the elastic plates can be modeled using the Euler-Bernoulli beam theory [28]:

$$EI\frac{\partial^2 y}{\partial x^2} = M \tag{9}$$

where y, I and M are the beam deformation, moment of inertia, and applied moment, respectively. The initial boundary conditions for rotation (θ) and displacement for the unstrained (initial) and strained (deformed) beams are:

$$\theta_{initial}(x = 0, L) = 0,\ y_{initial}(x = 0, L) = 0 \tag{10}$$

$$\theta_{(1),deformed}(x = 0) = \theta_1,\ y_{(1),deformed}(x = 0) = \Delta_1 \tag{11}$$

Using (Eq. 9), the deflection of beams (1) and (2) are derived as:

$$y_{(1),deformed} = \frac{M_2}{2EI}\left(x^2 - \frac{x^3}{3L}\right) - \frac{M_1}{6EIL}x^3 + \theta_1 x + \Delta_1 \tag{12}$$

$$y_{(2),deformed} = \frac{M_3}{2EI}\left(x^2 - \frac{x^3}{3L}\right) - \frac{M_4}{6EIL}x^3 + \theta_1 x + \Delta_3 + g_o \tag{13}$$

Therefore, the capacitive gap change can be calculated by taking the derivative of the displacement with respect to its lateral displacement, y:

$$\frac{\partial g}{\partial x} = \left(y_{(2),deformed} - y_{(1),deformed}\right) - g_o \tag{14}$$

Moreover, the lateral displacement of the electrodes will change the capacitive area. Eq. 12 and Eq. 13 can be simplified by inclusion of symmetry planes and imposing specific boundary conditions on the mechanical design. On the other

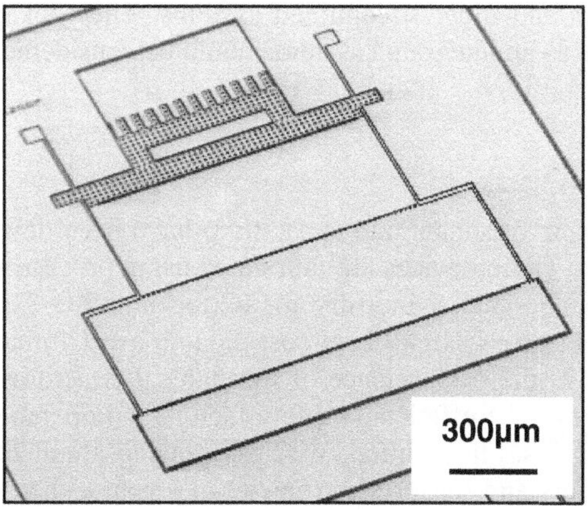

Fig. 8 High resolution capacitive strain gauge designed to attenuate cross-axis strain signals [29]

hand, any strain measurement may be influenced by both strain components ε_x and ε_y (Eq. 8) which makes it extremely difficult to monitor the field when detection in a single direction is interested. Therefore, it is preferred to attenuate the cross-axis strain through mechanical design to eliminate the need for complex circuitry. In addition to structural symmetry, special arrangements of parallel plate capacitors such as differential readout can assist with the rejection of undesired mechanical signals. Therefore, capacitive sensors (Fig. 8) can be designed as a robust means to measure strain in small ranges (1 με to 1000 με) while exhibiting nominal signal attenuation due to cross-axis sensitivity [22].

6 Packaging and Data Acquisition

As mentioned previously, the packaging of MEMS strain sensors is an important design consideration. This is due to the fact that the packaging itself could lead to device failure or performance drift. For example, if the sensor is not appropriately bonded or integrated into the material structure, delamination could occur leading to a failed sensor component or worse a failed structure. Furthermore, strain transfer from the mechanical structure to the sensor itself should be modelled and predicted to avoid signal biasing.

In addition, to ensure long term operation, the sensor should be protected from the external environment with packaging. For instance, extreme temperature excursions, particles and humidity can cause sensor drift and sensor housing (in vacuum) can mitigate these issues.

The electronics that interface with MEMS strain sensors can improve the performance of the sensor system. For example, the sensor itself converts mechanical deformations to electrical signals and those signals can be amplified or conditioned with external electronics. This leads to devices with signal drift compensation, thermal compensation and decreased noise. In addition, wireless telemetry of sensor data can be realized with the wireless sensor electronics which could lead to sensor networks and more streamlined systems. The packaging of the sensor and the electronics as an integrated system should be considered and developed.

7 Conclusion

MEMS strain sensors (resonant and capacitive) have been developed and studied by various groups. These devices are fabricated using processes and materials developed by the semiconductor industry for IC technology. The processes enable batch fabrication leading to significant cost reductions. Ultimately, MEMS strain sensing can improve the performance of mechanical structures and systems with real-time monitoring. The efficiency, safety factors and operation lifetimes can be increased with sensors. In addition, wireless sensing architectures composed of MEMS strain sensors and sensor electronics can enhance the design of buildings, automobiles and aircrafts.

References

1. Bustillo, J., Howe, R., Muller, S.: Surface micromachining for microelectromechanical systems. Proc. of the IEEE 86(8), 1552–1574 (1998)
2. Akyildiz, F., Su, W., Sankarasubramaniam, Y., Cayirci, E.: Wireless sensor networks: a survey. Computer Networks 38(4), 393–422 (2002)
3. Senesky, D., Jamshidi, B., Cheng, K., Pisano, A.: Harsh Environment Sili-con Carbide Sensors for Health and Performance Monitoring of Aerospace Systems: A Review. IEEE Sensors Journal 9(11), 1472–1478 (2009)
4. Chang, F.: Structural Health Monitoring: Current Status and Perspectives. CRC Press, Boca Raton (1998)
5. Ghezzo, F., Rye, P., Huang, Y., Nemat-Nasser, S.: Integration of sensing networks into laminated composites. In: Proc. of SPIE Int. Symp. on Smart Structures and Materials (2008)
6. Hautamaki, C., Zurn, S., Mantell, S., Polla, D.: Experimental evaluation of MEMS strain sensors embedded in composites. Journal of Microelectrome-chanical Systems 8(3), 272–279 (1999)
7. Mall, S.: Integrity of graphite/epoxy laminate embedded with piezoelectric sensor/actuator under monotonic and fatigue loads. Smart Materials and Structures 11, 527–533 (2002)
8. PolyMUMPS Design Handbook, `http://www.memscap.com`
9. Azevedo, R., Jones, D., Jog, A., Jamshidi, B., Myers, D., Chen, L., Fu, X., Mehregany, M., Wijesundara, M., Pisano, A.: A SiC MEMS Resonant Strain Sensor for Harsh Environment Application. IEEE Sensors Journal 7(4), 568–576 (2007)
10. Myers, D., Cheng, K., Jamshidi, B., Azevedo, R., Senesky, D., Chen, L., Mehregany, M., Wijesundara, M., Pisano, A.: Silicon carbide resonant tuning fork for microsensing applications in high-temperature and high G-shock environ-ments. Journal of Micro/Nanolithography, MEMS, and MOEMS 8(021116) (2009)
11. Saponara, V., Horsley, D., Lestari, W.: Structural Health Monitoring of Glass/Epoxy Composite Plates Using PZT and PMN-PT Transducers. Journal of Engineering Materials and Technology 133(011011) (2011)
12. Wojciechowski, K., Boser, B., Pisano, A.: A MEMS Resonant Strain Sensor in Air. In: Proc. 17th IEEE International Conference on Micro Electro Mechanical Systems, pp. 841–845 (2004)
13. Azevedo, R., Zhang, J., Jones, D., Myers, D., Jog, A., Jamshidi, B., Wijesundara, M., Maboudian, R., Pisano, A.: Silicon Carbide Coated Silicon MEMS Strain Sensor for Harsh Environment Applications. In: Proc. 20th IEEE International Conference on Micro Electro Mechanical Systems, Japan, pp. 643–646 (2007)
14. Wojciechowski, K., Boser, B., Pisano, A.: A MEMS resonant strain sensor with 33 nano-strain resolution in a 10 kHz bandwidth. In: Proc. IEEE Sensors Conference, USA, pp. 947–950 (2005)
15. Young, W., Budynas, R.: Roark's formulas for stress and strain, 7th edn., pp. 196–197. McGraw-Hill, New York (2002)
16. Roessig, T.: Integrated MEMS tuning fork oscillators for sensor applications. Ph.D. Thesis, Department of Mechanical Engineering, University of California, Berkeley (1998)
17. Wojciechowski, K.: Electronics for Resonant Sensors. Ph.D. Thesis, Department of Electrical Engineering, University of California, Berkeley (2005)

18. Myers, D., Pisano, A.: Torque Measurements of an Automotive Halfshaft Utilizing a MEMS Resonant Strain Gauge. In: Proc. of 15th International Conference on Solid-State Sensors, Actuators, & Microsystems, USA, pp. 1726–1729 (2009)
19. Filanc-Bowen, T., Kim, G., Shkel, Y.: Novel Sensor Technology for Shear and Normal Strain Detection with Generalized Electrostriction. Proceedings of IEEE Sensors 2(4), 1648–1653 (2002)
20. Arshak, K., McDonagh, D., Duran, M.: Development of New Capacitive Strain Sensors Based on Thick Film Polymer and Cement Technologies. Sensors and Actuators A. 79, 102–114 (2000)
21. Cockbain, A., Horrop, P.: The Temperature Coefficient of Capacitance. British Journal of Applied Physics 2(9), 1109–1115 (1968)
22. Jamshidi, B., Azevedo, R., Jog, A., Pisano, A.: Silicon Cross-Axis Rejection Capacitive Strain Gauge. In: Proc. of ASME International Mechanical Engineering Congress and Exposition, USA (2007)
23. Guo, J., Kuo, H., Young, D., Ko, W.: Buckled Beam Linear Output Capacitive Strain Sensor. In: Proc. of Solid State Sensor, Actuator and Microsystems Workshop, USA (2004)
24. Azevedo, R., Chen, I., O'Reilly, O., Pisano, A.: Influence of Sensor Substrate Geometry on the Sensitivity of MEMS Micro-Extensometers. In: Proc. of International Mechanical Engineering Congress and Exposition, USA (2005)
25. Aebersold, J., Walsh, K., Crain, M., Martin, M., Voor, M., Lin, J., Jackson, D., Hunt, W., Naber, J.: Design and Development of a MEMS Capacitive Bending Strain Sensor. Journal of Micromechanics and Microengineering 16, 935–942 (2006)
26. Guo, J., Suster, M., Young, D., Ko, W.: High-Gain Mechanically Amplified Capacitive Strain Sensors. In: Proc. of IEEE Annual Meeting, pp. 464–467 (2005)
27. Jamshidi, B.: Poly-Crystalline Silicon Carbide Passivated Capacitive MEMS Strain Gauge for Harsh Environments. Ph.D. Thesis, Department of Mechanical Engineering, University of California, Berkeley (2008)
28. Azevedo, R.: Design and Evaluation of a MEMS Offset Capacitive Comb Strain Sensor. M.Sc. Dissertation, Department of Mechanical Engineering, University of California, Berkeley (2003)
29. Jamshidi, B., Azevedo, R., Wijesundara, M., Pisano, A.: Corrosion Enhanced Capacitive Strain Gauge at 370°C. In: Proc. of the 6th Annual IEEE Conference on Sensors, USA (2007)

A Pattern-Based Framework for Developing Wireless Monitoring Applications

James Brusey[1], Elena Gaura[1], and Roger Hazelden[2]

[1] Cogent Computing Applied Research Centre, Coventry University, Coventry, UK
j.brusey@coventry.ac.uk
[2] TRW Conekt, Solihull, UK
roger.hazelden@trw.com

Summary. Development of application-specific wireless monitoring systems can benefit from *concept* reuse and design patterns can form the enabling medium for such reuse. This chapter presents a set of five fundamental node-level patterns that resolve common problems when programming low-power embedded wireless sensing devices. Although the design patterns proposed are not subjected to a quantitative evaluation, a qualitative evaluation is performed through examining examples of these patterns in existing published deployments and systems. This analysis demonstrates that key deployment lessons are codified in each pattern.The pattern set forms a framework that is aimed at ensuring simple and robust deployed systems.

1 Introduction

The need for distributed sensing for Structure Health Monitoring (SHM) is commonplace. Sensing both needs to be local to the phenomena (such as crack sensors on weld joints) and must cover a region (such as a structure with many weld joints). Distribution is often best served by wireless sensors:

1. They are quick to set up and tear down and the associated infrastructure is minimal.
2. Wireless sensors avoid the need for installing cabling for communication and power.
3. Individual sensing points can be added, moved, or removed at low cost.

The idea of automatically and wirelessly acquiring data from a distributed set of sensors is relatively recent—feasible wireless sensors have only been readily available for the last decade or so. Although the technology is beginning to move into the mainstream, developers are still faced with a technology that is hard to understand and difficult to make reliable.

A key difficulty, for example, is in powering sensors and wireless transmitters, thus optimising energy efficiency of a Wireless Sensor Network (WSN) can often be critical to the business case for their use. For SHM in aircraft, a minimum battery lifetime of about seven years is required to ensure that the wireless system is cost effective.

S.C. Mukhopadhyay (Ed.): New Developments in Sensing Technology for SHM, LNEE 96, pp. 75–91.
springerlink.com

Where distributed sensing is used for one application, there often arise multiple applications for the sensory data and thus the need for sensing and sensor-based actuation evolves over time. For this reason, a well-structured, systematic development and framework are required to ensure that new applications and additional sensors can be easily integrated as the system grows.

Some support exists for simplifying the development of wireless sensors (e.g. TinyOS, Embedded Linux). However, there is little work on guidelines or frameworks that establish best practice in this area. In particular, there appears to be a series of identifiable lessons that are being repeatedly rediscovered by programmers and research groups. Part of the difficulty is that WSN deployments are diverse. There appears to be little carry-over in terms of lessons learnt from one deployment to the next simply because many of the issues do not apply.

This chapter sets out a framework for reusable patterns for WSNs. Although no quantitative evaluation of the framework is provided here (and indeed may not be possible), a qualitative evaluation is performed by identifying key lessons from several deployed systems and linking these to elements of the framework.

This work builds on prior work [4] that formulated the framework mathematically. Although precise, the mathematical formulation may be less intuitive for some readers. In comparison, it is hoped that this presentation is more accessible while the mathematical formulation can be used for reference where clarification is needed. The presentation here is loosely based on design patterns [6] but without the emphasis on object-orientation.

The next section presents the framework and the associated five node-level patterns: the Filter pattern, the Event Detector pattern, the Priority Buffer pattern, the Nonpreemptive Scheduler pattern, and the Interval Listening pattern. Each pattern is described in terms of its aims, the triggers that indicate the need for it to be considered, collaborations that can occur with other patterns, possible extensions, and finally examples of pattern usage from the literature. The final section concludes the work and outlines how it might best be applied to aiding the development process of novel monitoring applications.

2 A Pattern-Based Framework

In this work, the term "framework" is used partly to refer to a form of proto-architecture where elements may be added, removed, or altered to suit an application and partly to encapsulate the collection of related design patterns. The design pattern literature is relatively well-established as a means of describing prototypical solutions for common object-oriented design problems. This work borrows the term "design pattern" but without the object-oriented undertones and associated requirements. Here, a design pattern is intended to be merely a template or guide for solving specific design problems with software development for WSN systems.

The framework presented here is based on two fundamental assumptions:

1. There are benefits to processing at the node in a wide variety of applications.
2. Benefits from sharing information between (leaf) nodes within a network are rare in practice and even less frequently worth the associated risks and complexity.

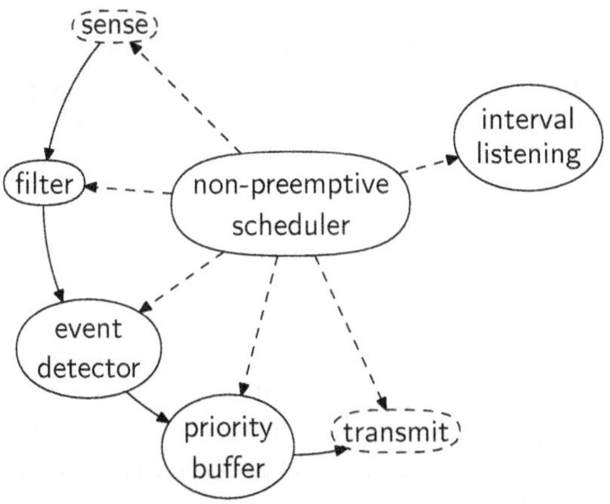

Fig. 1 Pattern-based Framework for nodes. A dashed box is drawn for elements that have no explicit pattern described here

This framework, then, focuses on a simple WSN where remotely stationed wireless nodes communicate directly (single hop) or indirectly (multi-hop) with a "sink" or base station.

This approach is aligned with Raman and Chebrolu [15] who argue that the WSN domain is divided into two main camps: Those devoted to devising algorithms and protocols and those pursuing application centric design and deploying systems "in the wild". They find that the sophisticated algorithms and protocols devised by the former group are rarely used by the latter group. Deployed systems tend to eschew complexity. Simpler, well understood MAC layers are favoured.

Werner Allen et al. [17] in their description of Lance also argue for keeping node interaction simple. In their volcano monitoring system, sufficient complexity (and frustration!) was introduced even by using the well known FTSP time synchronisation protocol, which at the time, had some unresolved bugs. The Lance architecture specifically assumes that remote nodes do not collaborate or share information.

Comprehensive arguments such as those above lead to the key elements of the node-level framework, which are summarised in Figure 1. The central task for the node begins with the "sense" operation. Noise is *filtered* and the original data is transformed into meaningful information. *Event detection* occurs next potentially leading to a message that must be transmitted. The message is *buffered* according to *priority* before being transmitted. These tasks must be interleaved along with sleeping and *listening at intervals* and this is the job of the *scheduler*.

It is usual, when developing a monitoring system, to include various data structures (or perhaps classes) that are specific to what is being measured. This framework describes the sensed data and the subsequent inferred state as simple vectors. The framework does not preclude using more complex structures but flattening the data structure in this way emphasises the generality of the approach to a wide variety of possible sensors, phenomena, and applications.

In the following sections each design pattern is described in more detail. A general description of each pattern is given, followed by its *Aims* (what is the intended function achieved by the pattern), *Triggers* (the reasons why the pattern might be used), *Collaborators* (which other patterns are often used with it), *Possible Extensions* (additional functionality) and *Examples* (some examples from the literature of successful use of the pattern).

2.1 Filter (or Model-Based Smoothing) Pattern

The Filter Pattern, which could also be termed the Model based Smoothing Pattern, is a node-level pattern to *smooth* the raw, sensed data and / or *infer the state* of the phenomena at the node. There are some specific reasons for performing filtering at the node rather than at the sink, as described in Section 2.1.2. Thus this approach is advantageous in some applications and not others.

The Filter Pattern is based roughly on the design of a Kalman Filter (see Welch and Bishop [16] for a introduction) and its structure is summarised in Figure 2. This is a recursive, on-line filter that takes as *input* a vector representing the estimate of prior state, the elapsed time, and a vector containing current sensor readings and produces as *output* an updated state estimate. Kalman Filters may be too computationally intensive or difficult to implement (due to the requirement for floating point arithmetic and matrix inversion) for most WSN applications, however the overall design is still applicable. A light weight alternative, which has a similar recursive structure, is the Exponentially Weighted Moving Average (EWMA) filter.

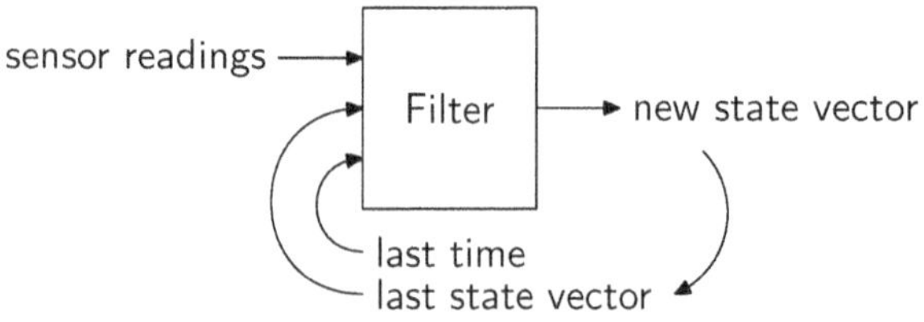

Fig. 2 Synopsis of the Filter pattern

2.1.1 Aims

A filter aims to do the following, based on a series of sensor readings:

- Reduce noise, and / or,
- Summarise a sensory "chunk", and / or,
- Infer state, possibly from sensors of differing modality.

Most sensor measurements incorporate some form of noise. The effect of noise can often be reduced by applying some form of low-pass filter such as an EWMA or Kalman Filter. Although the computation involved is typically more easily performed at the sink, filtering at the node helps to ensure that other processing, such as event detection, is affected minimally by noise.

Filters can also summarise a "chunk" of sensor measurements. A common application is processing audio data, where a large amount of data is being received by the sensor during each sampling period. Summarisation can substantially reduce the bandwidth required as the summaries are generally much smaller than the original data. Summarisation might be generic (such as finding the peak audio levels over the last second) or specific (is the call of a particular animal species being heard?). Summarisation might be final (a cane toad call is being heard) or tentative (possible earth tremor occurring currently). In the latter case, the unfiltered data might need to be stored for later analysis, perhaps when other nodes have confirmed that a tremor event occurred.

Note that it is important to keep distinct the two issues of:

1. *filtering*, which transforms data into an estimate or summary of the state, and
2. *event detection*, which detects whether the change in the state is significant.

Such separation ensures that the two distinct concerns of deriving a state representation and decision making based on that state are not confused.

Filters are often explicitly model-based, in which case, the filter attempts to derive an estimate of the state of the system based on past sensor readings. Often it is possible to assume that the system has the Markov property, which means that the most recent sensor reading and the last state estimate are all that are required to estimate the current state and that no better can be done by knowing the complete history of states. For example, when estimating the number of people in the room from a door sensor, it is only necessary to know the past state (how many people were previously in the room) and how many people exited or entered. A model-based approach is often useful to fuse data from several sensors of differing modalities. For example, there may be a Passive Infra-Red (PIR) sensor detecting overall occupancy alongside the exit sensor attached to the same node[1]. Information can be combined from the pair of sensors to give a more accurate estimate of the true occupancy.

2.1.2 Triggers

The Filter Pattern should be used when:

- Available bandwidth is low relative to the amount of data sensed.
- The relative cost of transmitting data is higher than processing it on the node
- Actual sensor readings are not necessarily required (or only contingently required).

Many wireless sensor deployments involve a set of individual sensors that in combination can provide much more data per unit time than the wireless transmission medium can sustain. High data rate sensing applications involving video, audio, or vibration sensors, in particular, are limited by the available wireless bandwidth. Such situations provide a strong motivation to attempt to process and summarise

[1] Fusion between sensors on different nodes might also be possible but the framework encourages us to first consider moving such sensor fusion to the sink.

sensor readings on the node. Further reductions in bandwidth requirements are possible by combining the Filter pattern with the Event Detection pattern.

Transmission costs tend to be an order of magnitude greater than the computational costs associated with filtering. Listening costs can also be a significant factor, however, if the node needs to act as a router (which is often needed in mesh networking).

Individual sensor readings may not be required. For example, an application may involve monitoring cupboard "opening" and "closing" events using a light sensor. It is not necessary to know how much light is falling on the sensor when the door is open, it is enough to know that the door is open. Filtering the data into a state variable of "open" or "closed" not only reduces the needed bandwidth but also better supports subsequent Event Detection by reducing the effect of noise and thus reducing spurious event detection.

2.1.3 Collaborators

The Filter pattern is often used in collaboration with the Event Detection pattern. There are several reasons why such a collaboration can be useful:

1. The process of filtering removes noise thus reducing spurious event detection.
2. Transforming the raw sensor data into a state vector simplifies the task of identifying whether the state has changed in a way that can be considered a meaningful event.
3. It supports avoiding a "slippery slope" problem where the event detection mechanism cannot detect a change if the change occurs slowly enough.

Further, combining the Filter pattern with the Interval Listening pattern can avoid the possibility that the energy gained from reduced transmissions is not then subsequently lost due to increased listening time.

2.1.4 Possible Extensions

Although the framework begins with the assumption that individual nodes do not share information and are not required to communicate directly with one another, for some applications, it may be useful to allow such communication. In this case, the state estimate produced by the Filter can take into account measurements from neighbouring nodes. For example, an intrusion detection system might consider a possible intrusion more likely if neighbouring nodes are also sensing a disturbance.

The Lance architecture suggests a useful extension that involves locally storing the original (unfiltered) data and providing it on-demand. This approach is particularly useful when local information is not sufficient to fully make a decision about how useful the data is.

The state vector need not be just about the phenomena. It is often useful to include management information or, in other words, information about the state of the sensors or the wireless node. For example, this could include local timestamps, battery voltages, estimates of uncertainty in measurement readings, link reliability statistics, and so forth.

2.1.5 Examples

On-node filters are quite common in the literature. Here are two examples:

- Lance [17] is an architecture built originally for volcano monitoring that made use of audio sensors. Transmitting all of the audio over a multi-hop network led to much contention and low yield. By sending summaries of the data instead, the bandwidth requirement was significantly reduced and the yield of useful data improved.
- The Cane Toad monitoring project [10] is another excellent example of successfully processing complex audio data on the node. Frog calls were collected in the wild and analysed in real-time using spectrograms and C4.5 decision trees to classify the frog species. The initial work required more sophisticated processors but the final systems were able to be deployed on Mica2 motes. Performing the conversion from raw audio to identified frog species on-board was critical in reducing the bandwidth requirement for this application and thus allowing it to be performed with inexpensive motes.

2.2 Event Detector Pattern

A fundamental and simple pattern for reducing the number and size of transmissions is based on detecting events at the node. The pattern is summarised in Figure 3. Event detectors typically work by comparing the current state with the last transmitted state. If the difference exceeds some threshold, then an event is detected. Comparing with the last transmitted state avoids the possibility of sending duplicate event messages while using the last *transmitted* state for comparison avoids a "slippery slope" effect where a slowly changing phenomena may appear to be uneventful (the gradient at any point is low) but the long term change is still significant.

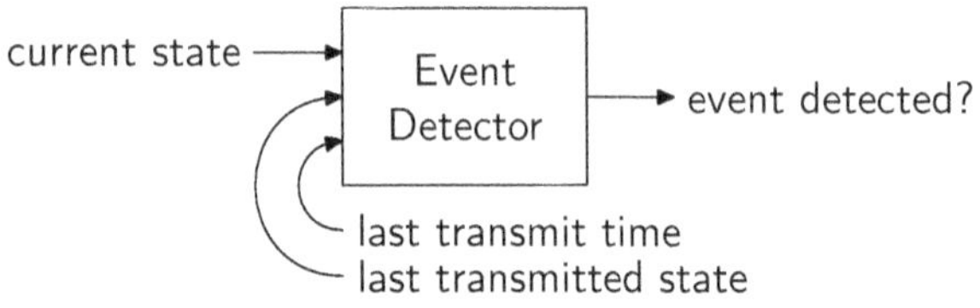

Fig. 3 Synopsis of the Event Detector Pattern

2.2.1 Aims

The Event Detector Pattern aims to:

- reduce the transmission of unnecessary data
- allow for increased rate of transmission of needed data

When performing initial investigation, it is often useful to acquire a large number of samples from a large array of sampling points. Once this initial phase has ended

and the phenomena is better understood, much of this data is not needed and continuing to acquire it is an unnecessary cost. Identifying which data is unnecessary will depend on the application however there are some common cases:

1. where the state maintains the same (or nearly the same) value over an extended period;
2. where the state is easily predictable over time (e.g. a linear trend); or,
3. where the state continues to stay within a set of expected values (but it is not necessary to know exactly which).

The term "state" is used above, rather than "sensor reading" since it is typically the case that the raw, unsmoothed, uncalibrated reading will first be processed into an application-specific state vector by a Filter prior to event detection. For example, it is simpler to design event detection based on a state vector that includes, say, an estimate of the residual life rather than one that gives wear sensor measurement readings.

To properly detect events for systems that are predictable over time, some prediction is needed. For example, if the last transmitted state was taken 5 minutes ago and indicated that the state was at 1 unit and rising linearly by half a unit every minute, then the predicted state is 3.5 units. If the new state estimate is close to this (within some threshold), then it is considered uneventful. In principle, arbitrarily complex models could be used here. In practice, however, simple linear regression is sufficient for most cases.

A further advantage of event detection is that it may save sufficient transmission energy and bandwidth to allow an increase in sensing frequency. This potentially allows detection of short-lived phenomena that might be missed otherwise.

2.2.2 Triggers

The Event Detector pattern should be considered when:

- the system being measured has a steady or easily predicted state for extended periods, and / or,
- transmission cost (say, in terms of energy or bandwidth use) is high.

Steady state systems are reasonably common and, for these systems, the use and benefit of the Event Detector pattern is more obvious. Less obvious is the application of event detection to systems that follow diurnal, periodic, or short term linear trends. Some examples include: temperatures within a building, water pressure within the water supply pipe network, wear on machine bearings, and so forth.

2.2.3 Collaborators

The Event Detector Pattern is often used in conjunction with the Filter Pattern (also see section 2.1.3). In fact, they are so often used jointly that it is easy to confuse them or not to know when to use one without the other.

Filters are used *without* event detection when the decision about whether or not an event has occurred must be deferred until more information is known. Perhaps

the decision can only be made at the sink, when summaries from other nodes have been heard.

Event detection is used *without* filtering when the sensor already provides a sufficiently clean signal. For example, an RFID tag reader provides tag-read messages that are free from noise. Event detection is needed to identify when tagged items appear or disappear. Even in this case, it may still be useful to have a "filter" to organise the incoming tag-read messages into an estimate of which items are present (i.e. a representation of state).

2.2.4 Possible Extensions

There are several ways in which to extend the basic Event Detector pattern:

- Incorporating a "heartbeat" message can ensure that the sink will eventually detect node failure. Without this, the node might not send any data for an indefinite period, if the phenomena is in a steady state. A simple method to incorporate a heartbeat is to signal an event if the last transmission time was long ago, even if the state is unchanged. (The exact definition of how long to wait before sending a heartbeat will depend on the application.)
- Model-based event detection (based on predicting from linear or other trends) can be further enhanced by assuming that the sink can also apply the same model-based prediction. The Spanish Inquisition Protocol [8] describes an event detector that makes use of dual prediction (on both node and sink).
- A useful assumption is that the state vector (used as input) has the Markov property. That is, a prediction based on the state vector would not be improved by knowing the complete history of states. This is a helpful consideration when deciding what features to include in the state vector. For example, rate of change is needed if one wants to predict based on a linear extrapolation of the trend.

2.2.5 Examples

The use of the Event Detector pattern is commonplace in the literature. Two interesting examples both begin with high data rate sensors.

- VoxNet is a deployed WSN that localises animal calls using a set of four microphones at each node [2,1]. Full trilateration of incoming audio signals could only be performed at the sink, however sending all of the audio signals tended to overload the 802.11 network used. Setting up an event detector that looked for the start and end times of possible animal calls meant that audio data could be sent much less frequently.
- Event detection for human activity monitoring systems can substantially reduce transmissions. In work elsewhere [3], a postural activity monitoring system was developed that classified posture based on 2 or more MEMS accelerometer sensors worn on various places on the body. A combination of on-board posture classification, an exponentially weighted voting filter and event detection reduced the transmissions from the original 10 Hz to about 600 event transmissions in 30 minutes (0.3 Hz) without the filter or around 100 in a 30 minute period with filtering included (0.06 Hz).

2.3 Priority Buffer Pattern

A synopsis of the Priority Buffer pattern is given in Figure 4. The priority of any message is determined by the contents of the message. This priority is used to determine ordering in the priority buffer along with the time of arrival. Transmission then proceeds from the head of the buffer.

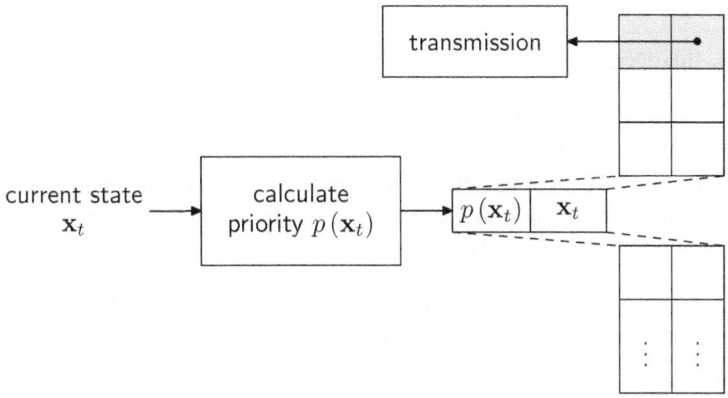

Fig. 4 Synopsis of the Priority Buffer Pattern

This simple pattern can be critical in ensuring that high priority messages are communicated successfully. The first part of the pattern consists of ordering the buffer according to priority. The second part consists of controlling the timing of transmission and, in particular, controlling when transmissions should be retried.

2.3.1 Aims

The aim of the Priority Buffer pattern is to:

- increase the likelihood that important packets are transmitted,
- reduce the contention for the transmission medium,
- gracefully handle extended periods without the ability to transmit.

Traditional wired networks assume that the probability of any given transmission failing is always the same. Wireless networks, however, suffer from variations in failure probability. For example, mobile wireless devices may be in range and able to communicate for some long period and then subsequently out of range or RF occluded from communicating for a period. Fixed devices can have similar variations in failure probability due to environmental factors such as rain or snow, the movement of occluding objects, and so forth. For this reason, when a transmission fails, particularly if it has already failed several times, it may not be best to retry immediately.

The Priority Buffer pattern responds to this problem by:

1. raising the communication buffer to an application level (rather than an operating system one),
2. allowing re-ordering of transmissions by priority even when a transmission has failed, and,
3. allowing control of when retries should occur.

Dealing with the communication buffer at an application level means that it is possible to support much larger buffers than usual, perhaps making use of flash memory. Furthermore, since message headers have not been added yet, the individual messages will be smaller. When communication is cut for an extended period, this application buffer may be sufficient to ensure that no information is lost.

Some communication messages are of high priority ("the building is on fire") while others are of low priority ("the temperature in the hallway was 20 °C"). Priority may also depend on time ("temperature was x, three hours ago" may be less important than "temperature is currently y"). If communication has been prevented for several hours, when communications returns it makes sense to ensure that high priority messages are sent first. Sending them first will also mean that it is more likely that they are transmitted successfully.

Where communication is failing because of contention for the transmission medium, reducing the number of attempts to transmit will help to reduce contention and this is an important consideration for the designer of a Priority Buffer.

Communication may also be failing due to a transient environmental effect (such as rain or snow) that will continue to prevent successful transmission for some time. An application-level strategy can balance the importance of timely transmission against the cost of many retries.

2.3.2 Triggers

The Priority Buffer pattern should be considered when:

- some messages are of higher priority than others,
- the likelihood of successful transmissions varies over time.

2.3.3 Collaborators

A critical question when devising a Priority Buffer is how to determine which messages are more important. In particular, the message should contain enough information to enable a decision about its priority to be made. This implies an interaction with the associated Filter. The Filter helps the Priority Buffer by placing sufficient context into the state vector. For example, in a patient health monitoring application, rather than just stating the vital signs (heart rate is 180, core temperature is 39 °C, etc), the Filter can help by interpreting the data somewhat ("likelihood of imminent cardiac arrest is 30%"). In principle, the burden of inference can lie in either place. In practice, however, it can be easier to encode the priority decision as a set of rules. Also, this ensures that any computed inference is encoded as part of the state vector and thus transmitted to the sink.

2.3.4 Examples

During the development of a glacier monitoring application, Martinez et al., [11] had the problem of wirelessly transmitting from the glacier to an Internet café several miles away. To save power, communication was reduced to a few transmissions per day. However, snow storms would severely disrupt communication. If the transmission was continuously retried throughout the storm, it would just drain the batteries. Therefore, a series of 3 failures caused the node to give up transmitting for several hours before retrying.

The above example illustrates how it is important to consider the application and its environment. It also shows how useful it is to elevate the question of when to retry to an application-level, rather than leaving this to the operating system, to avoid wasting battery power and to allow consideration of the priority of the message being communicated.

2.4 Nonpreemptive Scheduling Pattern

Nonpreemptive scheduling is a central component of simple, embedded operating systems such as TinyOS. There are two reasons for declaring this as a pattern. The first reason is that an understanding of the implications of this pattern will help developers understand how to best use TinyOS and similar systems. The second reason is that there are still many specialised applications that call for simpler hardware or more stripped down software than TinyOS or a similar system would allow but where task interleaving and timed operations are still required.

A synopsis of the Nonpreemptive Scheduling Pattern is given in Fig. 5. The scheduler maintains a "step schedule" or list of active "steps" and their associated start times. A *step* is a short-lived task. For example, beginning to send a message is a step, whereas the whole process of sending a message is a series of steps. The

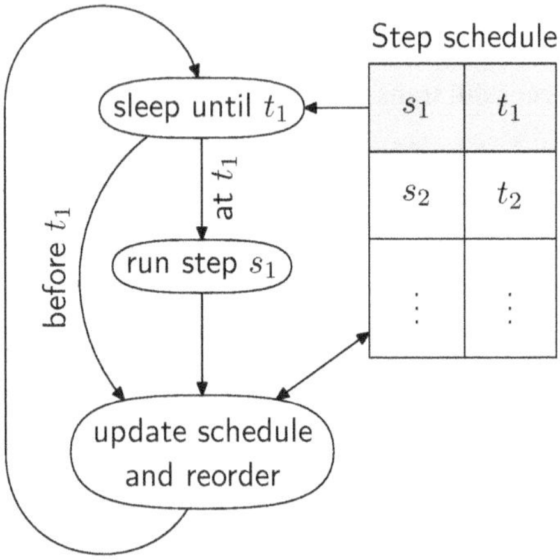

Fig. 5 Synopsis of the Nonpreemptive Scheduler Pattern (adapted from Cassandras and Lafortune [5])

schedule process begins by taking the first item from the list of steps and sleeping until its start time. If the start time has arrived, the step is executed. If the start time has not yet arrived, it may be due to waking for another reason such as an interrupt (and thus the schedule may need updating). The last step is to update the schedule and reorder according to start time. Updating the schedule involves asking each possible task whether they can (still) perform a step.

While preemptive scheduling is the norm in modern computers, low-power processors such as Texas Instrument's MSP430 or generic PIC processors, which are widely used for WSN applications, are limited in this regard. Nonetheless, hardware interrupts, due to timers and I/O, will interrupt other tasks and care is needed to ensure that there are no race conditions as a result for any buffers shared between the main process and interrupt routines.

In most programming idioms, each subroutine or module, once started, will run to completion. A program that calculates π to one million decimal places will hold the CPU captive for as long as the task requires. Multi-tasking operating systems avoid this problem by preemption. That is, they interrupt the task, save its state, and switch to a new task transparently. This allows other tasks to carry on working while the calculation is ongoing. preemptive multitasking, however, is expensive (in terms of memory and CPU overhead) and may be difficult to support on low-power processors.

2.4.1 Aims

The Nonpreemptive Scheduling pattern aims to:

- provide efficient interleaving of sleeping, sensing, listening, and transmitting cycles,
- allow for timed communication for listening and transmitting,
- support long running or slow external sensors with minimal CPU

One way to allow fine-grain interleaving of tasks *without preemption*, is to recode each module as a state machine. A simple example is shown below in terms of the original code in Figure 6 and the equivalent state machine in Figure 7. Note that recursive routines first need to be converted to iterative ones prior to conversion.

```
simple-stmt;
if (cond1)
  stmt2;
else
  stmt3;
while (cond2)
  stmt4;
```

Fig. 6 Original procedural psuedo-code

```
int state=1;
bool fsm1_feasible() { return state != 7; }
time_t fsm1_when() { return now(); }
void fsm1_step() {
  if (state==1) { simple-stmt; state++; }
  else if (state==2) { if (cond1) state=3; else state=4; }
  else if (state==3) {stmt2; state=5;}
  else if (state==4) {stmt3; state=5;}
  else if (state==5) {if (cond2) state=6; else state=7; }
  else if (state==6) {stmt4; state=5;}
  else state = 7;
}
```

Fig. 7 Reworked code as a state machine

For the example in Fig. 7, the finite state machine method `fsm1_step()` must then be called repeatedly (by the scheduler) until it is no longer feasible (specifically, `fsm1_feasible()` returns `FALSE`). Each method call instance is termed a *step*. This structure allows an arbitrarily large set of tasks to be interleaved without preemption.

Recoding as a state machine solves the problem of interleaving but to support operations that are triggered on a timer or a hardware interrupt, the scheduler must keep track of the list of pending tasks along with their associated execution time, ordered by earliest time first. Sleeping can occur until the earliest task time is reached or a hardware interrupt occurs. Cassandras and Lafortune provide a detailed example of the workings of such a scheduler in the context of discrete event simulation [5].

Correctly dealing with hardware interrupts is a key issue for this pattern. As pointed out by Pont [14], high priority interrupt service routines may mask lower priority interrupts from being serviced. Therefore, interrupt service routines must be minimalist—perhaps even just waking and setting a flag to note their occurrence. The scheduler must therefore be prepared to be woken before the next schedule step time and in this case, update the schedule according to which steps are now feasible.

For example, imagine a button press event handler `OnButtonRelease`. The button press triggers a hardware interrupt, possibly waking the system from sleep, that records that a button press has occurred. At this stage, the `OnButtonRelease_feasible` method will return "true". The schedule will be subsequently updated and the step method called until no longer feasible.

2.4.2 Triggers

- Multi-tasking operating system avoided or not feasible
- Need for more complex task interleaving than possible with a simple sense-process-send-sleep cycle
- Not possible to use an off-the-shelf nonpreemptive OS, such as TinyOS or Contiki, perhaps due to limits of microprocessor, or in an attempt to reduce the power budget.

2.4.3 Examples

The best known example of this type of scheduling pattern in the WSN domain is TinyOS. There are a number of other systems that use a similar approach (such as the JACK agent programming environment [9]). A common approach is to automatically rewrite the programmed code as a state machine (this is true for both NesC in TinyOS and the JACK compiler).

The Nonpreemptive Scheduler pattern derives much of its design from Pont's patterns for time-triggered architectures [14] and Cassandras and Lafortune's description of timed automata [5].

2.5 Interval Listening Pattern

2.5.1 Aims

The Interval Listening pattern has the following aims:

- support mesh-networking (most or all nodes act as routers),
- allow nodes to spend most of their time asleep but still not miss (most) messages,
- reduce the amount of time spent "idle listening".

To function as a mesh network, individual nodes must be capable of acting as routers. In principle, this means that they must be ready to receive messages at any time. In practice, such high alertness is generally only required when nodes are initially deployed or subsequently moved. For most installations, communication quickly stabilises into a predictable pattern based on regular sensing cycles and well established routing paths. Therefore, despite the need for nodes to act as routers, they can predict when the next message will arrive and revert to an ultra-low power mode until then.

2.5.2 Triggers

- Not all nodes are within communication range of the base station (and so mesh-networking is required)
- Nodes do not need to be actively sensing all the time

2.5.3 Examples

One form of the Interval Listening pattern is implemented as Low Power Listening (LPL) [12]. This protocol is a simple extension of standard TinyOS message transmission. It works by attaching a one second long prefix to transmitted messages. The receiver then only needs to wake up once per second to check for any transmissions. This simple modification substantially extends the life of each node.

The Time Synchronised Mesh Protocol (TSMP) [13] developed by Dust Networks is another approach to Interval Listening that is based on a combination of Time Division Multiplexing (TDM), where each node has a specific slot when it can transmit, and integrated time synchronisation that works by replying back to any sender how late or early their packet was. Note that the integrated time synchronisation is needed for two reasons: (a) to ensure that nodes wake at the right time to listen to neighbours, and (b) to avoid the need for top-down time synchronisation.

TSMP is potentially much more efficient than LPL since transmissions can be short and the node does not necessarily need to wake up as frequently as every second. TSMP is implemented in WirelessHART and is part of the ISA100 standard.

3 Conclusions

The WSN domain is transitioning in much the same way as Computer Science transitioned towards Software Engineering in the past: from being a research-only domain that focused on optimising algorithms to being one that included a greater focus on the problem of developing reliable, functionally correct, useful and *applicable* systems. This naturally includes a greater consideration of the task facing WSN developers. Design patterns have revolutionised the way software is engineered; a similar revolution is needed in WSN engineering.

The framework and patterns presented here should be taken as a work in progress. The WSN field continues to evolve. Nevertheless, they should also not be seen as untested. Examples throughout have shown that these patterns appear repeatedly in reports on functioning deployed systems.

The framework presented here is only one in a range of possible design frameworks. Some applications will require extremely simple nodes that cannot perform any processing on-board, while others will be able to incorporate much more sophisticated algorithms and patterns than those suggested here. Nonetheless, it is our strong belief that this framework will provide useful guidance to WSN developers across a broad range of applications.

References

1. Allen, M., Girod, L., Newton, R., Madden, S., Blumstein, D.T., Estrin, D.: Voxnet: An interactive, rapidly-deployable acoustic monitoring platform. In: International Conference on Information Processing in Sensor Networks, IPSN 2008, pp. 371–382 (2008)
2. Allen, M.: VoxNet: Reducing latency in high data-rate applications. In: Gaura, et al [7]
3. Brusey, J., Gaura, E., Rednic, R.: Classifying transition behaviour in postural activity monitoring. Sensors & Transducers Journal 7, 213–223 (2009), `http://www.sensorsportal.com/HTML/DIGEST/P_SI_98.htm`
4. Brusey, J., Gaura, E.I., Goldsmith, D., Shuttleworth, J.: FieldMAP: A spatio-temporal field monitoring application prototyping framework. IEEE Sensors 9(11) (November 2009), `http://dx.doi.org/10.1109/JSEN.2009.2021799`
5. Cassandras, C.G., Lafortune, S.: Introduction to Discrete Event Systems. Kluwer Academic Publishers, Dordrecht (1999)
6. Gamma, E., Helm, R., Johnson, R., Vlissides, J.: Design patterns: elements of reusable object-oriented software. Addison-Wesley Professional, Reading (1995)
7. Gaura, E.I., Girod, L., Brusey, J., Allen, M., Challen, G.W. (eds.): Wireless Sensor Networks: Deployments And Design Frameworks (Designing and Deploying Embedded Sensing Systems. Springer, Heidelberg (2010)

8. Goldsmith, D., Brusey, J.: The Spanish Inquisition Protocol: Model-based transmission reduction for wireless sensor networks. In: Proc. IEEE Sensors. IEEE, Los Alamitos (2010)
9. Howden, N., Rönnquist, R., Hodgson, A., Lucas, A.: JACK intelligent agents - summary of an agent infrastructure. In: Proceedings of the 5th International Conference on Autonomous Agents (Agents 2001) (2001)
10. Hu, W., Bulusu, N., Dang, T., Taylor, A., Chou, C.T., Jha, S., Tran, V.N.: Cane toad monitoring: Data reduction in a high rate application. In: Gaura, et al [7]
11. Martinez, K., Hart, J.K.: Glacier monitoring: Deploying custom hardware in harsh environments. In: Gaura, et al [7]
12. Moss, D., Hui, J., Klues, K.: Low power listening. Technical Report TEP 105, TinyOS Core Working Group (2007)
13. Pister, K.S.J., Doherty, L.: TSMP: Time synchronized mesh protocol. In: Proc. IASTED Intl. Symp. Distributed Sensor Networks (DSN 2008), pp. 391–398 (2008)
14. Pont, M.J.: Patterns for time-triggered embedded systems: building reliable applications with the 8051 family of microcontrollers. ACM Press/Addison-Wesley Publishing Co. (2001)
15. Raman, B., Chebrolu, K.: Censor networks: A critique of "sensor networks" from a systems perspective. ACM SIGCOMM Computer Communication Review 38(3), 75–78 (2008)
16. Welch, G., Bishop, G.: An introduction to the Kalman filter. Technical report, University of North Carolina at Chapel Hill (1995)
17. Allen, G.W., Dawson-Haggerty, S., Welsh, M.: Lance: Optimizing high-resolution signal collection in wireless sensor networks. In: Proc. 6th ACM conference on Embedded Network Sensor Systems (SenSys 2008), pp. 169–182. ACM, New York (2008)

Distributed Brillouin Sensor Application to Structural Failure Detection

F. Ravet

Omnisens,
Morges, Switzerland

Abstract. Disaster prevention in civil infrastructures requires the use of techniques that allow temperature and strain measurements in real time over lengths of a few meters to tens of kilometres. The distributed Brillouin sensor technique has the advantage to combine all these characteristics.

The sensing mechanism of the DBS involves the interaction of two counter-propagating lightwaves, the Stokes and the pump, in an optical fibre. Spatial information is obtained through time domain analysis. An analytical model describing the sensing mechanism based on stimulated Brillouin scattering (SBS) interaction is introduced and validated experimentally. This model development leads to the implementation of a signal processing method grounded in the physics of Brillouin scattering. An analytical approximation, valid for the optimum sensing region, reconstructs the Brillouin spectrum distribution from input sensing parameters and measured data. These data are obtained with a spectrum analysis methodology, based on three original tools: the Rayleigh equivalent criterion, the length-stress diagram, and the spectrum form factors. This methodology has been successfully used on experimental spectra.

The DBS and the signal processing approach were then used to monitor the structural changes of steel pipes, composite columns and concrete elements. The DBS measured the strain distribution of those structures while they were stressed. The DBS provided detailed information on the structure's health at local and global level, associated with deformations, cracks and buckling. This work demonstrates that the DBS is capable of extracting critical information useful to engineers: engineer's experience and judgement in conjunction with appropriate data processing methods make possible to anticipate structural failures.

1 Introduction

Structural health monitoring (SHM) is an important development of the civil engineering field. Recent events remind us that the cost of a bridge collapse is much more than economical; it touches people's life, as dramatically demonstrated by the collapses of the Laval's La Concorde overpass, in fall 2006, and, the Minneapolis bridge, in summer 2007. The implementation of comprehensive SHM in civil infrastructure is made possible by the use of optical fiber sensors and can substantially improve the safety of civil structures and help to manage them more efficiently. More specifically, distributed Brillouin-based sensing systems (DBS) are capable of measuring strain everywhere along a dedicated optical fiber cable

S.C. Mukhopadhyay (Ed.): New Developments in Sensing Technology for SHM, LNEE 96, pp. 93–136.
springerlink.com

attached to the structure to be monitored. Measurement readings can be taken every tenth of cm, which is a clear advantage when localized faults, such as cracks, need to be detected, but their position is not known beforehand.

Among the principal aims of SHM, the detection and localization of localized failures such buckling and cracks appear as an essential task as they can lead to lethal faults for the structure's life. The present work introduces a technique combining high resolution distributed strain measurements based on Brillouin scattering and advanced signal processing methodology to detect localized structural failures. The approach is validated by laboratory trials and field experiments.

2 Distributed Brillouin Sensor General Description

a. Brillouin frequency relationship with strain and temperature

The Brillouin effect is the scattering of a lightwave, called pump, by an acoustic wave [1]. In other words, the optical wave is scattered by a propagating periodic variation of the density of the medium. The scattered beam optical frequency experiences a Doppler shift known as Brillouin frequency shift (ν_B) which is expressed as

$$\nu_B = \frac{2nV_A}{\lambda_p}. \tag{1}$$

According to Eq.(1), the Brillouin frequency is proportional to the refractive index of the fiber (n) and to the acoustics wave velocity (V_A). It also depends on the pump signal wavelength (λ_p). Typically, the Brillouin frequency of ITU G.652 fibers [2] is about 12.80 GHz at 1.31 mm and 10.85 GHz at 1.55 μm. Figure 1 presents a typical Brillouin spectrum which is the product of a scattered lightwave at 1554nm.

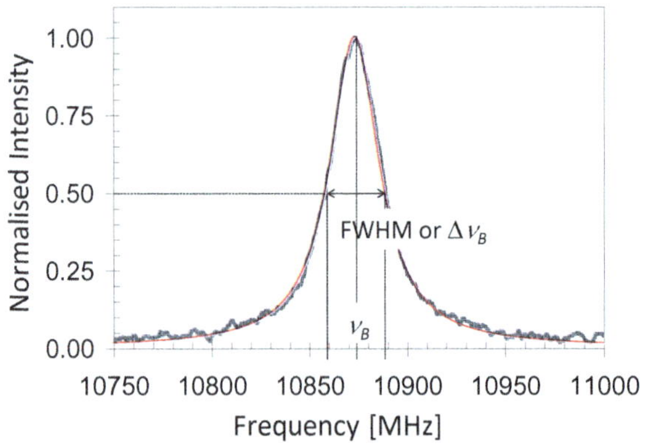

Fig. 1 Thick curve: Backscattered Stokes spectrum from an incident lightwave (λ_p = 1554 nm) in a 20 km long ITU G.652 fiber obtained by a heterodyne method (Nazarathy 1989, Derickson 1998); the incident power is 310 μW; Measured Brillouin frequency shift is 10873.6 MHz and linewidth is 31 MHz. Thin curve: Lorentzian distribution drawn with the measured Brillouin frequency and linewidth.

A sound wave propagates in bulk silica [3] and in optical fibers [4] over a few microns only, their attenuation coefficient (~ 10^6 m^{-1}) being much larger than the optical attenuation coefficient in the telecommunication window (~ 10^{-4} m^{-1}). The acoustic wave decay can not be neglected as it determines the Brillouin spectrum linewidth. It is commonly accepted in the literature that the decay follows an exponential law [5]. The exponential decay has the consequence that the Brillouin lines in the spontaneously backscattered spectrum must have a Lorentzian shape characterized by a full width at half maximum (FWHM or $\Delta\nu_B$) as shown in Figure 2. Typical linewidth value is 30 to 50 MHz dependending on the fiber type. The lorentzian distribution that models the product of the spontaneously scattered pump ligthwave is expressed as

$$g(\nu) = \frac{g_B}{1 + (2[\nu - \nu_B]/\Delta\nu_B)^2}, \tag{2}$$

where g_B is the Brillouin gain coefficient. For single-mode fibers, g_B varies from $1.12\text{x}10^{-11}$ to $5\text{x}10^{-11}$ m/W, depending on core doping and structure [6]. It is common that g be called the natural Brillouin gain of the fiber.

An estimate of the scattered power can be obtained by assuming that in spontaneous regime, the number of Stokes photons generated is proportional to the number of acoustic phonons (N_{ph}) present in the medium. At room temperature T, $N_{ph}{\approx}k_BT/h\nu_B$ which is an approximation of Bose-Einstein distribution (h is Planck constant and k_B is Boltzmann coefficient). The scattered power can then be evaluated by $P = Nh\nu_s\Delta\nu_B$. For the typical values of Figure 5, the power is about 0.5 nW.

Any temperature or mechanical stress would change the density of medium, and, in consequence, both n and V_A. The temperature variation relates to the Brillouin frequency as [7]

$$\nu_B(T) = \nu_B(T_r)[1 + C_T(T - T_r)], \tag{3}$$

where T is the temperature and T_r is the reference temperature. A typical value for the temperature coefficient C_T is 1.05 MHz/°C. Culverhouse demonstrated the feasibility of a temperature sensor based on the mechanism of Brillouin scattering [8] (Culverhouse 1989). When temperature remains constant, the Brillouin frequency shift $\nu_B(\varepsilon)$ relates to the applied strain as [7]

$$\nu_B(\varepsilon) = \nu_B(0)[1 + C_\varepsilon\varepsilon], \tag{4}$$

where $\nu_B(0)$ is the unstrained Brillouin frequency shift and C_ε is the strain proportionality coefficient. A typical value for C_ε is 0.0550 MHz/με.

b. Distributed measurement and sensor configuration

Distributed information is obtained by applying time, phase or frequency domain modulations of the measuring signals emitted by a laser. The distributed mode of operation can also be achieved by combining two or three of the modulation schemes. Two interrogator configurations can be implemented implying the use of two distinct regimes of Brillouin scattering which are known as spontaneous and stimulated Brillouin scattering (SBS).

Spontaneous scattering which relies on the detection and the analysis of the backscattering of a modulated pump signal (Figure 2); depending on the type of modulation, the interrogator is commonly called Brillouin Optical Time Domain Reflectometer (BOTDR), Optical Frequency Domain Reflectometer (BOFDR), Brillouin Optical Coherency Domain Reflectometer (BOCDR) etc…

Stimulated Brillouin Scattering (SBS) which relies on the detection and the analysis of a backscattered lightwave which is the product of the interaction of a pump and a probe signals (Figure 2); depending on the type of modulation, the interrogator is commonly called Brillouin Optical Time Domain Analyzer (BOTDA), Optical Frequency Domain Analyzer (BOFDA), Brillouin Optical Coherency Domain Analyzer (BOCDA) etc…

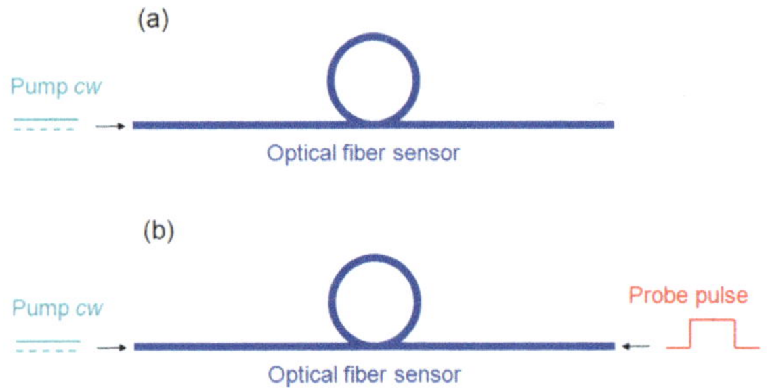

Fig. 2 Sensing configurations for spontaneous (a) and stimulated (b) Brillouin scattering. More specifically, BOTDR and BOTDA are presented here

BOTDR and BOTDA are the most commonly used configurations and are commercially available. They present inherent advantages in term of optoelectronics simplicity and measurement speed. The BOTDR requires access to only one fiber end. The launched lightwave is spontaneously scattered by the acoustic waves everywhere along the fiber length. The scattered light is then collected and analysed at the input end. Spatial information, and, hence, events location is given by measuring the round trip of a pulse propagating in the fiber. This configuration has been implemented by various research teams. In the BOTDA case, two lightwaves, the pump and the probe signals, are launched into the fiber in a counter-propagating configuration. The simultaneous presence of the Stokes and the pump waves generate a beat signal that reinforces the acoustic wave in the fiber when the beams frequency difference is equal to the Brillouin frequency. The coupling mechanism between the two lightwaves is electrostriction. The scattering of the pump is then enhanced, leading to its depletion and the input probe beam is amplified. The probe is also called Stokes as it corresponds to the frequency downshifted peak. The Brillouin spectrum can be recorded by tuning the frequency difference between pump and Stokes waves. One of the two lightwaves is pulsed and spatial information is obtained by the measuring the pulse round-trip [9].

Various parameters need to be considered when comparing BOTDR and BOTDA configurations. First, one has to keep in mind that the sensor must be implemented on the field. It must then be simple to install and complete the sensing operation as quickly as possible. Second, some of the sensor performances are critical. Those are the spatial resolution, which indicates the smallest detectable event size, the frequency resolution, which is the smallest Brillouin frequency shift that can be measured, and the measurement range, which is the longest length overwhich the sensor can make an accurate data acquisition. The BOTDR has obvious advantages over the BOTDA. First, it only requires access to one fiber end. Second, if the fiber breaks, which is common in the field when the fiber is heavily stressed, measurements can still be done along the remaining section. On the drawbacks side, the BOTDR approach relies on the emitted spontaneous intensity. These levels are usually low, necessitating long averaging time to achieve a satisfactory signal-to-noise ratio (SNR). That is not the case with the stimulated configuration where the intensity at the detector is significantly larger, reducing the overall measurement time and allowing the use of shorter pulses. If we keep in mind that a fiber sees its attenuation increase when it is heavily stressed, the BOTDA will still be able to continue the monitoring operation over the whole fiber while the BOTDR is blind or offer poor performance behind the strained point. Significant fiber loss increase are common in SHM applications making the BOTDA their technique of choice. The use of SBS based interrogator makes possible the compensation for fiber loss increase and strain resolution degradation.

A typical commercially available Brillouin interrogator system the DITEST which is an innovative high dynamic range laser-based monitoring system based on SBS [10]. The inherent stability of the system comes from the use of a single laser source and a high speed electro-optic modulator for the generation of both pump and probe signals. The intensity of both optical signals can be controlled in order to have the highest possible signal-to-noise ratio and reduce the acquisition time. The frequency difference between pump and probe signal is precisely controlled by the modulation frequency applied to the electro-optic modulator, leading to 10^{-5} precision on the frequency determination. Typically, the DITEST system performs strain profile measurement with a 10 $\mu\varepsilon$ resolution and a spatial resolution better than 1 m over the first 10 km. For SHM applications, the interrogator is designed to handle short distance and large, optical budget (over 20 dB). 50’000 distance points can be measured with a minimum sampling interval of 0.1 m. The acquisition time (time to get one complete profile) may vary from a second to 10 minutes depending on the application requirements.

c. Strategies for temperature compensation with the Brillouin sensor

In all laboratory tests, the temperature of the environment is controlled and variations are smaller than 1°C. Such situation is rarely encountered on the field where temperature variations are part of the measurement conditions. In fact, field implementation requires that the temperature influence on strain measurement must be compensated. Various strategies can be used involving the simultaneous monitoring of strain and temperature with the Brillouin sensor. The simplest consist in laying out an adjacent stress free fibre [11] or in gluing the jacket of a loose tube optical fibre cable. In that last case, all mechanical changes of the structure will only affect the cable while the fibre remains unstressed. This approach has led to the development of specialty cables which are specifically designed to measure temperature or strain [12]. It is also possible to measure simultaneously strain and temperature with a single fibre. Sensing can then be achieved by monitoring Brillouin frequency shift and Brillouin peak power[13]. Simultaneous temperature and strain can also be achieved by using fibres with multiple Brillouin peaks such as DSF, LEAF type [14] and PCF type fibers[1] [15]. Finally, the distinct Brillouin behaviour of the slow and fast axis of polarisation maintaining fibers is another approach to measure strain and temperature at once [16].

3 Sensing System Operation and Model

d. Performance definition

i. Spatial resolution

After Beller, "spatial resolution indicates instrument ability to resolve two adjacent events" (in Derickson 1998). In the case of the Brillouin sensor, the spatial resolution is the ability of the instrument to resolve two adjacent sections of distinct Brillouin frequencies, induced by either strain or temperature. The length over which the interaction between pump and Stokes wave occurs determines this parameter. This interaction length is the pulse length and it is defined as $v_g\Delta\tau$ where v_g is the pulse group velocity in the optical fiber and $\Delta\tau$ is the pulse width. The spatial resolution is then expressed as

$$w = v_g \Delta\tau / 2. \tag{5}$$

The factor ½ comes from the backscattered nature of the detected signal. It accounts for the round trip of the signal in the fiber [18]. Since in silica fiber the group velocity is $v_g \approx 2\text{x}10^8$ m/s the rule of thumb that 10 ns corresponds to 1 m spatial resolution can be used. Based on this definition, a given temperature/strain that spreads uniformly over a distance greater than the spatial resolution is measured with the lowest measurement uncertainty. If a local temperature/strain change occurs in a distance scale smaller than the preset spatial resolution, it might still be detected but the change will not be measured with the lowest uncertainty.

ii. Brillouin frequency resolution

The Brillouin frequency resolution is defined as the smallest Brillouin frequency that can be resolved at a given location along the fiber. It is directly related to the noise of the measurement. The noise includes spontaneous, short duration deviations in output (reading) about the mean output (reading), which are not caused by strain or temperatures changes. Noise is determined as the standard deviation about the mean and is expressed in frequency units. The measurement precision is a measure of the agreement between repeated measurements of the same property under identical, or substantially similar, conditions; the precision is defined. The frequency resolution is defined as twice the standard deviation of the noise (+/- twice the standard deviation includes 95.4% of the measurements). Once the fiber

---

[1] Dispersion Shifted Fiber, Large Effective Area Fiber, Photonics Crystal Fiber.

sensor is calibrated, it is always possible to display the measurement resolution in term of strain or temperature [19].

Horiguchi proposed a relation that gives an estimate of the minimum detectable frequency change [20]. The relation accounts for the measurement dependence to noise and Brillouin spectrum characteristics and is expressed as

$$\delta\nu_B = \frac{\Delta\nu_B}{\sqrt{2SNR}}, \tag{6}$$

where SNR_o is the signal-to-noise power ratios. As it appears in Eq.(6) Brillouin frequency resolution not only depends on the signal level but also on the spectrum width. Common distributed Brillouin sensors are then limited in frequency resolution when the pulse spectrum is larger or equal to $\Delta\nu_B$ which is the case when pulse width is shortened to achieve better spatial resolution [21]. For most of the Brillouin sensor configurations, there is clearly a trade-off between spatial and frequency resolution [22].

Both statistical and analytical definitions specifically apply to the minimum detectable change when the fiber Brillouin frequency is uniform over spatial resolution. It does not address the issue of the frequency resolution when ν_B is not uniform over w. A definition of the spatial resolution accounting for non-uniform ν_B distribution is discussed in detail in section 4.b.ii of the present work [23].

iii. Brillouin frequency accuracy

In general the term accuracy is a generic qualitative word. It should be associated with "uncertainty" or "calibration uncertainty". The measurement uncertainty depends on the calibration precision, i.e. on the quality of the calibration setup and procedure. For instance, the calibration of a piece of fiber as a temperature sensor requires that a traceable reference temperature sensor with given precision be available. It is therefore impossible to mention the instrument calibration uncertainty without including a given fiber sensor, that has been calibrated with a given precision [19].

iv. Dynamic range

The dynamic range (DR) expressed in dB is defined as the difference between the maximum input power to the photodetector and the smallest optical power level that can be detected. It is a measure of the total loss that can be accommodated by the instrument when performing a measurement [24]. The dynamic range is then a function of the power launched into the fiber, the Brillouin interaction, the loss of the components and the receiver characteristics [20]. It can be expressed as

$$DR = \frac{1}{2}\left\{P_{\max} - |G_p| - \alpha_{comp} - P_d - \frac{1}{2}SNR_{req} + \frac{1}{2}SNR_{imp}\right\}, \tag{7}$$

where P_{max} is the maximum fiber input power, G_p is the Brillouin loss, α_{comp} is the loss of any component located along the fiber, SNR_{req} is the signal-to-noise ratio required to achieve a target frequency resolution (Eq.(6)), and, SNR_{imp} is the signal-to-noise ratio improvement obtained by electrical signal processing (averaging, electrical amplifiers). Various causes limit the maximum fiber input power: 1)

P_{max} must be smaller than the SBS threshold for BOTDA configuration [25], [26]; 2) P_{max} has to be lower than the maximum power that the receiver can handle; 3) another technological constraint on P_{max} is determined by the available power at the laser output. The factor ½ in front of the bracket is introduced to account for the fact that the signal suffers twice the loss as it propagates in both directions before being measured [20], [24]. The other ½ factors account for the fact that these SNR's are expressed in electrical decibels.

4 System Operation and Model

The sensing configuration chosen is a BOTDA as illustrated in Figure 2 in which the pump is a *cw* and the probe is pulsed. From performance definition section it is obvious that temperature and strain accuracies are affected by the Brillouin spectrum shape. The Brillouin spectrum shape is influenced by the pulsewidth ($\Delta\tau$), shape, pulse power ($P_{\square}$) and pump *cw* power (P_{cw}), fiber length (L), and ON–OFF ratio of the optical pulse (or extinction ratio ER). The pulse power is always composed of an AC (P_{pk}) and a DC (P_b) component due to its finite ER as illustrated in Figure 3 due to the electro-optic modulator bias.

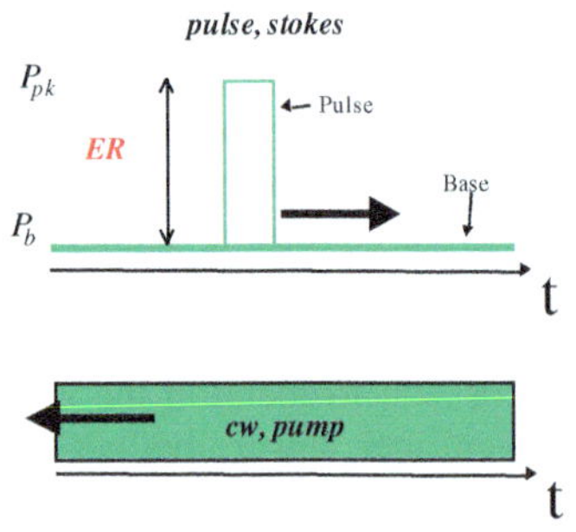

Fig. 3. Model of pump-stokes (pulse) interaction.

The interaction between probe and the pump lightwaves can be modelled by the steady-state-coupled intensity[2] equations [1], [5], which are

$$\frac{d}{dz}I_{cw} = -gI_pI_{cw} - \alpha I_{cw}, \tag{8}$$

[2] We need to introduce the relationship between the optical power in the fibre, P, and the total intensity distributed in the fibre cross-section. Assuming Gaussian radial distribution the $Power = I_0 A_{eff}$. As it appears in this relation, when the intensity has a Gaussian distribution, the power is the product of the peak intensity I_o with the effective area of fibre A_{eff}. The effective area can be interpreted as the area of the fibre cross section over which the peak of the intensity distribution is constant [5].

$$\frac{d}{dz}I_p = -gI_{cw}I_p + \alpha I_p. \tag{9}$$

where I_p is the Stokes intensity, which is pulsed; $I_{cw}$is the pump intensity; z is the position along the fiber in which the Stokes pulse is launched from z = 0and the pump from $z = L$; α is the fiber natural attenuation; and g is the natural Brillouin gain of the fiber. Rigorously, these equations can only be used to describe steady state or long pulses ($\Delta\tau$> 10 ns) interaction. We also assume that the gain coefficient g depends on position. The position dependence of g is attributed to the fact that fibers do not have a perfectly uniform Brillouin frequency distribution. In addition, the purpose of a sensor is to detect Brillouin frequency variations induced by the environment.

The coupled intensity equations can be solved under the weakly depleted approximation which can be applied to most of the sensing cases. Let us give two major reasons. First, the pulse length, and hence the Brillouin interaction length, exceeds rarely 100 m, in which case the pump depletion is always weak. Second, the DC component of the pulse can significantly deplete the pump if the fiber is longer than a few hundred meters. We then want to make sure that P_b is smaller than the SBS threshold for BOTDA configurations [25], [26]. Hopefully, it is in practice a fraction of the pulse peak power (e.g. a few tenth of mW at the very maximum). We make the assumption that pump is weakly depleted. If we choose to let the pulse enter into the fiber at $z = 0$ and to launch the pump from $z = L$, then initial conditions to Eqs.(8) and (9) are I_{P0} and I_{cwL}, for the Stokes and the *cw* pump lightwaves respectively. Solving Eqs. (9) leads to the following expression

$$I_P(\nu,z) = I_{P0}\exp\left[g(\nu,z)I_{cwL}\frac{e^{-\alpha L}}{\alpha}\left(e^{\alpha z}-1\right)-\alpha z\right]. \tag{10}$$

We now follow the assumption that the Stokes wave is constituted of two components [27], [28], [29]: one is time dependent (AC part of the pulse), which is characterized by the pulsewidth ($\Delta\tau$) and the peak intensity (I_{pk}); the other is the base (DC part) which is a continuous wave signal (*cw*) and determined by its intensity (I_b). Figure 3 describes this model. The Stokes intensity is then the sum of these two components $I_P=I_{pk}+I_b$. Solving Eq.(9) with these intensities, and their spatial dependence expressed as Eq.(10), we obtain the total Brillouin loss, which can be expressed in the following form for an arbitrary length l [31]

$$G_T(\nu,z) = \exp\left\{\alpha w - \int_z^{z+l} g(\nu,\zeta)\left(I_{pk}+I_b\right) \exp\left[g(\nu,\zeta)I_{cwL}\frac{e^{-\alpha L}}{\alpha}\left(e^{\alpha\zeta}-1\right)-\alpha\zeta\right]d\zeta\right\} \tag{11}$$

We see that the AC and DC components of the pulse can be separated leading to the following generic form of the Brillouin loss

$$G_T(\nu,z) = G_{pk}(\nu,z)G_b(\nu,z), \tag{12}$$

where G_{pk} is the Pump-AC Brillouin loss and G_b is the Pump-DC Brillouin loss. Due to their very distinct natures, we want to separate the calculation of these two interactions.

First, we consider the pump-AC interaction. The steady state approximation is valid for pulses larger than the phonon lifetime ($\Delta\tau > 10$ns), which is equivalent to a spatial resolution $w>1$m. We know that nanosecond pulses provoke the broadening of the Brillouin loss spectrum and then reduce the strain (temperature) measurement accuracy, while such pulses are required to achieve centimetre spatial resolution. As the broadening is induced by the wide spectrum of the pulse, we assume that each pulse spectrum component excites individually the phonon field whose spectrum is given by a Lorentzian distribution. These individual excitations are adding up over the pulse spectrum frequency range. That mechanism is described mathematically by a convolution product. Therefore, we account for the pulse effect in these equations by replacing g with the transient gain coefficient g_{pk}, defined as the convolution of the Brillouin natural gain $g(\nu,z)$ with the distribution $P_{pk}b(\nu)$ of the power spectrum of the pulse [22], [30].

$$g_{pk}(\nu,z) = g(\nu,z) * b(\nu). \tag{13}$$

If the pulse waveform has a rectangular shape, we can then calculate the convolution analytically [31].

Finally, we integrate equation II.45.b for the AC part of the Stokes wave at any position over the spatial resolution (w) [31]and obtain the Brillouin loss spectrum G_{pk} at z:

$$G_{pk}(\nu,z) = \exp\left\{\alpha w - \int_z^{z+w} g_{pk}(\nu,\zeta) I_{pk0} \exp\left[g_{pk}(\nu,\zeta) I_{cwL} \frac{e^{-\alpha L}}{\alpha}\left(e^{\alpha\zeta}-1\right) - \alpha\zeta\right] d\zeta\right\}, \tag{14}$$

Now, we want to evaluate the interaction between the base and the pump wave. Due to the DC nature of the base, we assume that its interaction with the pump can be modelled by the steady state equations without additional assumptions. Here the Stokes intensity reduces to $I_b=ERI_{pk}$ where ER is the extinction ratio of the optical pulse. The integration interval extends to the whole fiber length. The Brillouin loss spectrum contribution from the base-pump is then expressed as

$$G_b(\nu,z) = \exp\left\{\alpha(z-L) - ER\int_z^{L} g(\nu,\zeta) I_{pk0} \exp\left[g(\nu,\zeta) I_{cwL} \frac{e^{-\alpha L}}{\alpha}\left(e^{\alpha\zeta}-1\right) - \alpha\zeta\right] d\zeta\right\}. \tag{15}$$

When it is assumed that the Stokes pulse is the sum of two parts, DC and AC intensities, that are decoupled but interacting individually with the pump, the total Brillouin loss spectrum is the product of G_{pk} and G_b. G_T of a uniform Brillouin frequency distribution is characterized by a single peak spectrum whose FWHM, Γ, is close to $\Delta\nu_B$ when pump is weakly depleted and under steady state condition. In general, Γ varies with L, z, I_{pk0}, I_{cwL} and ER, which are the cause of spectrum distortion.

e. Model discussion – Unstressed fiber

We conducted a systematic study of the influence of pulse width, extinction ratio on the linewidth of the Brillouin loss. Brillouin frequency was assumed to be uniform along the fibers. Typical results for short and long fibers are presented in Figure 4. This agreement with exact solutions strengthens our confidence in the validity of the present approach. As shown in Figure 4, Γ increases when the pulse width decreases until it reaches a maximum. Then Γ drops to a value close to $\Delta\nu_B$. Small *ER* clearly limits the increase of the linewidth. When $\Delta\tau \approx$ 10 ns, the observed broadening must be attributed to the pulse spectrum widening. For nanosecond pulses, Γ drops due to the DC level dominating the Brillouin interaction over long fiber length and relative small contribution of the pulse portion. If large pulses are used ($\Delta\tau$>> 10 ns), the pulse spectrum is much narrower than $\Delta\nu_B$. The Brillouin loss spectrum tends to be similar to the spectrum resulting from the interaction of *cw* pump and Stokes lightwaves. The main difference between short and long fibers, respectively Figure 5.(a) and (b), must be attributed to increased influence of the base. Pump and base interaction extending over the whole fiber length, Γ tends to remain close to steady state value when the fiber is long as it appears in Figure 5.(b).

Γ also varies with position as shown in Figure 6(for a 2500 m long fiber and w = 1 m. In the *ER*=25dB case, it is observed that Γ first decreases. In the last kilometres, Γ starts to rise significantly. The increase of Γ is very weak when considering the *ER* = 10 dB situation. Similarly to Figure Figure 5, these curves confirm the role played by the base in mitigating the spectrum broadening. The effect of spectrum narrowing with increasing distance can be attributed to the enhancement of the scattering of Stokes spectral components near the peak of the resonance while the pulse is propagating along the fiber. Equivalently, a broader spectrum at the pulse input can be attributed to the effect of pump depletion. Spectrum widening observed at the fiber end can be understood by analysing Figure 5.(b) representing the base (G_b) contribution to the total Brillouin loss (G_T) as a function of position and *ER*. In the case of high spatial resolution sensor ($w \leq 1$ m), the change of G_{pk} as a function of z is small relative to G_b and does not depend on *ER*. Close to the pump input, the Brillouin loss is smaller ($G_b \rightarrow 1$ when $z \rightarrow L$). That effect is emphasized and affects G_b over the whole fiber length ($G_b \approx 1$) when the pulse extinction ratio is large. It is then possible to observe the pulse spectrum broadening in the last few hundred meters of the fiber. Spectrum narrowing with position can be experimentally evidenced as illustrated in Figure 6. The experiment was carried out with a Brillouin sensor using two DFB laser in the 1.55 μm region. The typical linewidth of these lasers is about 10 MHz and contributes to broaden the Brillouin loss spectrum. Under weak depletion condition, we measured that $\Gamma \approx \Delta\nu_B \approx$ 45 MHz. The phenomenological model is used to calculate the spectrum along the fiber. The FWHM of the reconstructed profile is plotted on Figure 6. It is obvious that the reconstruction matches the experimental trend, which is a confirmation that the model is capable to simulate the effect of moderate pump depletion that influences the spectrum shape.

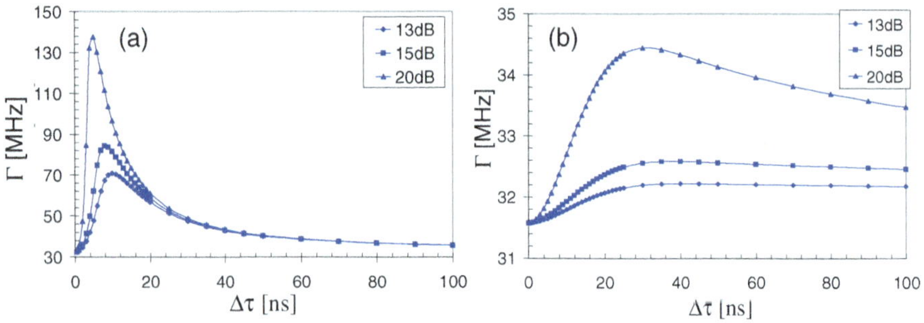

Fig. 4 Brillouin loss spectrum width as a function of pulsewidth and extinction ratio: (a) P_{p0} =10 mW, P_{cwL} =5 mW, L = 10 m, z = 5 m; (b) P_{p0} = 10 mW, P_{cwL} = 5 mW, L = 10000 m, z = 5000 m [33]

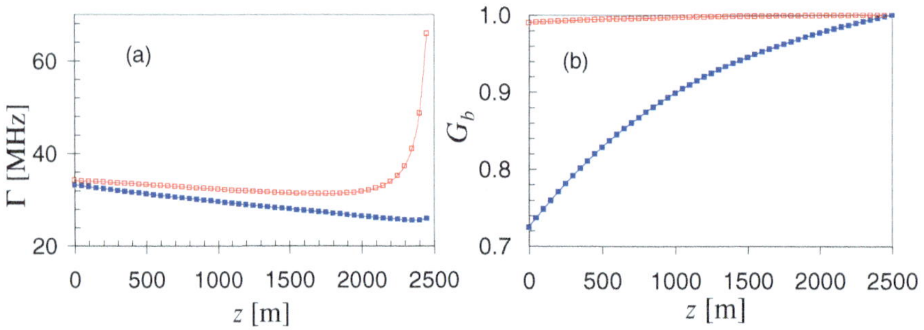

Fig. 5 (a) Brillouin loss spectrum width as a function of position and extinction ratio (filled symbols:ER = 10 dB; open symbols: ER = 25 dB); (b) base contribution to total Brillouin loss as a function of position and extinction ratio (filled symbols: ER = 10dB; open symbols: ER = 25dB), these values are calculated at the Brillouin frequency; Simulation parameters are: $\nu = \nu_B$, P_{p0} = 25 mW, P_{cwL} = 5 mW, $\Delta\tau$= 10 ns, L = 2500 m [33]

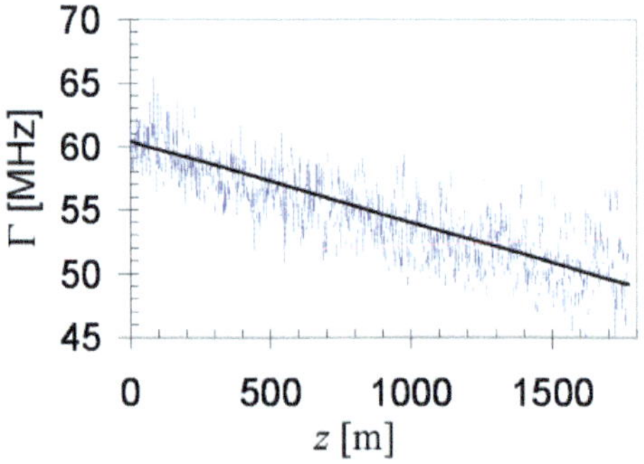

Fig. 6 Measured (light grey line) and calculated (dark line) Brillouin loss spectrum width, Γ, as a function of position for a uniform fiber; experimental and simulation parameters are P_{p0} = 20 mW, P_{cwL} = 5 mW, L = 1800m, $\Delta\tau$ = 10 ns, ER = 10 dB, $\Delta\nu_B$ = 45 MHz [33]

f. Model discussion – Stressed fiber

To study the effect of changing stress length and strength on the spectrum shape, we assume that the sensing fiber has a uniform Brillouin frequency (ν_B) over its whole length (L) except for a short section at distance z whose spatial extension δl is smaller than the spatial resolution ($\delta l \leq w$) and has a different Brillouin frequency shift (ν_{Bs}). As appearing in Figure 7, within the spatial resolution at z, the Brillouin frequency shift (ν_{Bs}) is constant over δl, while the rest of the pulse covers w- δl with a Brillouin frequency shift of ν_B. We use the phenomenological model for $w > 1$ m to generate composite spectra for various combinations of ν_B, ν_{Bs} and δl. Smaller spatial resolution could be considered but the analysis would be more complex without bringing useful information. We introduce the normalized Brillouin frequency shift $\Omega_{Bs}=(\nu_{Bs}-\nu_B)/\Gamma$ where Γ is the FWHM of the normalized Brillouin loss spectrum for given sensing parameters.

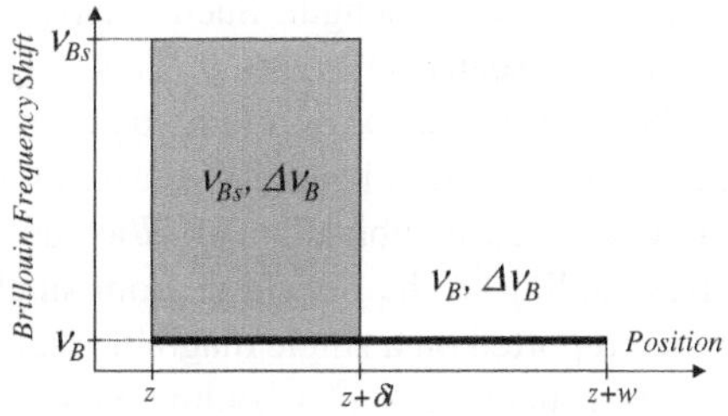

Fig. 7 Brillouin Frequency distribution within the length of the spatial resolution. Both sections have the same Brillouin linewidth but have a distinct Brillouin frequency [34]

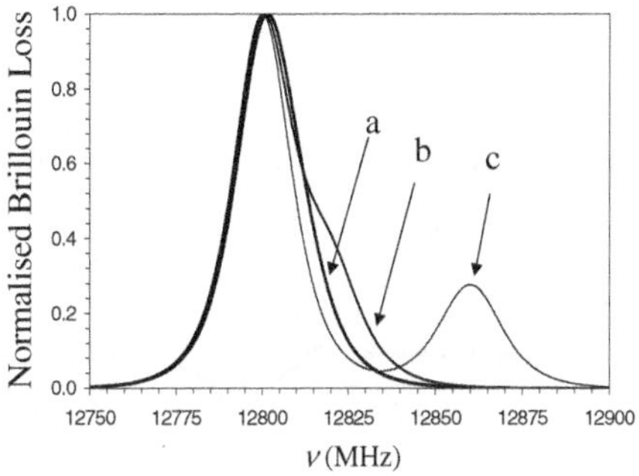

Fig. 8 Composite spectra for three distinct Brillouin frequency shift. Spectra a, b, and c are respectively associated with a Brillouin frequency of 12810MHz, 12820MHz and 12860MHz. The unstressed Brillouin Frequency shift is 12800MHz. The simulation parameters are P_{pk0} = 30 mW, P_{cwL} = 5 mW, L = 1000 m, z = 500 m, w = 20 m, δl= 5 m [34]

Figure 8 illustrates how the Brillouin spectrum shape changes when ν_B, ν_{Bs} and δl are varied. In this case, we have that δl = 5 m, ν_B = 12800 MHz while ν_{Bs} is 12810MHz (curve a), 12820MHz (curve b) and 12860MHz (curve c). Curve (a) is a single-peak distribution but lightly distorted. Curve (b) is still a single-peak distribution but it appears to be skewed. The central frequencies in Curves (a) and (b) are shifted from stress-free frequency (12800MHz), even if δl (stress section) is only 25% of the spatial resolution. The curve (c) has two peaks at 12800MHz and 12860MHz respectively due to the loose part of the fiber and the stressed section. The curves in Figure 8 clearly show the influence of the both stress length and strength on the spectrum shape. There is a transition from a single peak spectrum to a dual peak spectrum, which is depending on the stressed length.

i. Length-Strength diagram

The spectrum shape is driven by the combination of the normalised Brillouin frequency shift and the stressed section length. Such behaviour is summarised in a Length-Strength diagram represented in Figure 9. This diagram is the result of a systematic analysis of the spectrum shape as a function of the normalised Brillouin frequency shift and the stressed section length. We search for the number of peaks present in the spectrum for each combination of $\delta l/w$ and Ω_{Bs}. We record each couple ($\delta l/w$,Ω_{Bs}) corresponding to the transition from single to dual peak spectrum. The values are then reported on a single diagram (Figure V.4) in the form of a curve that shows Ω_{Bs} as a function of $\delta l/w$. Below the curve, only one peak can be seen; above the curve, two peaks are present. When the normalized Brillouin frequency shift is below 0.65, only one peak is observed whatever the value of

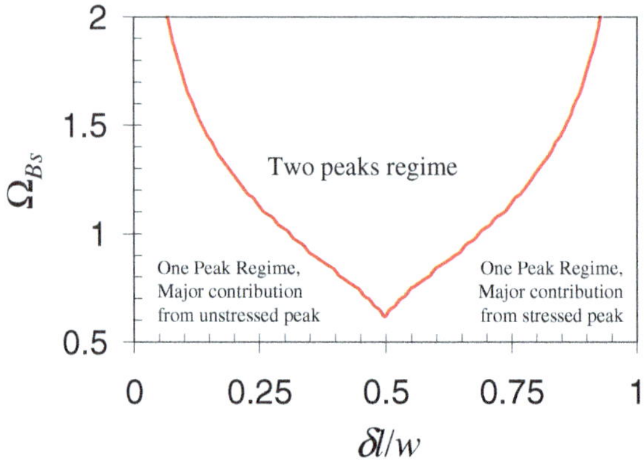

Fig. 9 Length-Strength diagram: this figure reports the normalized Brillouin frequency shift at which two peaks start to be observed as a function of $\delta l/w$. Below the curve, only one peak can be seen. Above the curve, two peaks are present. The simulation parameters are P_{pk0} = 30 mW, P_{cwL} = 5 mW, L = 1000 m, z = 500 m, w = 20 m [34].

$\delta l/w$. It is clear that there is a threshold frequency Ω^{th} that governs the number of peaks in the spectrum and that is determined by the Length-Strength diagram (LS).

ii. Rayleigh Equivalent Criterion

There are two frequency regimes characterized by single and two-peaks Brillouin loss spectra. A frequency threshold Ω^{th} sets the border between the two regions. As long as Ω_{Bs} is very different from Ω^{th}, there is no ambiguity in finding peak frequency. This claim is not valid when $\Omega_{Bs} \approx \Omega^{th}$, because the discrimination of the two peaks requires the peak search to be very precise. Besides, experimental data are contaminated with noise. That makes it more difficult to distinguish the two regimes. We want to introduce a practical and reproducible criterion that allows the unambiguous detection of multiple peaks and to determine the smallest resolvable frequency shift (Ω_{res}) using Rayleigh criterion[3] [37].

An equivalent criterion that applies to Brillouin Spectrum can be derived by making the assumption that both the normalised Brillouin spectrum and I must have the same FWHM [35]. If we define the normalised frequency in I to be $\beta = \upsilon\pi\nu/\Gamma$, it is easy to find that $\upsilon = 1.7718$ for Brillouin spectra that are Lorentzian like. Figure 10 shows Brillouin loss spectrum obtained by simulation of the phenomenological model. The dip amplitude (minimum of the Brillouin loss spectrum comprised between the two peaks) is 0.75 corresponding to $\Omega_{obs} = \Omega_{res} = 1.13$. We propose to define the dip amplitude as the Rayleigh Equivalent Criterion (REC).

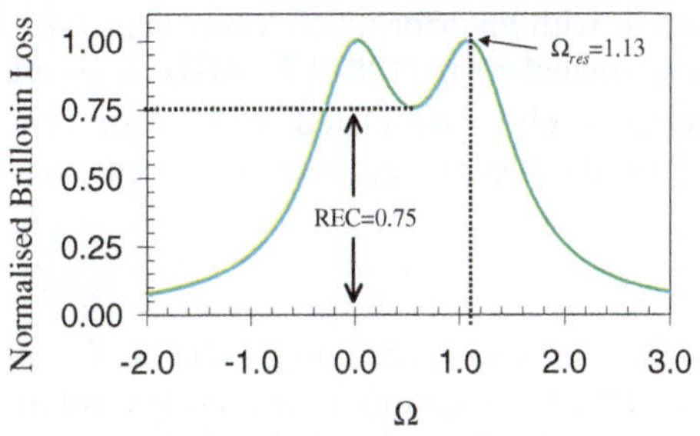

Fig. 10 Definition of the Rayleigh Equivalent Criterion for simulated Brillouin loss spectrum with the following parameters L=1000m, z=0, P_{p0}=30mW, P_{cwL}=5mW, w=20m [34][35]

[3] Rayleigh criterion is known to be a criterion that allows the determination of the smallest resolvable frequency difference. It applies to two distributions of equal intensity whose equations have the generic shape $I = \mathrm{sinc}^2(\beta)$ where β is the normalized frequency. The criterion assumes that these two peaks can be resolved as soon as the maximum intensity of the first peak coincides with the first minimum of the second peak, which happens for $\beta = \pi$. The distance between these two peaks is then the smallest resolvable frequency difference. The minimum between the two peaks has an intensity of $8/\pi^2$.

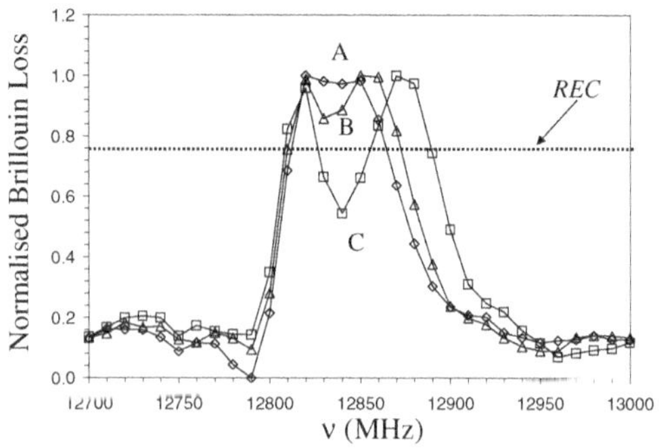

Fig. 11 Experimental Brillouin loss spectra measured at 20m at the boundary between the strained and unstrained sections for three strain values (A: 510με; B: 638 με; C: 893 με) [35]

Figure 11 illustrates how the REC can be used in measuring stresses that are shorter than the spatial resolution. These spectra come from the same experiment that illustrates the REC dependence against the normalised Brillouin frequency shift. The discussion focuses on the location at the boundary between the strained and unstrained sections. Profiles A (510 με) and B (638 με) show that the pulse covers more than one stress. According to the REC they are not distinguishable. Note that spectrum B clearly experiences two peaks and then the stress could be measured but an uncertainty much larger than 5% must be expected. The same criterion states that Spectrum C (893 με) has a stressed section that can be clearly identified and measured, with an error much lower than 1%. The stressed contribution frequency is estimated to be 12873.33 MHz when the peak frequency is measured. The frequency shift associated with a strain of 893 με is actually12878.90 MHz. Also the location accuracy has been reduced to ½ of the pulse length.

iii. Form Factors

When two peaks can not be resolved according to the REC (i.e. the spectrum lies in the single peak region of the LS diagram), further analysis of the spectrum shape can be carried out and then useful information deduced. That is possible by introducing two form factors, asymmetric (F_A) and broadening (F_B) Factors that describe the distortion of single peak spectrum [36]. The form factors are defined as

$$F_A = \frac{\Gamma_+}{\Gamma_-} \tag{16}$$

$$F_B = \frac{\Gamma_s}{\Gamma} \tag{17}$$

where F_A is the asymmetric factor and F_B the broadening factors, Γ_+ is the half width at half maximum of the right side of the spectrum, Γ_- is the half width at half maximum of the left side of the spectrum and Γ_s is the FWHM of the stressed fiber spectrum. Brillouin spectra measured at each location are analysed to extract these three parameters as illustrated in Figure 12.

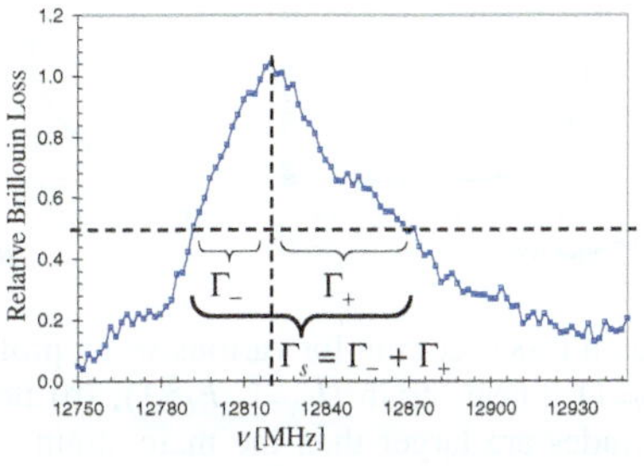

Fig. 12 Definition of the width parameters on an experimental Brillouin loss spectrum of a strained section of a single-mode optical fiber [36]

The asymmetric parameter, F_A, indicates the presence of large but short strain components. F_B describes the broadening of the Brillouin loss spectrum induced by non-uniform strain distribution. Let us discuss various strain regimes associated with the form factors value. Figure 13shows various cases with the same peak frequency but different strain distributions. When $F_A = 1$ and $F_B = 1$, the strain distribution is uniform. The spectrum is simply shifted and a peak finding approach is enough to characterize the status of the structure (Figure 13.(a)). If the spectrum is still symmetric ($F_A = 1$) but $F_B > 1$, then the distribution is non-uniform [38]. Peak finding technique describes the global behaviour of the structure but it fails to detect the presence of strain over section shorter than the pulse-width. The strain distribution becomes asymmetric when $F_A \neq 1$ as shown in Figure 13.(b), which is an indication that the strain distribution is non-linear [39]. For $F_A > 1$, the strain distribution is non-uniform over the pulse length: a short length strain component, whose amplitude is large, and, a long strain component, whose amplitude is small, are covered by the pulse. In other words, the spectrum presents a broadening happening on the right of the peak frequency. It indicates that small defects inducing large strain start to build up in the structure. In the case of $F_A < 1$, a strain component, whose amplitude is large, is longer than the weaker strain components. When *FA* value becomes smaller than unity, strains induced by local defects are expanding and becoming the dominant contribution to the spectrum asymmetry. It means that the structure is in jeopardy because the defect starts to expand. Apparently, the use of F_A and F_B introduces two advantages: 1) even if the peak Brillouin frequency is the same, they show distinct stress distribution; 2) it provides a complete picture compared to average strain detection or peak analysis (when only distorted spectrum is measured).

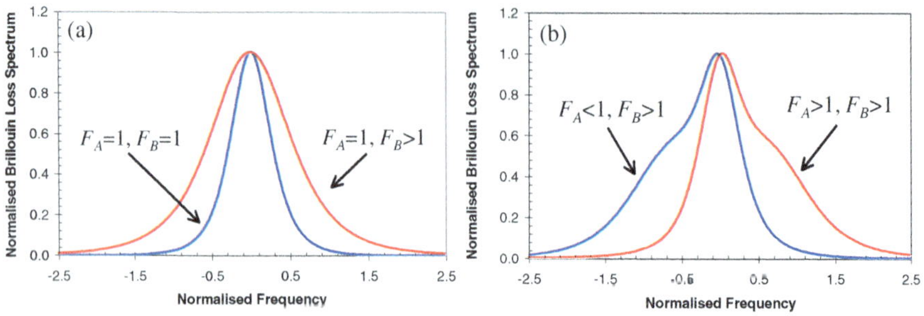

Fig. 13 Normalised Brillouin loss spectrum for various strain profiles included within w: (a) uniform strain (F_A=1, F_B=1), linear strain (F_A=1, F_B>1); (b) non-linear strain with short components whose amplitudes are larger than the main strain contribution (F_A>1, F_B>1), non-linear strain with short components whose amplitudes are smaller than the main strain contribution (F_A<1, F_B>1) [36]

5 Data Analysis Methodology

g. Proposed methodology

The model introduced previously not only explains the physics behind the instrumentation. It can also be used in a spectrum reconstruction scheme where the spatial distribution of ν_B is unknown which is the most common situation encountered on the field. The useful information is extracted from a careful analysis of the spectrum shape using the tools introduced in previous section. The first step would consist in determining to what part of the LS diagram the spectrum belongs. As mentioned, two types of spectrum shape are observed depending on the Brillouin frequency difference between stressed and unstressed components, as well as stressed section length. One type of spectrum has a single distorted peak which is broadened and asymmetric in most of the cases. The other type of spectrum has two peaks. Because the spectrum type is a function of Ω_{Bs} and $\delta l/w$, the classification in these two categories according to their dependence in stress value and length can be done as illustrated in Figure 14 by the LS diagram. There is a clear border (shown as a line in Figure 14.(a)) between the region where a single distorted peak is present (Figure 14.(b)) and the region where two peaks can be identified (Figure 14.(c)). The profile is then influenced by stress length and amplitude.

When two peaks are clearly identified, as shown on the spectrum of Figure 14.(c), stressed section length and amplitude are translated respectively in relative peak height, γ, and peak frequency. The relationship between γ, Ω_{Bs} and $\delta l/w$ is shown in Figure 15. Handling multiple integrations at each position, as the phenomenological model would require, is not necessary. Instead we propose to calculate G_T , assuming that g is constant over w but composite i.e. g at z is a linear combination of Lorentzian shape distributions defined as

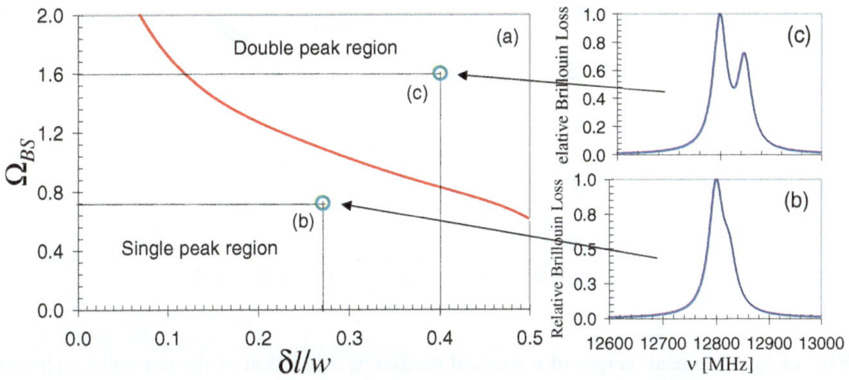

Fig. 14 (a) Length-Stress diagram for non-uniform Brillouin frequency over pulse length: the continuous line is the border between (b) single peak spectrum ($\delta l/w$ = 0.28, Ω_{Bs} = 0.72) and (c) two peaks spectrum ($\delta l/w$ = 0.40, Ω_{Bs} = 1.60). Simulation parameters are P_{pk0} = 10 mW, P_{cwL} = 8 mW, L = 100 m, w = 1 m, ER < 20 dB [33].

$$g(\nu, z) = \frac{1}{N(z)} \sum_{i=1}^{N(z)} \frac{\gamma_i(z) g_B}{\left(2\frac{\nu_i(z)-\nu}{\Delta\nu_B}\right)^2 + 1}, \tag{18}$$

where γ_i is the height and ν_i the peak frequency of the ith peak in spectrum, N is the number of peaks. As it appears in Eq.(17), γ_i, ν_i and N depend on the location in the fiber. The combination of these parameters is unique as it is based on the analysis of the spectrum shape, as it will appear in the following sections.

When the Brillouin spectrum is composed of multiple peaks, the present signal processing approach does not require to know the exact relationship between γ and $\delta l/w$ as shown in Figure 15. Here we would implement a peak search routine and associate each detected maximum with a pair (γ_i,ν_i). Near the borderline as defined in Figure 14, the distinction between single and double peak is not always unambiguous, particularly when the experimental data are contaminated with noise. To overcome that difficulty we introduce the Rayleigh Equivalent Criterion (REC). It states that two peaks are resolved if the minimum between two apparent maxima is lower than 75% of the lowest of the two peaks. We will use this criterion to separate the single peak region from the double peak region without ambiguity.

In the two peaks region, the identification of the various components is easier and the pair (γ_i,ν_i), (i=1,2), are determined without ambiguity, being the height and the frequency of the detected peak. When the spectrum only experiences one but distorted peak as shown in Figure 14.(b), the estimation of (γ_i,ν_i), (i=1,2), is more complicated. It is clear that in that case, the spectrum appears broadened and

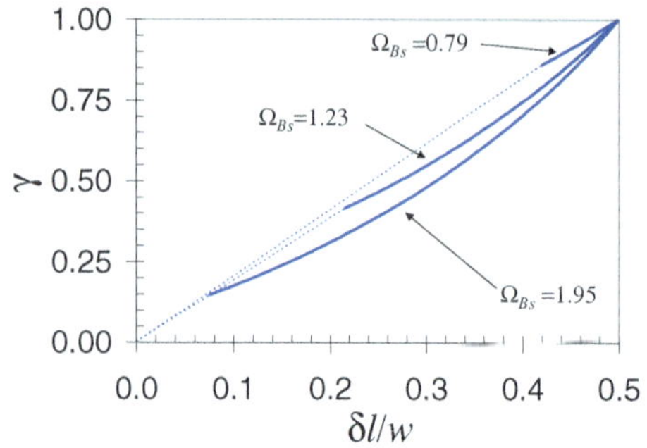

Fig. 15 Relative peak height of a stressed section as a function of the normalized stressed section length and Brillouin frequency shift. The solid line is the peak height when two peaks can be observed in the spectrum (all these points are in the double peak region of the LS diagram). The dotted line is a linear extrapolation of the stressed section peak height when the stressed contribution is buried in the single peak spectrum (all these points are in the single peak region of the LS diagram). Simulation parameters: P_{pk0} = 10 mW, P_{cwL} = 8 mW, L=100m, w=1m, ER<20dB [33], [34].

asymmetric. In that case, spectrum distortion can be analyzed further with the help of the two form factors, F_A and F_B. These parameters are a measure of the strain amplitude and the strained section length. We generated curves of constant form factors on the LS diagram for various practical sensing cases. They are also named iso-form factor curves, and more specifically, these curves are of two types: iso-FA (IF_A) and iso-FB (IF_B). Each of these curves drawn in a LS diagram is composed of two branches as shown in Figure 16. Curve fitting shows that the upper branch behaves as an arc of hyperbola while the lower branch is similar to an arc of ellipse. The intersection between one IF_A and one IF_B gives a couple ($\delta l/w$, Ω_{Bs}) from which the two Brillouin frequencies and the respective stressed section length can be extracted. In order to use the composite gain $g(\nu,z)$ with the reconstruction model, we need to convert $\delta l/w$ into γ. The relationship between $\delta l/w$ and γ is not known when the spectrum has a single peak as it appears in Figure 16. Nevertheless, Figure 16can be used to extrapolate that relationship. We make three assumptions: 1) γ must increase monotonically with $\delta l/w$; 2) γ=0 when $\delta l/w$ =0; 3) the transition from one to two peaks is continuous so that γ var ies continuously with $\delta l/w$. We simply suppose that γ is proportional to $\delta l/w$. After Figure 15, the proportionality coefficient, a, varies with Ω_{Bs} and is not significantly affected by other sensor parameters. We computed γ as a function of $\delta l/w$ for $\Delta\nu_s = \Omega_{Bs}\Gamma$ varying from 10MHz to 80 MHz. We obtain a large set of curves that are extrapolated linearly as shown in Figure 15 (dotted lines) and according to assumptions 1) to 3). Applying curve fitting to the numerical values of a (R^2 = 0.8577), we obtain that for $\Omega_{Bs} \leq 1$, $a \approx 2$, which represent most of the practical cases encountered.

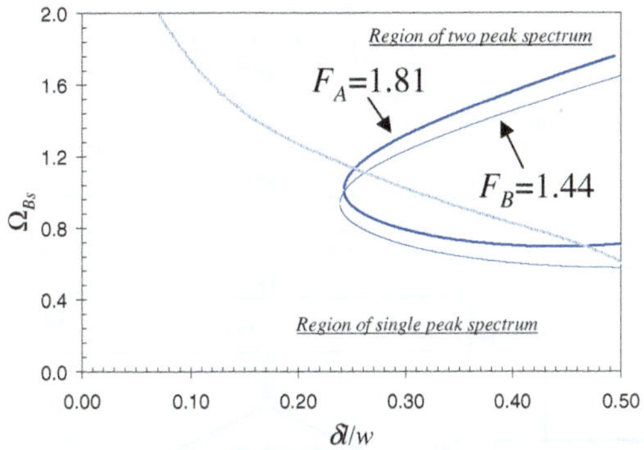

Fig. 16 Iso-form factor curves in Length-Stress diagram (LS) for non-uniform Brillouin frequency over pulse length; the continuous line is the border between single peak and two peak spectra. Simulation parameters are P_{pk0} = 10 mW, P_{cwL} = 8 mW, L=100m, w=1m, ER<20dB [33], [34].

Once ν_1 of the peak is determined by the extrema search routine, and, the couple ($\delta l/w$, Ω_{Bs}) found by searching the intersection of IF_A and IF_B, we can calculate $\nu_2=\nu_1+\Delta\nu_s$, $\gamma_1=a(1-\delta l/w)$ and $\gamma_2=a\delta l/w$. These values can then be used by Eq.(17) which in turn is used in the model to reconstruct the composite spectrum.

Any practical implementation require a calibration step. Strain being proportional to the variation of the Brillouin frequency, it is important to know its distribution all along the unstressed fiber which will be the reference measurement. Moreover, the signal processing approach implies that Γ is known as a function of position. Once the fiber is laid on the structure, a measurement over the frequency range of interest is carried out to set a baseline of ν_B and Γ. These values will then be used to detect any changes in the spectrum shape when the structure is stressed.

Figure 17 is a flowchart representing the various steps used to reconstruct the spectrum from experimental data. At a given position, we normalize the measured spectrum and then apply a filter to smooth the noise of the measured spectrum $S(\nu,z)$. We then set a threshold to the smallest peak detected that will be kept. An extrema search routine is applied to find all the peaks (γ_i,ν_i), $(i=1...M)$, and the minimum between two adjacent peaks (γ'_i,ν'_i). γ'_i and ν'_i are defined respectively as the amplitude and the frequency of the minimum between peaks i and i+1. The detected extrema are then subjected to a test: the amplitude of the maximum i must be larger than the peak threshold to be counted as a peak; the minimum must be lower than the *REC* criterion to have maxima i and i+1 counted as peaks. We then have a first set of (γ_i,ν_i), $(i=1...N_{pk})$. We now analyze the shape of each peak by estimating their *FA* and *FB*. Every time *FA* and *FB* are different from 1, the intersection of *IFA* and *IFB* must be calculated and the corresponding $(\gamma_1=a(1-\delta l/w), \nu_1)$ and $(\gamma_2=a\delta l/w, \nu_2)$ estimated increasing the total number of peaks (N_{pk} is updated). Eqs.(12) and (17) are then used to build the composite

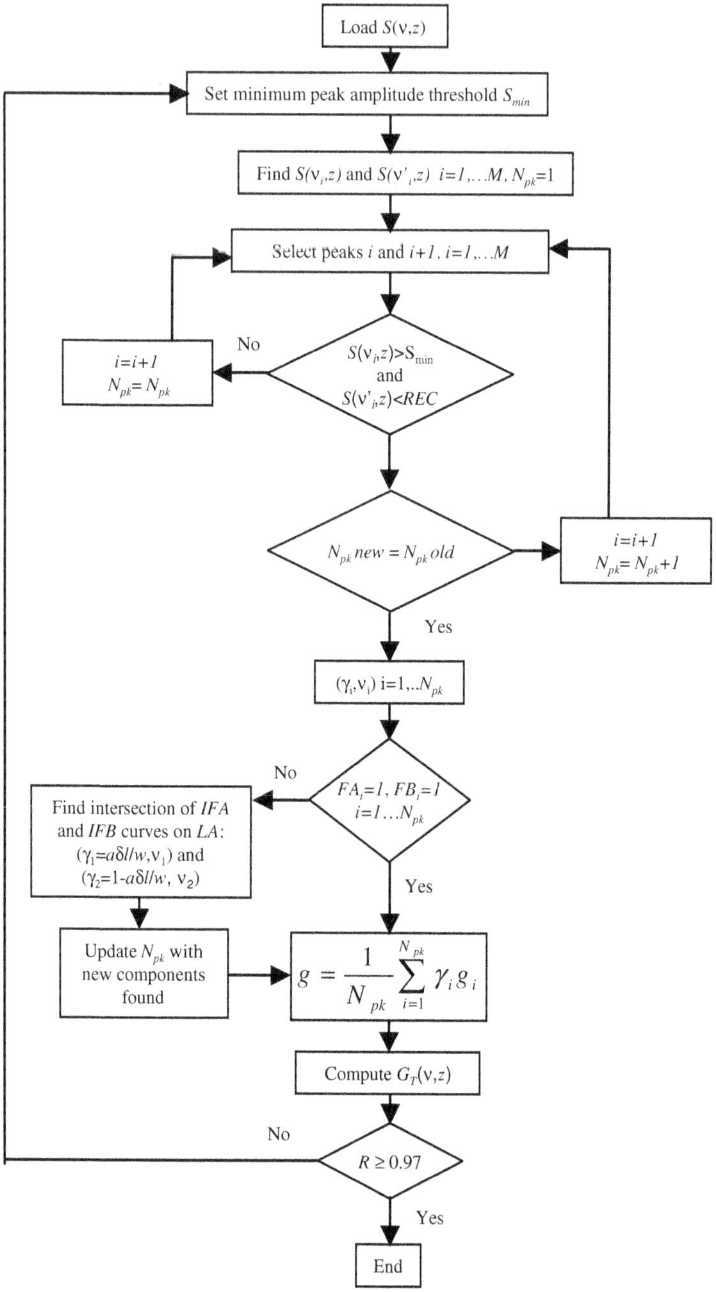

Fig. 17 Flowchart of the spectrum reconstruction procedure [33]

spectrum that is fed into the model. The reconstructed Brillouin loss spectrum is compared to the measured spectrum by computing the correlation coefficient [40] defined as

$$R = \frac{\sum_{i=1}^{N_d} \{S(\nu_i, z) - \langle S(z) \rangle\}\{G_T(\nu_i, z) - \langle G_T(z) \rangle\}}{\sqrt{\sum_{i=1}^{N_d} \{S(\nu_i, z) - \langle S(z) \rangle\}^2} \sqrt{\sum_{i=1}^{N_d} \{G_T(\nu_i, z) - \langle G_T(z) \rangle\}^2}} \tag{19}$$

where N_d is the number of measured data in the spectrum and the angular brackets refer to the average of the spectrum, measured or reconstructed, over the sample size. When $R = 1$, measured and reconstructed spectra match exactly and a diagram reporting $S(\nu,z)$ vs. and $G_T(\nu,z)$ would be aligned on a straight line whose coefficient is 1 and intercepting the origin. Pseudo-Voigt distribution curve fitting [41] on Brillouin spectra using the Levenberg-Marquhardt algorithm [40] normally requires that the correlation coefficient for the pseudo-Voigt distribution R_{pV} is larger than 0.97. We then expect that the reconstructed spectra using our signal processing approach should definitely give R values larger than 0.97. As a consequence, if $R \geq 0.97$, the routine ends the reconstruction of the spectrum at that location and starts to analyze the experimental profile of the next position. If $R<0.97$, the minimum peak amplitude threshold is decreased to account for peaks that were neglected in the previous reconstruction. The whole process is then repeated until $R \geq 0.97$.

Typically, the processing time for the reconstruction of spectra extending from 10750 to 11000MHz with a frequency step size of 4 MHz, and, acquired every 40 cm on a 2 km long single-mode fiber, is less than 5 minutes with a standard desktop computer (Intel Celeron processor, 847 MHz, 256 MB of RAM).

Because our approach uses a peak finding technique based on an extrema search routine, it can be argued that multiple distribution fitting can yield more accurate peak frequencies. Nevertheless such approach requires that the number of stress components building the spectrum is known in advance. Multiple trials are needed to obtain that information. That contributes to increase the processing time, which is not the case with our approach. In fact, distortions of the spectrum that are actually due to the sensor settings can wrongly be interpreted as additional stress components. With our approach, the spectrum shape is first determined by the sensor settings. Any difference between loose and stressed fibers spectra can then be attributed to the occurrence of an event as the sensor parameters are accounted for. The peak finding method is then faster. Moreover, the use of the REC criterion guarantees that the errors are lower than 2%, which is acceptable for applications were fault detection is critical [34], [35].

b. Application to experimental data

Figure 18 and Figure 19 show four measured Brillouin spectra and their respective reconstructed profiles. These spectra are measured at the same location, for different ε, in the transition region between the stressed and the pre-strained sections. It is clear that the reconstructed profiles match well the measured data (note that the correlation coefficient R between measured and reconstructed profiles is larger than 0.97. Figure 18.(a) is the unstressed case and single peak reconstruction is successful (R = 0.9889). Note that the pseudo-Voigt has a lower correlation parameter (R_{pV} = 0.9814). Figure V.19(b) still lies in the single peak region and appears lightly distorted. We have to compute the *IFA* and *IFB* from the experimental spectrum and extract the relevant hidden strain information from LS diagram embedded in the Figure 18.(b): $\Delta\nu \approx$ 19.75 MHz, $\delta l \approx$ 0.34 cm, R = 0.9916. Here too, R_{pV} = 0.9780 < R. The effect of the load increase becomes evident in Figure 19.(a) where a distortion of the measured profile is obvious. Analysis of *IFA* and *IFB* suggests that the strain condition is such that the spectrum must be at the edge of the single peak region. That is what the reconstructed profile states as a very small peak on the right part of the distribution is visible. The Form Factor analysis give $\Delta\nu \approx$ 29.41 MHz and $\delta l \approx$ 0.34 cm, and R = 0.9922 (R_{pV} = 0.9796). Finally, two peaks are clearly distinguishable in Figure 19.(b). We find that $\Delta\nu \approx$ 75.08 MHz, $\delta l \approx$ 0.34 cm, R = 0.9946 (R_{pV} = 0.9880).

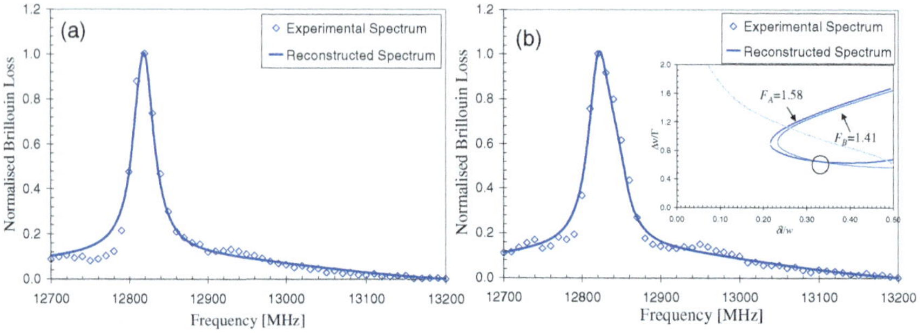

Fig. 18 Measured and reconstructed Brillouin loss spectrum for L = 40m and z = 16 m; measurement and computation parameters are P_{pk0} = 10 mW, P_{cwL} = 7.8 mW, ER =25dB, $\Delta\nu_B$ = 45 MHz, w = 20 cm; applied strain are 0 με (a) and 303 με (b) [33]

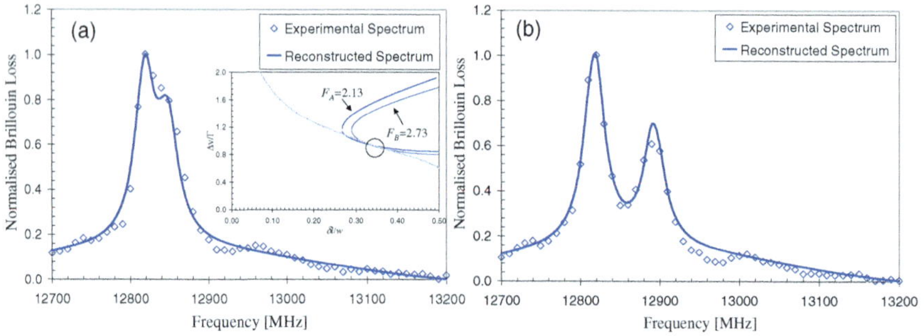

Fig. 19 Measured and reconstructed Brillouin loss spectrum for L = 40 m and z = 16 m; measurement and computation parameters are P_{pk0} = 10 mW, P_{cwL} = 7.8 mW, ER = 25 dB, $\Delta\nu_B$= 45 MHz, w = 20 cm; applied strain are 452 με (a) and 1138 με (b) [33]

6 Detection of Macroscopic Structural Failures

i. Detection of distribution pipe buckling

The tested specimen was a steel pipe of 1 m with a diameter of 18cm and square end caps (20cm side length). The location of buckling was controlled by thinning a small area of the specimen inner wall at the mid-length, which induced weakness in the structure for buckling to occur at this region when an axial load was applied. Moreover the test bench was designed to only exert vertical forces. Typical data acquisition time is 10 minutes.

The specimen was instrumented with strain gauges and distributed Brillouin sensor. Figure 20 shows the location of the fibres and strain gauges. The fibre was looped 8 times on the pipeline with 1m loose fibre separations. In order to avoid irregularities, the specimen surface was smoothed by using sandpaper. The fibres were attached to the prepared surface using a professional construction glue requiring three hours drying. The strain gauges are distributed symmetrically about the mid-length of the specimen.

Once placed on the test bench (Figure 20.(b)), the pipeline was subjected to a gradual load increase from 0 to 730kN. The buckling happened after 730kN and the fibre was broken due to the small bending radius and rigid glue (Figure 21). At the same time as the pipe was compressed, the deformations were continuously monitored with the strain gauges and the Brillouin sensor. The experiment was finished when the buckling happened, which is a very fast phenomenon when the steel starts to yield. The buckling could be visually observed as illustrated by Figure 21.

Two load levels (350 and 700kN) were kept constant for less than 15 minutes in order to capture the Brillouin spectra distributions along the whole fibre and over a frequency range broad enough to capture all possible strain components. Figure 22 represents the Brillouin loss spectra measured in section c. The three curves show the effect of the load increase: without load the Brillouin peak located at 12805MHz is higher than the loose fibre Brillouin frequency. That is induced by the

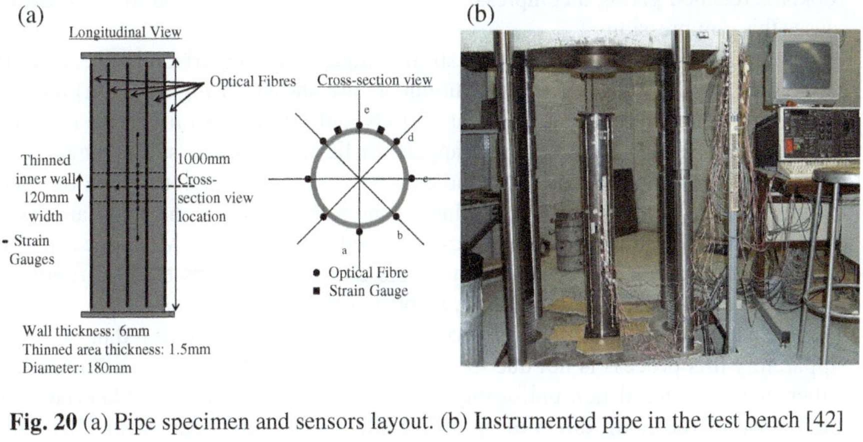

Fig. 20 (a) Pipe specimen and sensors layout. (b) Instrumented pipe in the test bench [42]

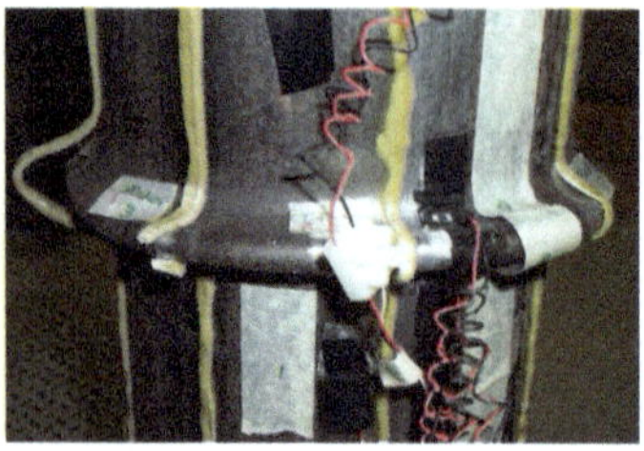

Fig. 21 Buckling of the pipeline. The deformation was obviously identified after the load was increased over 700kN [42].

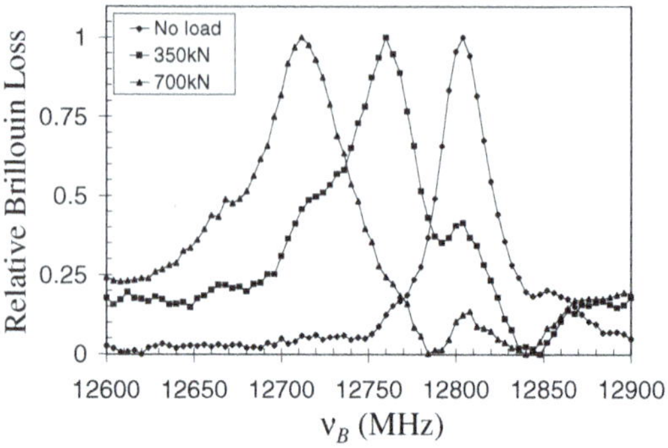

Fig. 22 Brillouin Loss Spectra for three distinct loads measured at 350 mm from the beginning of glued section c. The main peak is downshifted in frequency indicating that the pipe is compressed [42].

combination of small stresses during the fibre installation and the drying of the glue. The peak frequency at 350kN configuration is downshifted from 12805MHz to 12760MHz corresponding to -548 $\mu\varepsilon$. The peak frequency is further reduced when 700kN is reached giving a compression of -1390 $\mu\varepsilon$. The axial load to the structure causes this compression.

Pipe compression is confirmed by strain gauge, and comparison between strain gauge and the Brillouin sensor measurements are shown in Figure 23.(a) and (b) for various strips along the pipeline at 350 kN and 700 kN. Strain gauge readings and Brillouin sensor measurements appear to lie in the same strain range for a given load. In addition, the results indicate a consistent behaviour when the load increases from 350 kN to 700 kN. Material non-uniformity along hoop and axial directions are other interesting features observed in Figure 23.. More specifically, in the axial direction, it appears from Figure 23.(b) that curves e and d represent increased and decreased compression, respectively, while sections a, b, and c have a uniform compressive strain. The maximum compression is measured at 800 mm. Apparently this process is not due to wall thinning as the location is different. It is rather due to material non-uniformity enhanced by heavy loading. Material non-uniformity in the hoop direction is also evident when considering the Brillouin

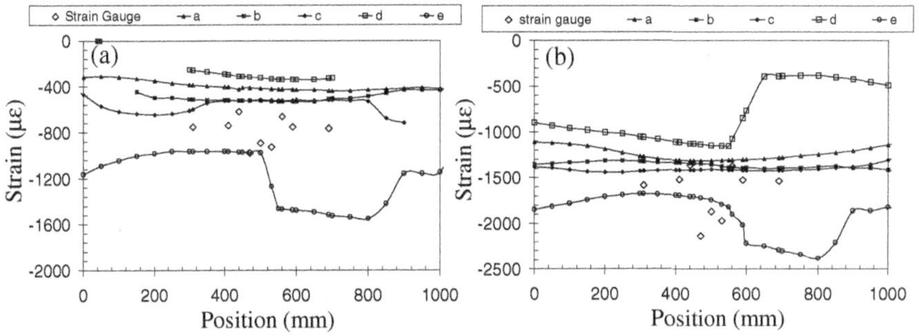

Fig. 23 Pipeline Strain profiles obtained by Brillouin sensor and strain gauges measurement for (a) the 350 kN load applied and (b) the700kN load applied. Labels a, b, c, d and e report the measurements obtained with the Brillouin sensor on fibers a, b, c, d and e [42].

sensor measurements and strain gauge readings at a fixed position. The largest strain variation happens in the region comprised between fibre section c and e. It is in the same region that the strain gauges are laid and show that their readings are comprised between Brillouin sensor measurements on fibres d and e. The fact that these values are not matching exactly is not unexpected. It accounts for two reasons. First, the material non-uniformity can be invoked because all the measured values, obtained with strain gauges and Brillouin sensor, show a monotonic transition from section d to e. Second, Figure VI.3 reveals that the spectra measured on the stressed pipe are broadened and asymmetric. This is not a surprise as the spatial resolution is 15 cm. As the induced strain by a heavy load is rarely uniform, the Brillouin sensor detects the average strain while the strain gauges measure localised strain.

Compression is not the only effect that we detected with the Brillouin sensor. In fact, we noticed the presence of a second peak in the Brillouin spectrum, which has a lower relative peak power (30% and smaller) than the highest peak associated with compression. It means that this smaller peak comes from a strained section within the pulse width that is shorter than the major contribution, due to compression. Resulting compressive and tensile strain profiles in Figure 23 and Figure 24, respectively, show the variations of these two strain components. Elongation increases as the applied load is raised as shown by the strain profiles in Figure 24. We interpret such behaviour as a signature of the buckling formation. We have two confirmation of this intuition. First, the location of the highest strain value suggests that it lies in the thinned wall region. Second, the location also coincides with the buckling position estimated by visual inspection (Figure 24). The whole pipeline suffers compression but a tiny part, axially distributed, must be extruded to elongate locally. At that stage of the experiment, the deformation is still too small to be seen visually, but can be felt by pressing the hand on the surface.

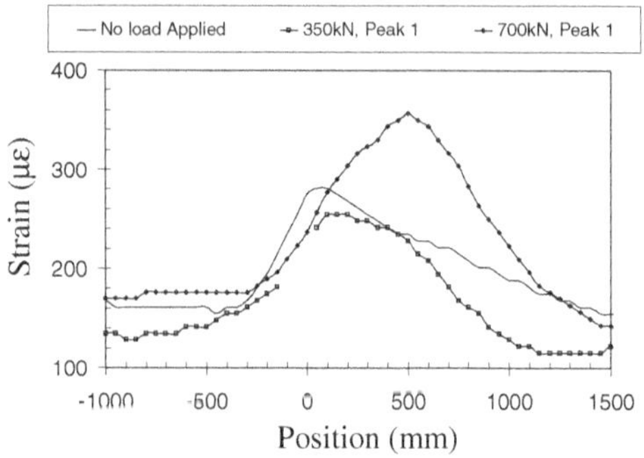

Fig. 24 Strain profiles along fiber section c extracted from Brillouin sensor measurements. 700kN (diamond), 350kN (square) and unloaded (plain curve) cases are reported

j. Detection of transmission pipe buckling

The tested pipe is a section of a real natural gas transmission steel pipeline of the type shown in Figure 25(a). The pipe was sealed on both ends. To simulate a real condition of operation of a natural gas pipe, the inner pressure was kept at 18.4 MPa during the whole buckling experiment. Longitudinal directions at 6 and 12 o'clock positives along the pipe were subjected to tension and compression, respectively, by applying simultaneous vertical and lateral forces. Typical data acquisition time is 10 minutes.

A 29 m acrylate buffered SMF-28 optical fibre was used to measure the strain along the pipe. 10 fibre sections located from 6 to 12 o'clock around the pipe were glued on the external surface to measure strain changes on the outer surface, as illustrated in Figure 25.(b). Each glued section is connected by 1 meter of loose fibre.Figure 25.(b) also shows the instrumentation of the pipe with strain gauges. These devices are glued in parallel with fibre sections 1 and 5.

Strain distributions along section 5 (tension side) under two vertical and bending loads conditions are presented in Figure 26. It appears that for both load conditions, the largest tensile strain occurs around 140 cm from the bottom of the specimen. The evolution from lower load (Figure 26.(a)) to higher load levels (Figure 26.(b)) emphasized the strain increase at that location. Assuming that the compressive strain coefficient is the same as that of the tensile strain, we drawn the strain profile of the compression side (section 1) in Figure 27. As in the tension case, the largest compressive strain (largest in absolute value) is observed at 140 cm. Again the compressive strain increases significantly when the load is stronger. The behaviours illustrated by Figure 26 and Figure 27indicate that the largest values of compressive and tensile strains observed at ~140 cm are the signature of the buckling formation, which is confirmed by visual inspection (Figure 28). When vertical and bending loads were further increased, the sensing fibre glued on the compression side of the pipe (section 1) ruptured terminating further measurements with the Brillouin sensor.

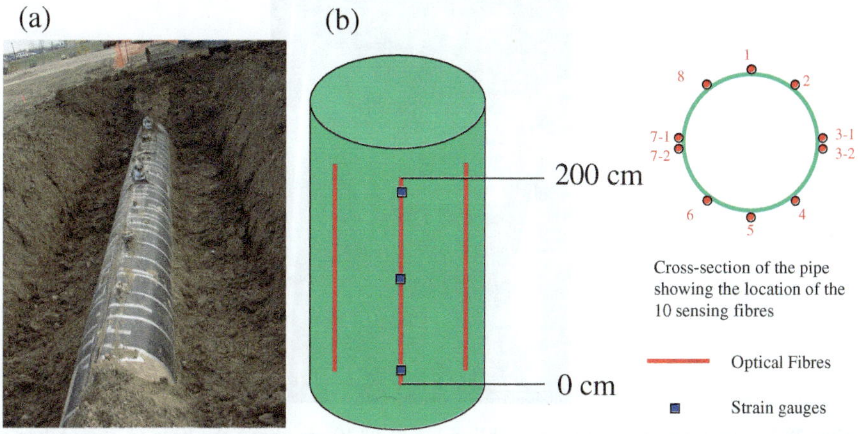

Fig. 25 (a) Example of a transmission pipe in its trench (picture taken at TransCanada PipeLine plant of Spruce Groove, Alberta). (b) Axial layout of the sensing fibre; the 10 sections are glued and connected to each other by 1 metre long of loose fibre.

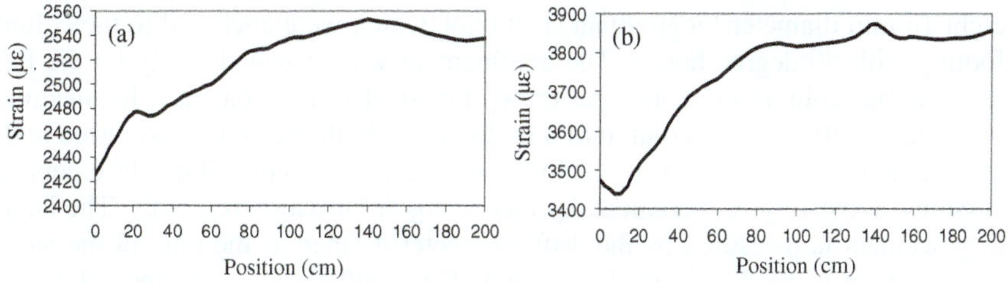

Fig. 26 Strain distributions along section 5 of the pipe: (a) Vertical load of 8799 kN and horizontal load of 979 kN; (b) vertical Load of 8954 kN and bending load of 1334 kN [43], [44]

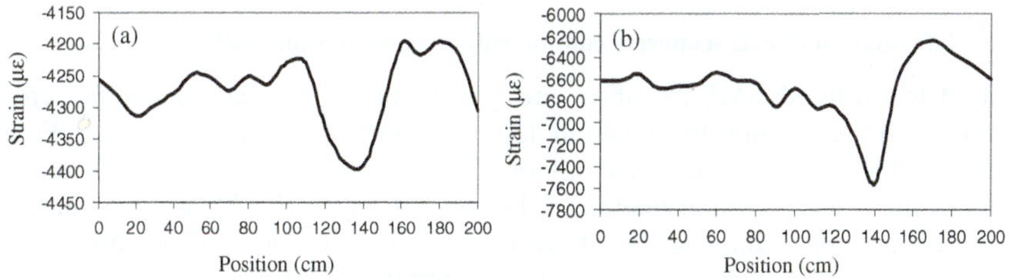

Fig. 27 Strain distribution along section 1 of the pipe: (a) Vertical load of 8799 kN and horizontal load of 979 kN; (b) Load of 8954 kN and bending load of 1334 kN ([43], [44]

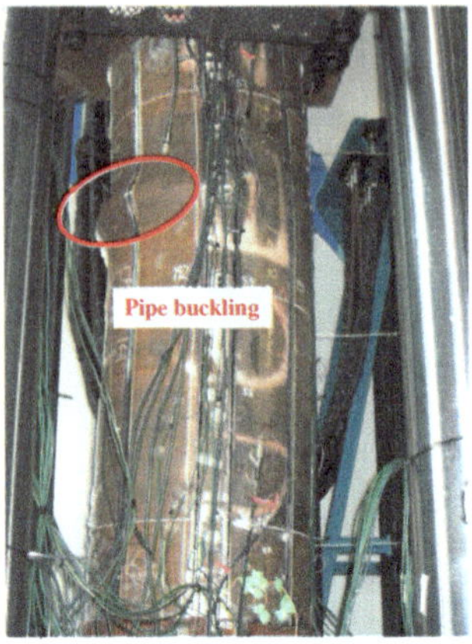

Fig. 28 Visual inspection of with buckling located 140 cm above the base (picture taken at CFER structural laboratory in Edmonton, Alberta) [43], [44]

A large steel reinforced concrete building column, encased in FRP[4] casing, was constructed and tested under simulated seismic loading (Figure 29). The column had a 270 mm square cross-section and a 1.72 m height. The column contained eight 16 mm diameter longitudinal steel bars, which were anchored to the column footing with 90-degree hooks. The confinement was provided solely by the FRP tube, as the column contained no transverse steel reinforcement. The specimen represented a first storey column of a multi-storey building and it was tested under an axial load of 1880 kN. The specimen was subjected to lateral displacement excursions, consisting of incrementally increasing deformation reversals. The lateral displacement is measured by the drift parameter defined as the ratio of the lateral displacement to the height of the column. Three full cycles were applied at each deformation level, starting with drift value of 0.5%, then 1%, 2%, 3% etc, in the deformation control mode of the horizontal actuator. Lateral loading continued until the specimen was unable to maintain a significant fraction of its maximum lateral load resistance. In the rest of this section, the lateral displacement will be associated with push and pull configurations, push and pull referring to the relative location of the observatory. Typical data acquisition time is 10 minutes.

k. Deformation of FRP-concrete column subjected to seismic load

Acrylate buffered SMF-28 fibres are glued horizontally at 10 distinct cross-sections of the column (from bottom, layer 1, to the top, layer 10) shown in Figure 29.(b), which is separated by 1m of loose fibre. An optical pulse is launched at the end of the fibre located at the top of the column (layer 10). Measured strain data with strain gauges and distributed sensors were used to monitor the column's response to seismic loading at each drift step. Strain gauges were also placed on the surface of the FRP casing, oriented in the direction of the carbon fibres. These devices are symmetrically glued on both pull and push sides of the column close to each level determined by a glued fibre optic (Figure 30).

[4] Fiber Reinforced Polymer.

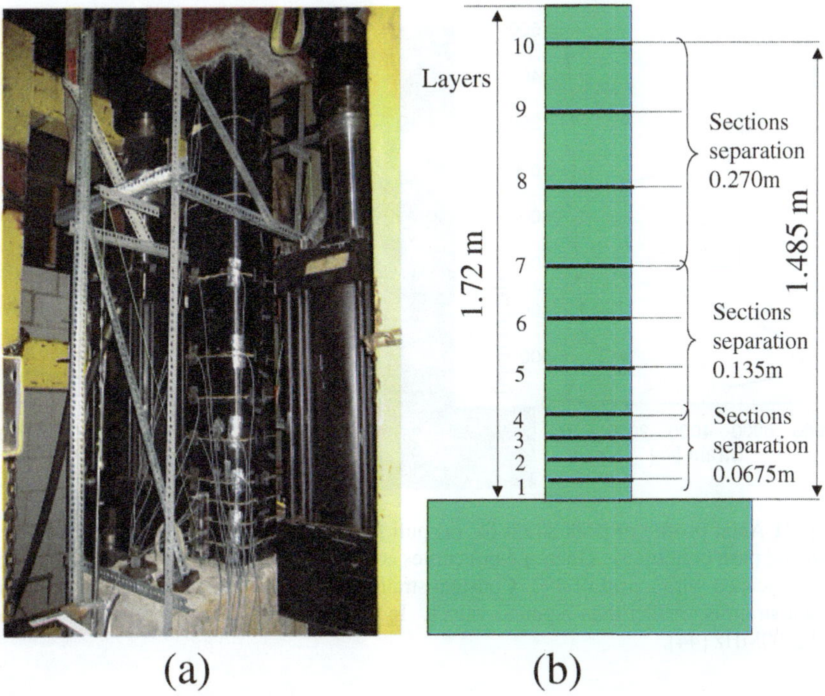

Fig. 29 (a) Instrumented FRP/concrete column in test set-up; (b) Column dimensions and fibre optic layout kN [36], [44]

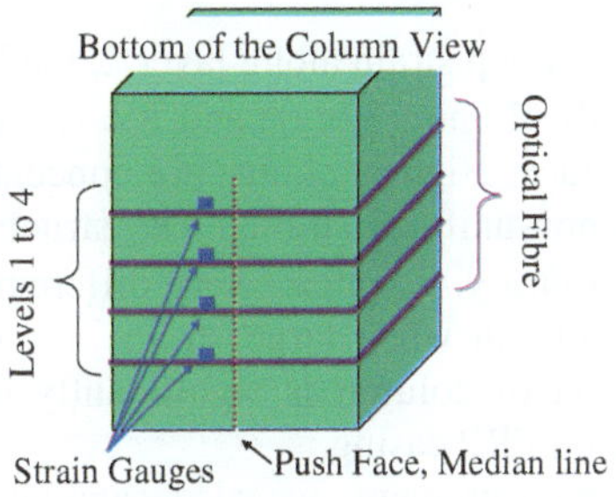

Fig. 30 Detailed view of the bottom of the column kN [36], [44])

Peak frequencies are extracted from the spectra in order to obtain hoop strain distributions. The peak strains for the push and pull conditions at drifts 4 and 8% are presented in Figure 31. Large strains are concentrated at the bottom of the column (levels 1 to 5) with a peak value at level 2. This was supported by the recorded strain gauge data, which were reported elsewhere [45]. The most extensive damage occurred at approximately 100 mm to 160 mm above the column-footing interface, which coincided with the location of first fibre rupture in all columns.

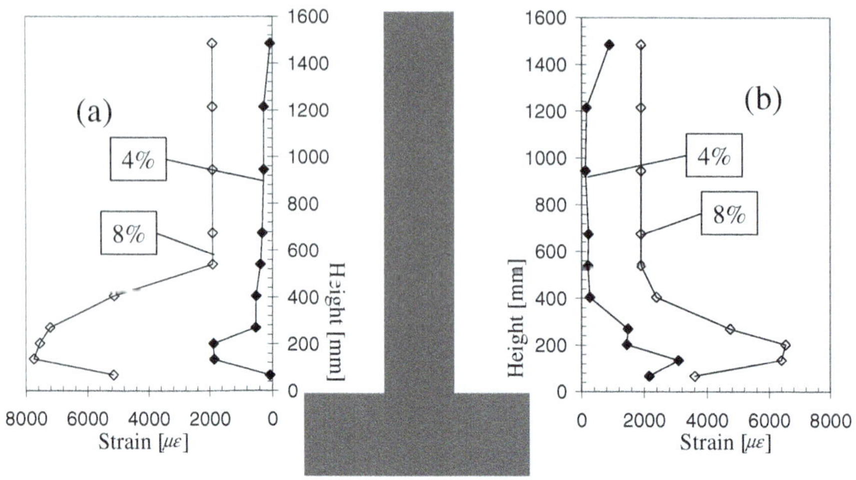

Fig. 31 Axial profile of peak strain for (a) pull face and (b) push faces under respectively pull and push conditions. Open symbol curves correspond to a drift of 8% and full symbols are associated with a drift of 4%. Constant strain for 8% cases (Layers 6 to 10) means that actual strain is smaller than reported values. In this case, Brillouin frequency span started at 12900MHz [44].

The shifting of the critical section from the interface was attributed to the confining effect of the footing as previously reported [45], [46], [47]. Note that strain that appears to be constant at 8% for levels 6 to 10 means that the actual strain is smaller than these reported values. In this case, Brillouin frequency span started at 12900MHz.

Figure 32 represents the hoop strain along layer 2, the layer of largest strain, for pull case with drifts of 3% (Figure 32.(a)) and 8% (Figure 32.(b)). ε'_{pk} is maximum at 3% drift on pull face. Highest strains are concentrated on pull side of the column with maximum non-uniform strains. The structure is capable to absorb stresses locally. On the contrary, it appears very different in 8% case: ε'_{pk} is high everywhere around the column when large strains dominate. This suggests that concrete at critical section of column is significantly damaged and generating large amount of pressure on FRP casing.

From each Brillouin measurement, we also calculated F_A and F_B. We then drawn ε_{pk} and the two form factors as a function of the drift amplitude for both push and pull condition. We concentrated our analysis on two fibre sections located on the median of layers 2 and 4 of push side (Figure 30). We also analysed the median point of layer 4 of pull (i.e. symmetric of layer 4 push side).

The progressive column degradation can be viewed closely using e'_{pk}, e'_{SG} (readings from strain gauges shown in Figure 30) and the form factors. detailed analysis of the median line of levels 4 and 2 of the push side is provided (Figure 33). Most of these graphs show that ε'_{pk}, ε'_{SG} and F_B experience a monotonic increase with a slope rise at larger drifts. The slope change happens when $F_A \approx 2$ and $F_B \approx 3$. At larger drifts, F_B tends to saturate or to fluctuate. F_A increases above 2

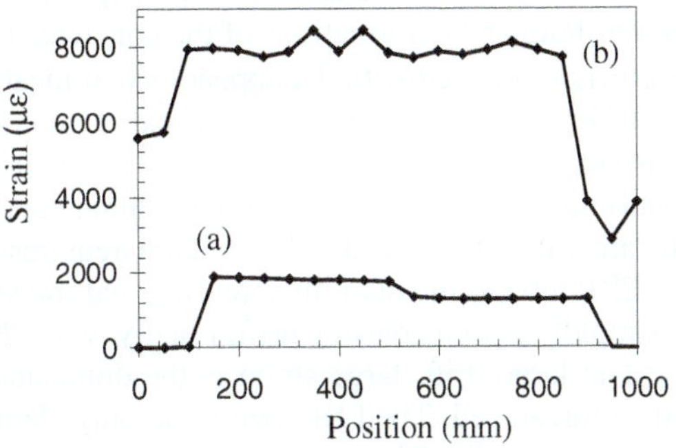

Fig. 32 Hoop strain profiles for layer 2 under pull condition with drifts of 3% (a) and 8% [44]

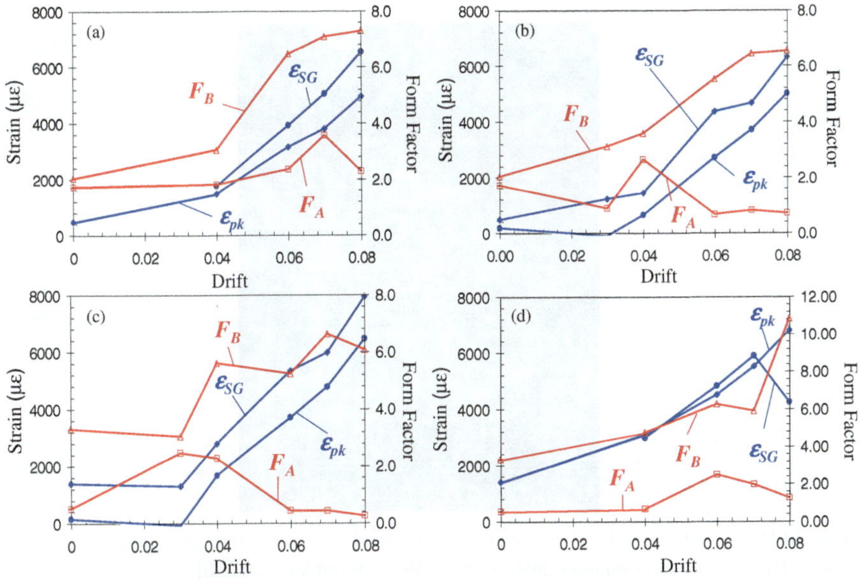

Fig. 33 Peak frequency (left y axis) and form factors (right y axis) as a function of column drift: (a) push side, Layer 4, median point, push condition; (b) push side, Layer 4, median point, pull condition; (c) push side, Layer 2, median point, push condition; (d) push side, Layer 2, median point, pull condition [36], [44].

(it can reach a maximum of 4) and then drops below 1 and becomes steady. The behaviour of these four parameters can be associated with the column degradation. The region of smaller ε'_{pk} slope corresponds to the elastic condition. At that stage, the damage in the concrete is not significant and it is still capable of resisting the applied loads without a significant contribution from the FRP casing to maintain the column. Moreover the concrete and FRP are still holding together. The increase of F_A and F_B values are associated with the appearance of local stresses, contributing to the crushing and deformations of the concrete. The slope change of ε'_{pk} at $F_A \approx 2$ and $F_B \approx 3$ is associated with the appearance of local stresses indicating the start of local crushing of the concrete at the critical region of the column. Concrete crushing is visually evident as shown in Figure 34. The increase of ε'_{pk} slope is then a manifestation of extensive damage in the column concrete. At this point, FRP and concrete are fully de-bonded. The column requires high confinement pressures from the FRP tube to maintain its integrity, and transverse strains in the FRP tube increases rapidly with increasing drift. Finally, when F_B saturates (and/or fluctuates) and $F_A \leq 1$ at large drift, large strain is the dominant contribution. The column safety is then threatened. The FRP, being the only element supporting the structure, starts to rupture locally. These ruptures release locally the tension inducing a local strain reduction (ε'_{SG} drops as shown in Figure 33.(d)), mitigating the spectrum broadening but ε'_{pk} increases, meaning that the structure continues to degrade.

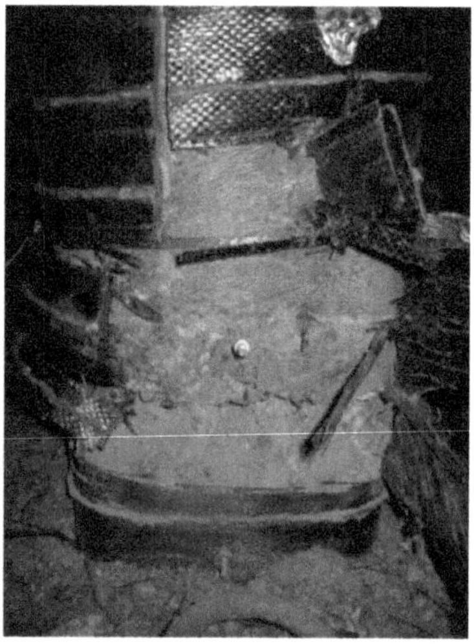

Fig. 34 Post-mortem analysis of the column: concrete at the bottom part has been crushed; once FRP is removed, concrete dust flown on the column support [36]

Table 1 summarizes the relationship of the structure behaviour with the three parameters variation. Monitoring the changes of these values can predict the early sign of collapse. The conclusions drawn in Table 1 are valid for 1.7 ns pulses but should not be affected by pulse width of the same order of magnitude, which is the best spatial resolution that could be achieved.

The spectrum shape analysis is then a powerful approach when their static and dynamic variations are considered. First, global structure deformation is monitored through the Brillouin peak frequency. Second, form factors are the signature of local defects induced by non-uniform strains, which cause the spectrum broadening and/or asymmetry. Third, the plot of their change as a function of stress to get the metric/load slope change indicates non-linearity of these parameters

Table 1 Signature of structure failure with form factors [36], [44].

Strain Observation	F_A	F_B	ε_{pk} Slope	Structure Status
Uniform	<2	<3 Small slope	Constant, small	Elastic regime, good shape
Non-uniform, low strain dominates	>2 Peak value	>3 Large slope	Increase	Deformation, local cracks, local de-bonding
Non-uniform, large strain dominates	<1 Stationary	>>3 Constant and large slope	Constant, Large	Full FRP/concrete de-bonding
Reduced non-uniformity, large strain dominates	<1 Stationary	>>3 Stationary	Constant, Large	FRP cracks

change. The relationship between load and strain is expected to be linear as long as localised defects are absent. The tracking of slope variation would give us an indication on local defects apparition, such as de-bonding and cracks (or crushed concrete).

7 Detection of Microscopic Structural Failures

In crack detection, several issues can be identified. First of all, such faults have a very small width (δl_c), usually $\delta l_c < 1$ mm, which means that a large strain concentration is induced leading quickly to the fiber sensor break. Second, should the sensor survive, the peak would be buried in the noise of the measurement as the spectrum peak powers are roughly proportional to the length of the events as illustrated in Figure 15. One efficient way to detect a crack consists in transferring the stress to a longer section of the sensor, defined as the delaminated length (δl_g), such that there is no risk of breakage and the peak height is high enough to be measured. That approach is illustrated in Figure 35. Nevertheless, there are limits to large δl_g. In fact, the debonding can be so long that the induced strain is small. A small strain has the consequence to hide the crack information in the main peak, making the fault detection more difficult. Moreover, there is also another upper limit to δl_g. In fact, we want to keep it as short as possible so that deformation monitoring and crack detection capabilities elsewhere in the structure are not jeopardized. Obviously there is a need for the estimation of an optimum delaminating length δl_g.

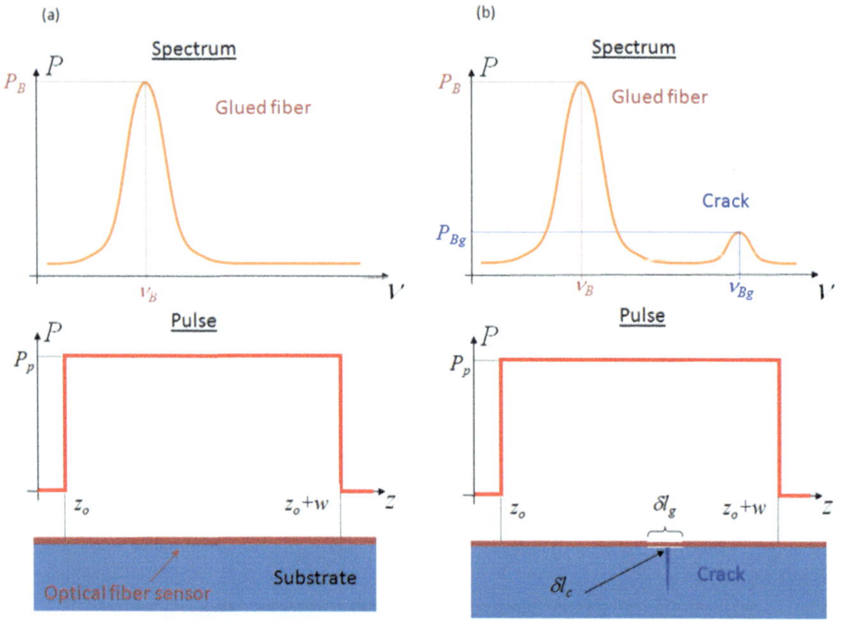

Fig. 35 (a) An optical fiber sensor is bonded at the surface of a substrate. A pump pulse of peak power P_p and spatial resolution w propagates down the sensor and interacts with the *cw* probe. The result of the interaction is a Brillouin spectrum that is characteristic of unstressed fiber as schematized. (b) A crack occurs and delaminate the sensor over a length of δl_g, crack size length at surface is $\delta l_c < \delta l_g$. At the crack location, pump-probe interaction leads to the measurement of a new spectrum experiencing an additional peak, which is a signature of the fault formation [48].

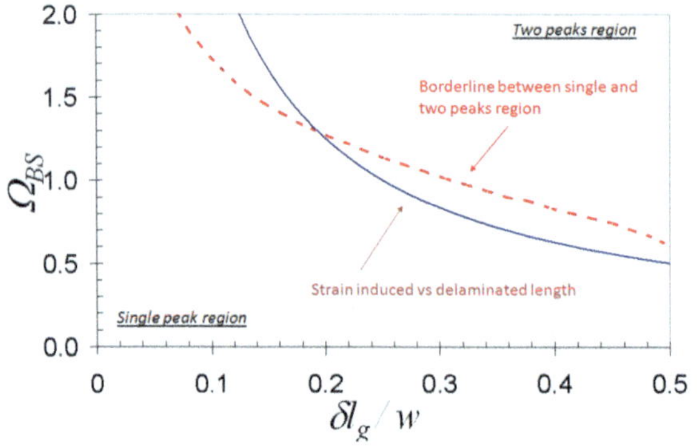

Fig. 36 LS diagram showing the borderline between single and two peaks region (dashed curve) and the curve representing the induced strain as a function of the delaminated section length (plain curve) [48]

The *LS* diagram is used in order to estimate the optimum δl_g. It is interesting to note that the strain induced Brillouin frequency shift $\Delta\nu$ is a simple function of the delaminated length δl_g. It is expressed as $\Delta\nu=(\delta l_c C_\varepsilon)/\delta l_g$ when it is remembered that the strain induced by the crack is given by $\varepsilon=\delta l_c/\delta l_g$. When drawing this function on the *LS* diagram (plain curve), after normalization, it is obvious that the strain induced decreases with the increasing delaminated length. Figure 36 shows that the curve crosses the border for $\delta l/w\approx0.2$. We then conclude that the delaminating approach can be used for $\delta l_g/w<0.2$. According to Figure 15 when $\delta w_g/w\approx0.1$, the peak associated with the crack is about a fifth of the main peak. Such signal level guarantees a crack detection capability for most of the practical cases. The fiber sensor packaging and bonding procedure must then be carefully selected to delaminate over an optimum delaminating length that is about one tenth of the spatial resolution, typically 10 cm when $w = 1$ m.

The approach is validated by using specialty optical fiber sensor cable, the SMARTape [12] dedicated to the measurement of strain, with a BOTDA based interrogator unit, the Omnisens DITEST. Both components have proven track of uninterrupted and reliable field operations [49], [50], [51].

The SMARTape was developed because strain measurement on a structure requires an excellent bonding between the sensor and the substrate surface. Optimum strain transfer occurs when the fiber optic is embedded in a thermoplastic tape in the similar manner as the reinforcing fibers are integrated in composite materials. To produce such a tape, a glass fiber reinforced thermoplastic with PPS matrix is used. This material has excellent mechanical and chemical resistance properties. Since its production involves heating to high temperatures (in order to melt the matrix of the composite material) it is necessary for the fiber to withstand this temperature without damage. In addition, the bonding between the optical fiber coating and the matrix has to be guaranteed. Polyimide-coated optical fibers fit these requirements and were therefore selected for this design. The typical cross-section width of the thermoplastic composite tape that is used for manufacturing composite structures is in the range of ten to twenty millimeters. As a consequence, it is not critical for optical fiber integration. The thickness of the tape can be as low as 0.2 mm, and this dimension is more critical since the external diameter of polyimide-coated optical fiber is of 0.145 mm approximately. Hence, only less than 0.03 mm of tape material remains on top or bottom of the optical fiber, with the risk that the optical fiber will emerge from the tape. The scheme of the sensing tape cross-section, with typical dimensions, is presented in Figure 37. The use of the SMARTape is twofold: it can be used externally, attached to the structure, or embedded between the composite laminates, having also a structural role.

Important optical losses, ranging between 25 and 30dB/km, are generated in optical fibers during the production of the SMARTape. These losses are induced by micro-bending and matrix shrinkage which limit maximal length of a single sensor to 200-250 m approximately. Functionality of sensors with such losses is guaranteed by extraordinary high power budget of the reading unit (20dB). Several laboratory and on-site tests were performed in order to assess the performance of the SMARTape [50]. Axial Young modulus was determined to be approximately 31 GPa, while the rupture strain was higher than 3%. Such high Young

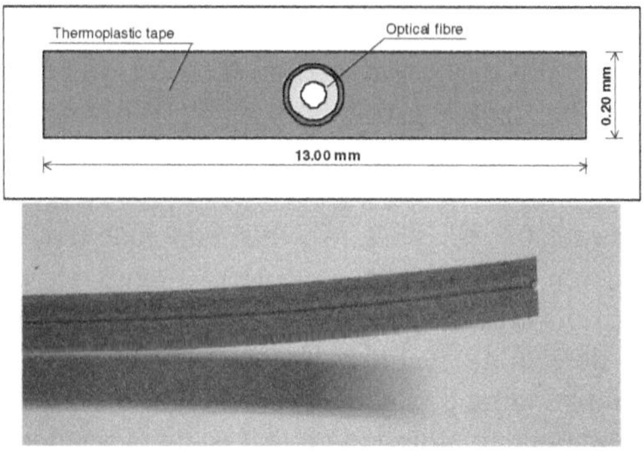

Fig. 37 Fiber optic sensing cable characteristics (SMARTape) [48]

modulus and strength provide the necessary stiffness to ensure safe installation of long sensors and delamination of sensor in area surrounding the crack. Comparisons of strain measurement obtained by SMARTape with those obtained by traditional micrometer had linearity error of 0.3% and correlation coefficient square R^2=0.99992.

The glue used to install the SMARTape is carefully selected in order to both ensure good transfer of strain from the structure to the sensor and make possible delamination in case of crack opening. The selection was made after consulting several suppliers and testing different types of glue. The tests included shear-strength and peel tests, and exposure to extremely low temperatures, down to -30°C. Once the glue selected, the installation procedure was fully developed and tested in laboratory and on-site.

The test is performed on rails loaded by wagon where the SMARTape is compared with other interferometric optical fiber sensors. Installation is performed following the pre-established installation procedures and the differences between two types of sensors were in range of resolution of interferometric interrogator ($2\mu\varepsilon=2\cdot10^{-6}$ m/m), confirming applicability and good field measurement performance of the SMARTape. The installed SMARTapes were left on the rails in order to assess the performance in long-term and after nearly five years were still in a good condition. These tests included verification of installation procedures, mid-term performance, comparison with mechanical gages, crack detection and parameterization and temperature compensation.

Validation of our approach requires a test set-up in which cracks are produced in a controlled manner. In order to achieve that goal we built a special set-up. Two flat and smooth metallic supports were assembled. One of them is fixed while the other can be moved. As an initial step, the two supports were joined and the SMARTape was glued on their surface (Figure 38). The metallic supports were then exposed to a relative translation movement simulating crack opening. The relative translation movement was ensured by special metallic holders that prevented relative rotations and forced the metallic supports to slide over straight lines. The translation motion was imposed by a micrometric screw. The relative

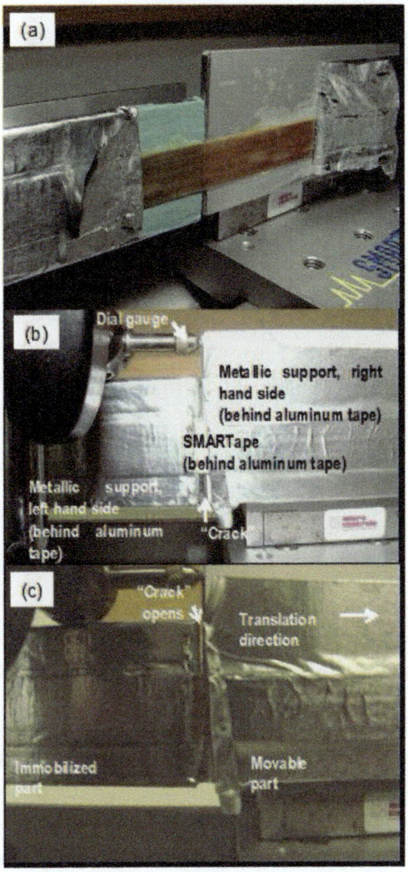

Fig. 38 (a) SMARTape glued on the metallic supports. (b) Test set-up before the "crack" is formed. (c) Test set-up after the "crack" is formed [48].

displacement between the two metallic supports is strictly monitored by using a dial gauge (Figure 38).

The crack opening was also monitored by measuring the SMARTape behavior with the Brillouin interrogator. Figure 39.(a) shows the Brillouin frequency distribution once a 0.56 mm "crack" was formed. As it appears in Figure 39.(b), the spectrum off the "crack" region is typical of a fiber not subjected to a localized stress i.e. the Brillouin frequency is uniform over the *w*. When we examine Figure 39.(c), it is obvious that in the "crack" region the spectrum presents a composite structure. Two peaks are observed, the highest being related to the unstressed part of the fiber while the tiniest is a signature of the "crack". It is not a surprise that the detected crack section seems to extend roughly over a distance $w/2 > \delta l_g$. The measurement interval is a fraction of *w* such that there is much more than one digitized position in which the crack appears. In other words, the event has an apparent length of about *w*. Nevertheless, crack actual location can be estimated

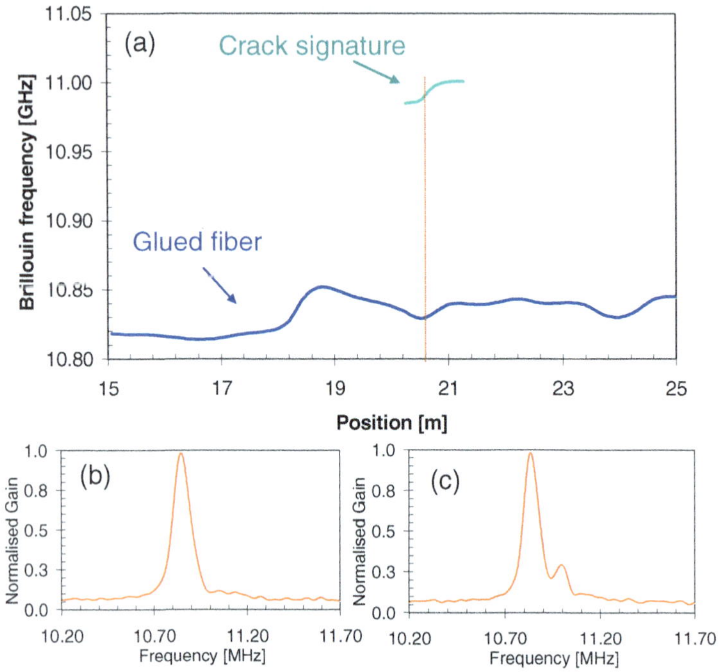

Fig. 39 (a) Brillouin frequency distribution near the crack location derived from the measured spectra. (b) Brillouin spectrum at 20.5 m, off the "crack" region. (c) Brillouin spectrum at 20.6 m, in the "crack" region [48].

more accurately thanks to the following reasoning. According to Figure 39.(a), delaminated section is comprised between 20.2 and 21.2 m which is the crack signature interval. That interval can be sampled into 10 cm segments due the instrument sampling resolution. Moreover, delaminated section is centered on the middle of the crack signature interval that is to say at 20.80 m. As crack is located within the delaminated section, it is estimated to be localized between 20.75 and 20.85 m as the instrument sampling resolution is 0.1 m.

8 Real World Implementations

Full scale implementation on Brillouin based sensors is now a reality. Bridges are currently being monitored for structural stability monitoring as well as crack detection. Fiber optic sensing cables are integrated to the structure and the described monitoring approach is implemented for continuous monitoring [52], [53], [54]. The sensing technology is used in geotechnical engineering to monitor landslide on a continuous mode and hence generate alarms when populated areas, building or roads are threatened [55]. Distributed Brillouin sensor installations for structural or integrity monitoring are not limited to civil engineering structures. The energy domain and in particular the oil and gas industries are making use of fiber optic sensors for offshore facilities [56] and pipelines[57], [58].

References

[1] Boyd, R.W.: Nonlinear optics, 2nd edn. Academic Press, London (2003)

[2] ITU-T G.652, Series G: Transmission Systems and Media, Digital Systems and Networks. International Telecommunication Union (2000)

[3] Vacher, R., Pelous, J.: Behavior of thermal phonons in amorphous media from 4 to 300 K. Physical Review B 14, 823–828 (1976)

[4] Rowell, N.L., Thomas, P.J., van Driel, H.M., Stegeman, G.I.: Brillouin spectrum of single-mode optical fibers. Applied Physics Letters 34, 139–141 (1979)

[5] Agrawal, G.P.: Nonlinear fibre optics, 2nd edn. Academic Press, London (1995)

[6] Niklès, M., Thévenaz, L., Robert, P.A.: Brillouin gain spectrum characterization in single-mode optical fibers. Journal of Lightwave Lightwave Technology 15, 1842–1851 (1997)

[7] Horiguchi, T., Kurashima, T., Tateda, M.: Tensile strain of Brillouin frequency shift in silica optical fibers. IEEE Photonics Technology Letters 1, 107–108 (1989)

[8] Culverhouse, D., Frahi, F., Pannell, C.N., Jackson, D.A.: Potential of stimulated Brillouin scattering as sensing mechanism for distributed temperature sensor. Electronics Letters 25, 913–915 (1989)

[9] Horiguchi, T., Tateda, M.Y.: BOTDA-nondestructive measurement of single-mode optical fibers attenuation characteristics using Brillouin interaction: theory. Journal of Lightwave Technology 7, 1170–1176 (1989)

[10] Niklès, M., Thévenaz, L., Robert, P.A.: Simple distributed fiber sensor based on Brillouin gain spectrum analysis. Optics Letters 21, 758–760 (1996)

[11] Bao, X., Webb, D.J., Jackson, D.A.: Combined distributed temperature and strain sensor based on Brillouin loss in an optical fiber. Optics Letters 19, 141–143 (1994)

[12] Inaudi, D., Glisic, B.: Development of distributed strain and temperature sensing cables. In: Proceedings of SPIE 17th International Conference on Opical Fibre Sensors, vol. 5855, pp. 222–225 (2005)

[13] Smith, J., DeMerchant, M., Brown, A., Bao, X.: Simultaneous distributed strain and temperature measurement. Applied Optics 38, 5372–5377 (1999)

[14] Lee, C.C., Chiang, P.W., Chi, S.: Utilization of a dispersion-Shifted fiber for simultaneous measurement of distributed strain and temperature through Brillouin frequency shift. IEEE Photonics Technology Letters 13, 1094–1096 (2001)

[15] Zou, L., Bao, X., Chen, L.: Brillouin scattering spectrum in photonic crystal fiber with a partially germanium-doped core. Optics Letters 28, 2222–2224 (2003)

[16] Bao, X., Yu, Q., Chen, L.: Simultaneous strain and temperature measurements with polarization-maintaining fibers and their error analysis by use of a distributed Brillouin loss system. Optical Letters 29, 1342–1344 (2004)

[17] Derickson, D.: Fiber Optic Tests and Measurements. Prentice-Hall, Englewood Cliffs (1998)

[18] Hartog, A.H., Gold, M.P.: On the theory of backscattering in single-mode optical fibers. Journal of Lightwave Technology 2, 76–84 (1984)

[19] Nikles, M.: Fibre optic distributed scattering sensing system: perspectives and challenges for high performance applications. In: Proceedings of SPIE 3rd European Workshop on Optical Fibre Sensors, vol. 6619 (2007)
[20] Horiguchi, T., Shimizu, K., Kurashima, T., Tateda, M., Koyamada, Y.: Development of a distributed sensing technique using Brillouin scattering. Journal of Lightwave Technology 13, 1296–1302 (1995)
[21] Fellay, A., Thévenaz, L., Facchini, M., Niklès, M., Robert, P.: Distributed sensing using stimulated Brillouin scattering: towards ultimate resolution. Optical Fiber Sensors, Optical Society of America Technical Digest Series 16, 324–325 (1997)
[22] Naruse, H., Tateda, M.: Trade-off between the spatial and the frequency resolutions in measuring the power spectrum of the Brillouin backscattered light in an optical fiber. Applied Optics 38, 6516–6521 (1999)
[23] Ravet, F., Bao, X., Yu, Q., Chen, L.: Criterion for Sub-Pulse-Length Resolution and Minimum Frequency Shift in Distributed Brillouin Sensors. IEEE Photonics Technology. Letters 17, 1504–1506 (2005)
[24] Danielson, B.L.: Optical time-domain reflectometer specifications and performance testing. Applied Optics 24, 2313–2322 (1985)
[25] Ravet, F., Bao, X., Snoddy, J., Li, Y., Chen, L.: Characterization of Brillouin fiber generator and amplifier for optimized working condition of distributed sensors. Optical Fiber Technology 15, 304–309 (2009)
[26] Ravet, F., Bao, X., Snoddy, J., Chen, L.: Power Thresholds and Pump Depletion in Brillouin Fiber Amplifiers. The Open Optics Journal 2, 1–5 (2008)
[27] Afshar, S.V., Ferrier, G.A., Bao, X., Chen, L.: Effect of the finite extinction ratio of an electrooptic modulator on the performance of distributed probe-pump Brillouin sensor systems. Optics Letters 28, 1418–1420 (2003)
[28] Kalosha, V.P., Ponomarev, E., Chen, L., Bao, X.: How to obtain high spectral resolution of SBS-based distributed sensing by using nanosecond pulses. Optics Express 14, 2071–2078 (2006)
[29] Lecoeuche, V., Webb, D.J., Pannell, C.N., Jackson, D.A.: Transient response in high-resolution Brillouin-based distributed sensing using probe pulses shorter than the acoustic relaxation time. Optics Letters 25, 156–158 (2000)
[30] Smith, J., Brown, A., DeMerchant, M., Bao, X.: Pulse width dependence of the Brillouin loss spectrum. Optics Communications 168, 393–398 (1999)
[31] Bao, X., Dhliwayo, J., Heron, N., Webb, D.J., Jackson, D.A.: Experimental and theoretical studies on a distributed temperature sensor based on Brillouin scattering. Journal of Lightwave Technology 13, 1340–1348 (1995)
[32] Ravet, F., Bao, X., Zou, L., Yu, Q., Li, Y., Kalosha, V., Chen, L.: Accurate strain detection and localization with the distributed Brillouin sensor based on a phenomenological signal processing approach. In: 13th International Symposium on Smart Structures and Materials and NDE for Health Monitoring and Diagnostics, Proceedings of SPIE, vol. 6176 (2006)
[33] Ravet, F., Bao, X., Li, Y., Yu, Q., Yale, A., Kalosha, V.P., Chen, L.: Signal processing technique for distributed Brillouin sensing at centimetre spatial resolution. Journal of Lightwave Technology 25, 3610–3618 (2007)
[34] Ravet, F., Bao, X., Yu, Q., Chen, L.: A simple approach to determine minimum measurable stress length and stress measurement accuracy in distributed Brillouin sensing. Applied Optics 44, 5204–5310 (2005)

[35] Ravet, F., Bao, X., Yu, Q., Chen, L.: Criterion for Sub-Pulse-Length Resolution and Minimum Frequency Shift in Distributed Brillouin Sensors. IEEE Photonics Technology Letters 17, 1504–1506 (2005)
[36] Ravet, F., Bao, X., Ozbakaloglu, T., Saatcioglu, M.: Signature of structure failure using asymmetric and broadening factors of Brillouin Spectrum. IEEE Photonics Technology Letters 18, 394–396 (2006)
[37] Born, M., Wolf, E.: Principles of Optics. Cambridge University Press, London (1999)
[38] Naruse, H., Tateda, M., Ohno, H., Shimada, A.: Dependence of the Brillouin gain spectrum on linear strain distribution on optical time-domain reflectometer-type strain sensors. Applied Optics 41, 7212–7217 (2002)
[39] Naruse, H., Tateda, M., Ohno, H., Shimada, A.: Deformation of the Brillouin gain spectrum caused by parabolic strain distribution and resulting measurement error in BOTDR strain measurement system. IEICE Transactions in Electronics E86-C, 2111–2121 (2003)
[40] Press, W.H., Flannery, B.P., Teukolsky, S.A., Vetterling, W.T.: Numerical recipes in C: the art of scientific computing, Cambridge, New York, New Rochelle, Melbourne, Sydney (1999)
[41] DeMerchant, M.D., Brown, A., Bao, X., Bremner, T.W.: Signal processing for a high-spatial-resolution distributed sensor. Optical Engineering 39, 1632–1635 (2000)
[42] Ravet, F., Zou, L., Bao, X., Chen, L., Huang, R.F., Khoo, H.A.: Detection of buckling in steel pipeline and beam by the distributed Brillouin sensor. Optical Fiber Technology 12, 305–311 (2006)
[43] Zou, L., Bao, X., Ravet, F., Chen, L.: Distributed Brillouin fiber sensor for detecting pipeline buckling in an energy pipe under internal pressure. Applied Optics 45, 372–375 (2006)
[44] Ravet, F., Zou, L., Bao, X., Ozbakkaloglu, T., Saatcioglu, M., Zhou, J.: Distributed Brillouin sensor for structural health monitoring. Canadian Journal of Civil Engineering 34, 291–297 (2007)
[45] Ozbakkaloglu, T., Saatcioglu, M.: Seismic performance of square high-strength concrete columns in FRP stay-in-Place formwork. Journal of Structural Engineering 133, 44–56 (2007)
[46] Sheikh, S.A., Khoury, S.S.: Confined concrete columns with stubs. ACI Structural Journal 90, 414–431 (1993)
[47] Ozbakkaloglu, T., Saatcioglu, M.: Seismic performance of high-strength concrete columns confined by fiber-reinforced polymer tubes. Journal of Composites for Construction 10, 538–549 (2006)
[48] Ravet, F., Briffod, F., Glišić, B., Niklès, M., Inaudi, D.: Submillimeter Crack Detection With Brillouin-Based Fiber-Optic Sensors. IEEE Sensors Journal 9, 1391–1396 (2009)
[49] Inaudi, D., Glişić, B.: Realiability and field testing of distributed strain and temperature sensors. In: 13th International Symposium on Smart Structures and Matrials and NDE for Health Monitoring and Diagnostics, Proceedings of SPIE, vol. 6167, pp. 3167ID (2006)
[50] Glišić, B., Inaudi, D.: Integration of long-gage fiber-optic sensor into a fiber-reinforced composite sensing tape. In: Proceedings of SPIE, Smart Structures and Materials 2003, vol. 5050, pp. 179–186 (2003)
[51] Glišić, B., Inaudi, D.: Fibre Optic Methods for Structural Health Monitoring. John Wiley & Sons, Chichester (2007)

[52] Enckell, M.: Structural health monitoring of bridges in Sweden. In: The 3rd International Conference on Structural Health Monitoring of Intelligent Infrastructure (2007)
[53] Glišić, B., Posenato, D., Inaudi, D.: Integrity monitoring of old steel bridge using fiber optic distributed sensors based on Brillouin scattering. In: 14thInternational Symposium on Smart Structures and Materials and NDE for Health Monitoring and Diag-nostics. Proceedings of SPIE, vol. 6531, pp. 65310P (2007)
[54] Glišić, B., Enckell, M., Myrvoll, F., Tuvert, J.: Distributed sensors for damage detection and localization. In: 4 thInternational Conference on Structural Health Monitoring on Intelligent Infrastructure (2009)
[55] Iten, M., Ravet, F., Niklès, M., Facchini, M., Hertig, T., Hauswirth, D., Puzrin, A.M.: Soil-embedded fiber optic strain sensors for detection of differential soil displacements. In: 4 thInternational Conference on Structural Health Monitoring on Intelligent Infrastructure (2009)
[56] Niklès, M., Ravet, F.: Depth and sensitivity. Nature Photonics, Tech. Focus. 4, 231–232 (2010)
[57] Niklès, M., Vogel, B., Briffod, F., Grosswig, S., Sauser, F., Luebbecke, S., Bals, A., Pfeiffer, T.: Leakage detection using fiber optics distributed temperature monitoring. In: Proceedings of SPIE Smart Structures and Materials, vol. 5384, pp. 18–25 (2004)
[58] Ravet, F., Briffod, F., Niklès, M.: Extended distance fiber optic monitoring for pipeline leak and ground movement detection. In: 7th International Pipeline Conference, IPC 2008, p. 64521 (2008)

Sensing Network Paradigms for Structural Health Monitoring

C.R. Farrar[1], G. Park[1], and M.D. Todd[2]

[1] The Engineering Institute
Los Alamos National Laboratory
Los Alamos, NM 87545, USA
[2] Department of Structural Engineering
University of California, San Diego
La Jolla, CA 92093, USA

Abstract. The process of structural health monitoring (SHM) requires an integrated paradigm of networked sensing and actuation, data interrogation (signal processing and feature extraction), and statistical assessment (classification of damage existence, location, and/or type) that treats structural health assessments in a systematic way. An appropriate sensor network is always required in observing the structural system behaviour in such a way that suitable signal processing and damage-sensitive feature extraction on the measured data can be performed efficiently. Consequently, several sensing network paradigms for SHM have emerged in the past, and this chapter is intended to provide an overview of these paradigms. Various parameters of SHM sensing systems that must be considered in its design and subsequent field deployment are also summarized.

1 Introduction

Structural health monitoring (SHM) is the process of detecting damage in structures. The goal of SHM is to improve the safety and reliability of aerospace, civil, and mechanical infrastructure by detecting damage before it reaches a critical state. These processes are implemented using both hardware and software with the intent of achieving more cost-effective condition-based maintenance.

The authors believe that all approaches to SHM, as well as all traditional non-destructive evaluation procedures, can be cast in the context of a statistical pattern recognition problem [1]. Solutions to this problem require the four steps of 1. Operational evaluation, 2. Data acquisition, 3. Feature extraction, and 4. Statistical model development for feature classification. Within this process, the first line of attack for SHM is clearly the establishment of an appropriate sensor network that can adequately observe the system dynamics for suitable signal processing and feature extraction. To date, however, almost all such SHM sensing system designs are done somewhat in an *ad hoc* manner where the engineer picks a sensing system that is readily available and/or that they are familiar with, and then attempts to demonstrate that a specific type of damage can be detected with that system. If an appropriate level of damage detection fidelity cannot be obtained,

S.C. Mukhopadhyay (Ed.): New Developments in Sensing Technology for SHM, LNEE 96, pp. 137–157.
springerlink.com

then the system is modified in some empirical manner with the hopes that the fidelity is improved. Alternatively, as new sensing systems are developed by engineers outside the SHM field, researchers in this field will apply these new systems to their respective SHM studies in an effort to see if these systems provide an enhanced damage detection capability. Through these approaches, several sensor network paradigms for SHM have emerged, and this chapter will summarize and compare these paradigms. When making such a comparison, it should be noted that the authors do not believe there is one sensor network paradigm that is optimal for all SHM problems. All of these paradigms have relative advantages and disadvantages. Also, the paradigms described are not at the same level of maturity and, hence, some may require more development to obtain a field-deployable system, while others are readily available with commercial off-the-shelf solutions.

This chapter will first provide a brief summary of the sensing modalities that have been typically employed for SHM applications with particular attention given to power requirement. Next, several design parameters of SHM sensing systems are briefly summarized. Several sensor systems that have been developed specifically for SHM are then discussed in terms of these parameters. These sensor systems lead to the definition of four general SHM sensor network paradigms that are described along with a summary of their relative attributes and deficiencies. The chapter concludes by summarizing the practical implementation issues of the SHM sensor system in an effort to suggest a more physically rigorous approach to future SHM sensing system design.

2 Sensor Modalities in Current SHM System Use

The sensing component (transducer) refers to the actual transduction mechanism that converts a physical field (such as acceleration) into a measurable form (usually an electrical potential difference). If the sensing system involves actuation, then the opposite is required, i.e., a voltage command is converted into a physical field (usually displacement). The most common measurements currently made for SHM purposes by far are, in order of use:

- acceleration (with piezoelectric, piezoresisitve, piezoceramic, capacitive or fiber optic accelerometers)
- strain (resistive foil, fiber optic, or piezoelectric patch gages)
- high frequency waves/impedance (piezoelectric patches)

This section provides a brief summary of these sensing modalities.

Acceleration

Making local acceleration measurements using some form of accelerometer is by far the most common approach today. This situation is primarily the result of the relative maturity and commercial availability of accelerometer hardware, such as a piezoelectric accelerometer. These accelerometers are originally designed to be used within a conventional wired network, and each individual sensor output voltage must be transferred to a centralized data acquisition unit containing appropriate charge amplification, analog-to-digital (A/D) converters, signal processing (e.g., anti-aliasing filtering), and demultiplexing. There are two general designs for the piezoelectric sensor: high and low impedance [2]. High-impedance designs require a charge amplifier or external impedance converter for charge-to-voltage conversion. The charge amplifier consists of a high-gain inverting voltage amplifier with a field–effect transistor at its input for high insulation resistance. Low-impedance designs use the same piezoelectric sensing element as high-impedance units, but they also incorporate a miniaturized built-in charge-to-voltage converter. They also require an external power supply coupler, which provides the constant current excitation required for linear operation over a wide voltage range and also decouples the bias voltage from the output. Both the power into and the signal out of the sensor are transmitted over this cable. The energy consumed by the accelerometers themselves is very small because of their passive nature, but the centralized multiplexing, amplification, and signal conditioning units required to obtain usable raw data can often have power requirements that approach 1 W. A typical 4-channel power supply delivers 3-30 mA of current at 30 V, equating to 0.9 W in the largest case; power requirements go up with large channel counts so that very large (~100) accelerometer arrays may have power requirements measuring tens of watts.

Accelerometer designs have also taken advantage of manufacturing, fabrication, and microelectronics developments at the micrometer scale that have led to the micro-electromechanical systems (MEMS) revolution. MEMS accelerometers have clearly capitalized on the most widely-developed MEMS system-on-a-chip modality, with millions used per year by the automotive industry alone for airbag deployment systems. MEMS accelerometers consist of the same basic components as any accelerometer, namely a proof (inertial) mass suspended somehow by elastic elements (springs). Often a wafer layer (or subset thereof) itself is the proof mass, coupled by thin 'beams' (the springs) to small capacitive plates that transform deflection-induced capacitance shifts to a voltage. This capacitive design is by the far the most widely-used, although other MEMS accelerometer designs include piezoresistive, ferroelectric, optical, and tunneling [3]. Performance characteristics for MEMS accelerometers are comparable to those of conventional accelerometers. By tuning the resonant frequency and damping characteristics, MEMS accelerometers have performed with wide dynamic ranges (nano-g to hundreds of kilo-g in shock-specific designs), noise floors approaching 25 $ng/Hz^{1/2}$, and bandwidths into the kHz range (prior to first resonance). This performance is typically achieved with power usage in the mW range, depending on signal conditioning. Nonetheless, MEMS accelerometer use in SHM applications is significantly less than conventional accelerometer use, primarily because of the comparative lack of commercialization (availability) and ruggedness/robustness issues for many field applications.

Strain

Second to measurements of acceleration for SHM is the measurement of strain. Strain is a non-dimensional measure of an objects deformation resulting from an applied stress. More formally, strain is defined as the displacement per unit length of the object, and strain gages have a finite gage length that serves as this normalizing factor. As such, the strain gage actually gives an average strain reading over the length of the gage. Like accelerometers, strain gages are a mature technology. The most common strain gage technology is the resistive kind: Lord Kelvin in 1856 first noted that some metallic conductors' resistive properties change as a function of applied strain, and this effect was put into practical use by the 1930s. In practice, other properties such as capacitance or inductance also change with applied strain, and variations on the resistive theme have been commercialized as well, but their sensitivity to other measurands, mounting requirements, and complex circuitry have limited their application. Bulk optical methods, taking advantage of interference patterns produced by optical flats, are very accurate and highly sensitive, but the technique is delicate and cannot withstand industrial applications in many cases.

Foil gage systems consume power at a level very commensurate with piezoelectric accelerometers; this is typically about 1 W for 3-4 channels, although the number depends on the specific input impedance of the bridge circuit being used.

Fiber optic strain sensing

Although foil resistive gages dominate current market usage, the last several years have witnessed an explosion of commercially-available fiber optic solutions to strain measurement. The fiber optic communications revolution of the late 1990s led to great improvement in component technologies at lower costs, and the sensor development community piggy-backed on these advances. The two dominant fiber optic technologies are direct fiber interferometry and fiber Bragg gratings (FBGs) [4]. The former method is older, but it's relative complexity (despite several orders of magnitude sensitivity improvement over foil gages) and low multiplexing capability has rendered its use to specialized military (and some industrial) applications. Most commercial systems today take advantage of FBG technology. The resolution of FBG systems is several orders of magnitude better than the best foil resistive gage, but the costs of FBG systems (and specifically, the FBGs themselves, which are ~$150 per sensor) have limited deep market penetration. However, because FBG systems are insensitive to electromagnetic interference, do not create a spark source, are extremely lightweight and non-intrusive, and are highly-multiplexible, many application areas, particularly in aerospace structural monitoring, are emerging. Furthermore, FBGs may be coupled with mechanical transducers to measure other fields such as acceleration, pressure, velocity, or temperature. Power requirements for fiber optic systems are usually larger than for conventional strain gage systems. The largest consumer in the fiber system is the thermoelectric cooler. This device is used to temperature-control the Fabry-Perot filter to ensure accurate voltage-to-wavelength conversion. While it is not required for some applications, in those for which it is required, it consumes energy at the rate of approximately 3-5 watts, depending on control demands imposed by the environment. The filter and SLED optical source used typically require power levels below 1 W.

Piezoelectric Sensor/Actuators

The piezoelectric effect works both ways. The direct effect refers to a charge being produced when the material is strained, and the converse effect refers to, when a voltage is applied to the material, the material will deform proportionally to the applied potential difference. This electromechanically coupled effect allows such materials to be used as both sensors (direct effect) and actuators (converse effect). These materials, usually ceramic- or polymer-based, may be fabricated into a variety of shapes amenable for various applications. The devices discussed in the previous sections cannot be used as an excitation source, but piezoelectric devices may be used to create local excitation to actively probe a structure. Arrays of these devices may be configured to induce local motion, and the same array is also used to measure the response. In the actuation mode, the free strain levels produced in typical piezoelectric materials such as Lead Zirconate Titanate (PZT) are on the order of 0.1%-0.2%, although newer relaxor ferroelectric crystals may produce strains on the order of 1% [5].

The electromechanical coupling property of piezoelectric materials allows one to design and deploy active-sensing sensing systems whereby the structure in question is locally excited by a known and repeatable input, and the corresponding responses are measured by the same excitation source. The employment of a known input facilitates subsequent signal processing of the measured output data in SHM. Examples of using piezoelectric materials in the areas of active and local SHM sensing are Lamb wave propagations [6,7,8] and the impedance-based structural health monitoring methods [9]. Compared to passive sensing systems, an active-sensing SHM system, however, requires additional components including a digital-to-analog converter (D/A) and a waveform generator. Because of the local-excitation and local-sensing nature, this system puts further demands on the use of much higher speed A/D converters, additional memory, and possibly multiplexers in order to control and manage a network of piezoelectric transducers. These extra components would inevitably demand more energy to complete an active-sensing SHM process.

In the passive sensing mode, piezoelectric transducers would consume much less energy, compared to accelerometers or strain gauges, because they do not require any electrical peripherals such as signal conditioning and amplification units. Any A/D converters could measure the charge output from a piezoelectric transducer, although this low power consumption characteristic will be modified if one needs to use charge amplifiers or voltage follower circuits to improve the signal to noise ratio depending on applications or frequency range of interest.

For actuation, the average power requirement for the piezoelectric capacitive loading can be readily derived from lumped equivalent circuits. Typical Lamb wave propagation approaches using a 6-mm-disc-type piezoelectric patch (approximately 1 nF) would require around 300 mW of average power to launch 500 kHz Lamb waves, although the overall power demand will become much higher if one considers the peak power requirement or the energy consumed by a waveform generator with a D/A converter. It should also be noted that this amount is dedicated to the actuation only, hence this level of power will be an additional energy requirement to the typical power consumption of passive sensing systems.

3 SHM Sensing System Design Consideration

Sensor networks, generally speaking, contain three main components: the sensing unit itself, communications, and computation (hardware and, as appropriate, software control and processing algorithms) [10]. The goal of any SHM sensor network system is to make the sensor reading as directly correlated with, and as sensitive to, damage as possible. At the same time, one also strives to make the sensors as independent as possible from all other sources of environmental and operational variability, and, in fact, independent from each other (in an information sense) to provide maximal data for minimal sensor array outlay. To best meet these requirements, the following design parameters must be defined, as much as possible, *a priori*:

- Types of data to be acquired,
- Sensor types, number and locations,
- Bandwidth, sensitivity and dynamic range,
- Data acquisition/telemetry/storage system,
- Power requirements,
- Sampling intervals (continuous monitoring versus monitoring only after extreme events or at periodic intervals),
- Processor/memory requirements, and
- Excitation source needs (for active sensing).

Fundamentally, there are five issues that control the selection of hardware to address these sensor system design parameters:

- The length scales on which damage is to be detected,
- The time scale on which damage evolves,
- Effect of varying and/or adverse operational and environmental conditions on the sensing system,
- Power availability, and
- Cost.

In addition, the feature extraction, data normalization and statistical modeling portions of the process can greatly influence the definition of the sensing system properties. Before such decisions can be made two important questions must be addressed. First, one must answer the question, "What is the damage to be detected?" The answer to this question must be provided in as quantifiable a manner as possible and address issues such as (i) type of damage (e.g. crack, loose connection, corrosion); (ii) threshold damage size that must be detected; (iii) probable damage locations; and (iv) anticipated damage growth rates. The more specific and quantifiable this definition, the more likely it is that one will optimize their sensor budget to produce a system that has the greatest possible fidelity for damage detection. Second, an answer must be provided to the question, "What are the environmental and operational sources of variability that must be accounted?" To answer this question, one will not only have to have some ideas about the physical sources *per se*, but one will also have to have thought about how to accomplish data normalization. Typically, data normalization will be accomplished through some combination of sensing system hardware and data interrogation software. However, these hardware and software approaches will not be optimal if they are not done in a coupled manner.

In summary, from the discussion in this section it becomes clear that the ability to convert sensor data into structural health information is directly related to the coupling of the sensor system hardware development with the data interrogation procedures.

4 Current SHM Systems

A very generalized sensor network paradigm is shown in Figure 1. The most common general approach in this function is a conventional wired sensor network, where some number of a given transducer type (e.g., accelerometers) are connected via conductive cabling to a centralized data processing and multiplexing unit. Each sensor is effectively independent of other sensors in the network—each sensor has its own cabling—and controlled synchronized interrogation of the entire network is achieved only through the central unit. This interrogation is typically only passive as well, meaning that the sensors individually provide information to the central unit, but the central unit cannot pass information back to an individual sensor. In applications demanding control or feedback, then actuator arrays (e.g., piezoelectric actuators) can take the place of some of the passive sensor arrays, but typically each node (sensor or actuator) is still individually wired and connected to a central unit.

While the majority of sensor networks in use today employ a wired architecture, development and deployment of wireless sensor networks has exploded in recent years. Wireless communication protocols are now standardized with such protocols as IEEE 802.11 through 802.15, and bandwidths are now approaching that of conventional wired networks. Furthermore, increases in chip real estate and processor production capability have reduced the power requirements for both computing and communication. In fact, sensing, communication, and computing can now be performed on a single chip, reducing the cost further and permitting economically viable high-density sensor networks. All of these advances have yielded wireless sensor networks that increasingly meet the original visions for these networks: (1) a large number of individual sensor nodes, densely deployed in possibly random configurations in the sensing environment; (2) the capability for self-organization and near-neighbor awareness so that information exchange between an individual node and a user may be achieved via point-to-point hopping protocols; (3) cooperation between sensor nodes, where they use local processing capability to perform data fusion or other computational duties and then only transmit required or partially processed onward.

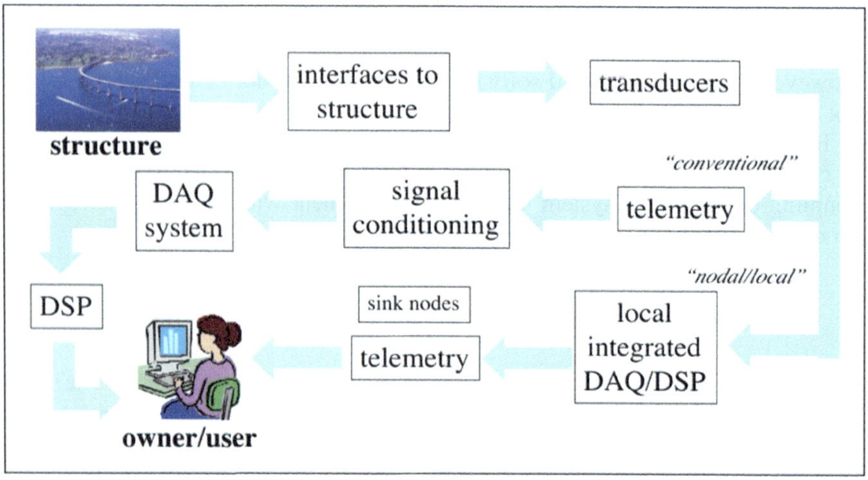

Fig. 1 General sensor network architecture

Sensing systems for SHM consist of some or all of the following components.

1. Transducers that converts changes in the field variable of interest (e.g. acceleration, strain, temperature) to changes in an electrical signal (e.g. voltage, impedance, resistance).
2. Actuators that can be used to apply a prescribed input to the system (e.g. Lead-Zirconium Titanate (PZT) bonded to the surface of a structure)
3. Analog-to-digital (A/D) converters that transfer the analog electrical signal into a digital signal that can subsequently be processed on a computer. For the case where actuators are used a digital-to-analog (D/A) converter will also be needed to change the prescribed digital signal to an analog voltage that can be used to control the actuator
4. Signal conditioning
5. Power
6. Telemetry
7. Processing
8. Memory for data storage

The number of sensing systems available for SHM is enormous and these systems vary quite a bit depending upon the specific SHM activity. Two general types of SHM sensing systems are described below.

Wired System

Here wired SHM are defined as ones that telemeter data over direct wire connection from the transducer to the central data analysis facility, as shown schematically in Figure 2. In some cases the central data analysis facility is then connected to the internet such that the processed information can be monitored at a subsequent remote location. There are a wide variety of such systems. At one extreme is peak-strain or peak-acceleration sensing devices that notify the user when a certain threshold in the measured quantity has been exceeded. A more sophisticated system often used for condition monitoring of rotating machinery is a piezoelectric accelerometer with built-in charge amplifier connected directly to a hand-held, single-channel fast-Fourier-transform (FFT) analyzer. Here the central data storage and analysis facility is the hand-held FFT analyzer. Such systems cost on the order of a few thousand dollars. At the other extreme is custom designed systems with hundred of data channels containing numerous types of sensors that cost on the order of multiple millions of dollars such as that deployed on the Tsing Ma bridge in China [11].

There are a wide range of commercially available wired systems, some of which have been developed for general purposed data acquisition and other which have been specifically developed for SHM applications. Those designed for general purpose data acquisition typically can interface with wide variety of transducers and also have the capability to drive actuators. The majority of these systems have integrated signal conditioning, data processing and data storage capabilities. The majority of these systems run off of AC power. Those designed to run off of batteries typically have a limited number of channels and they are limited in their ability to operate for long periods of time.

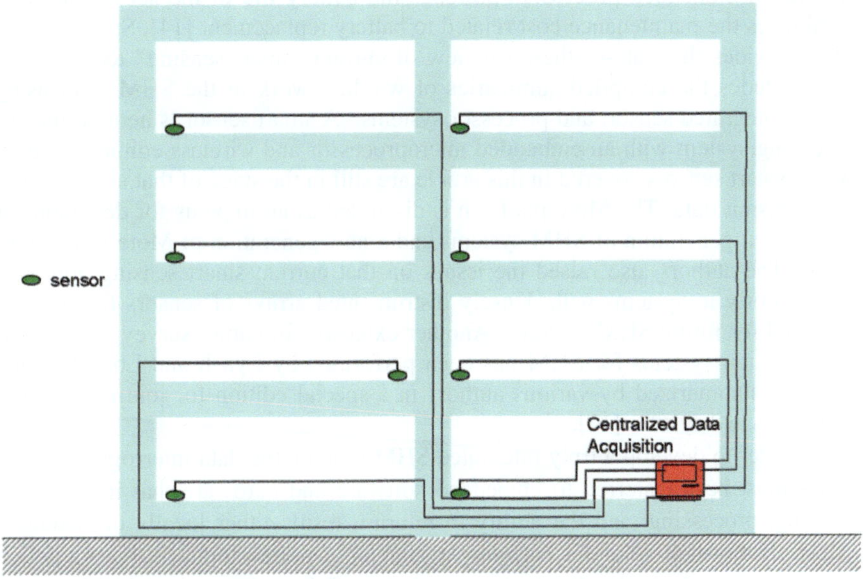

Fig. 2 Conventional wired data acquisition system

Wireless Transmission systems

The integration of wireless communication technologies into SHM methods has been widely investigated. Straser [12] was the first to propose the integration of wireless radios with sensors to reduce the cost of structural monitoring systems. Lynch et al. [13] presented hardware for a wireless peer-to-peer SHM system and subsequently improved the capability for various structural applications. Using off the shelf components, the authors couple sensing circuits and wireless transmission with a computational core allowing a decentralized collection, analysis, and broadcast of a structure's health. The final hardware platform includes two microcontrollers for data collection and computation connected to a spread spectrum wireless modem. The software is tightly integrated with the hardware and includes the wireless transmission module, the sensing module, and application module. The application module implements the time series based SHM algorithm. This integrated data interrogation process requires communication with a centralized sever to retrieve model coefficients. The object of the close integration of hardware and software with the dual microcontrollers strives for a power efficient design. Tanner, et al. [14] adapted an SHM algorithm to the limitations of off-the-shelf wireless sensing and data processing hardware because of the focus towards a proof of concept rather than designing a field installable product. A wireless sensing system of "Motes" running TinyOS operating system developed at UC Berkeley was chosen because of their ready-made wireless communication capabilities. A Mote consists of modular circuit boards integrating a sensor, microprocessor, A/D converter, and wireless transmitter all of which run off of two AA batteries. Because one byte of data transmission consumes the same energy as approximately 11,000 cycles of computation in the employed hardware platform, the use of embedded processors prolongs the battery life of the sensor unit and minimizes the maintenance cost related to battery replacement [14]. Spencer et al. [15] provides the state-of-the-art review of current "smart sensing" technologies that includes the compiled summaries of wireless work in the SHM field using small, integrated sensor, and processor systems. A smart sensor is here defined as a sensing system with an embedded microprocessor and wireless communication. Many smart sensors covered in this article are still in the stage of that simply sense and transmit data. The Mote platform is discussed as an impetus for development of the next generation of SHM systems and a new generation of Mote is also outlined. The authors also raised the issues on that current smart sensing approach scale poorly to systems with densely instrumented arrays of sensors that will be required for future SHM systems. Another extensive literature survey on wireless transmission systems for SHM has been performed by Lynch and Loh [16], and recently summarized by various authors in a special edition for journal of smart structures and systems[17].

In order to develop a truly integrated SHM system, the data interrogation processes must be transferred to embedded software and hardware that incorporates sensing, processing, and the ability to return a result either locally or remotely. Most off-the-shelf solutions currently available, or in development, have a deficit in processing power that limits the complexity of the software and SHM process that can be implemented. Also, many integrated systems are inflexible because of tight integration between the embedded software, the hardware, and sensing. To implement computationally intensive SHM processes, Farrar et al. selected a single board computer as a compact form of true processing power [18]. Also included in the integrated system is a digital signal processing board with six A/D converters providing the interface to a variety of sensing modalities. Finally, a wireless network board is integrated to provide the ability for the system to relay structural information to a central host, across a network, or through local hardware. Figure 3 shows the prototype of this sensing system. Each of these hardware parts are built in a modular fashion and loosely coupled through transmission control protocol over the internet. By implementing a common interface, changing or replacing a single component does not require a redesign of the entire system. By allowing processes developed in the Graphical Linking and Assembly of Syntax Structure (GLASS) client to be downloaded and run directly in the GLASS node software, this system becomes the first hardware solution where new processes can be created and loaded dynamically. This modular nature does not lead to the most power-optimized design, but instead achieves a flexible development platform that is used to find the most effective combination of algorithms and hardware for a specific SHM problem. Optimization for power is of secondary concern and will be the focus of follow-on efforts.

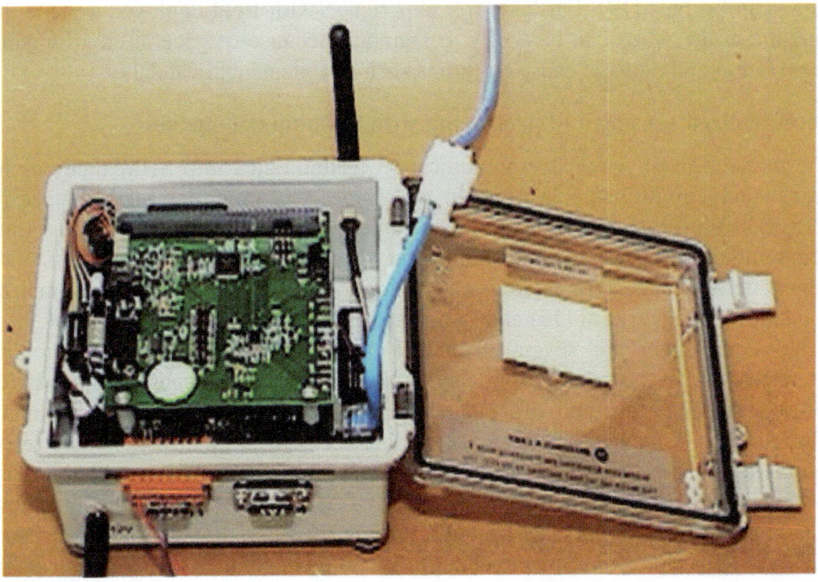

Fig. 3 The wireless communication board displayed on the prototype SHM system [18]

5 Sensor Network Paradigms

The sensor systems discussed in the previous section have lead to three types of sensor network paradigms that are either currently being used for structural health monitoring or are the focus of current research efforts in this field. These paradigms are described below. Note that the illustrations of these systems show them applied to a building structure. However, these paradigms can be applied to a wide variety of aerospace, civil and mechanical system and the building structure is simply used for comparison purposes.

Sensor arrays directly connected to central processing hardware

Figure 2 shows a sensor network directly connected to the central processing hardware. Such a system is the most common one used for structural health monitoring studies. The advantage of this system is the wide variety of commercially available off-the-shelf systems that can be used for this type of monitoring and the wide variety of transducers that can typically be interfaced with such a system. For SHM applications, these systems have been used in both a passive and active sensing manner. Limitations of such systems are that they are difficult to deploy in a retrofit mode because they usually require AC power, which is not always available. Also, these systems are one-point failure sensitive as one wire can be as long as a few hundred meters. In addition, the deployment of such system can be challenging with potentially over 75% of the installation time attributed to the installation of system wires and cables for larger scale structures such as those used for long-span bridges [19]. Furthermore, experience with field-deployed systems has shown that the wires can be costly to maintain because of general environmental degradation and damage cause by things such as rodents and vandals.

Decentralized sensing and processing with hopping connection

The integration of wireless communication technologies into SHM methods has been widely investigated in order to overcome the limitations of wired sensing networks. Wireless communication can remedy the cabling problem of the traditional monitoring system and significantly reduce the maintenance cost. The schematic of the de-centralized wireless monitoring system, which is summarized in detail by Spencer et al [15] and Lynch and Loh [16], is shown in Figure 4.

However, there are several technical challenges and requirements for the intended wireless network applications just described because of bandwidth restrictions, uncertain and often harsh deployment environments, and dynamic configuration demands. For example, the networks must be autonomously reconfigurable, meaning that each node, after deployment, must detect, identify, and locate its neighbor nodes. Of course, planned networks eliminate this challenge, but such ad hoc networks are becoming the norm since they can update periodically as both the environment changes or as nodes fail. Because there is no planned connectivity in ad hoc networking, the software must provide this information as necessary. It must autonomously consider communications distance and energy demands in an effort to for identify the right routing. The network must know how to optimally determine collaborative computations, balancing energy, latency, and robustness. Processing data from many sensors results in better performance and robustness, but at the cost of more network resources. Similarly, network losses are lower when information is communicated at an unprocessed level, but at the expense of higher bandwidth. Furthermore, as individual nodes receive neighboring information, they must intelligently fuse it with local information. Data fusion algorithms must be able to identify, classify, and accept or reject data packets all within the constraints of limited energy resources. Finally, the network, depending on the application, may have to deal with issues such as data security and seamless communication between mobile and fixed platforms.

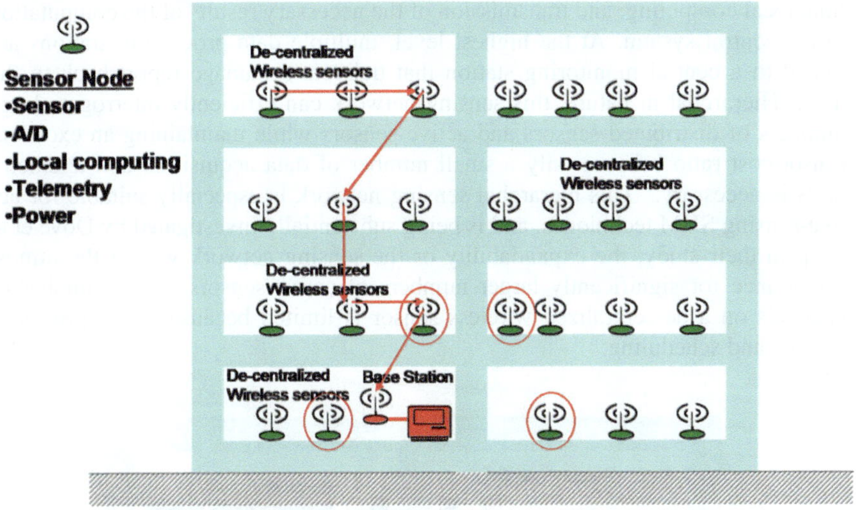

Fig. 4 De-centralized wireless SHM system employing hopping communications protocol

Another major consideration in deploying a dense wireless sensor array is the problem of providing power to the sensor nodes. This demand leads to the concept of "information as a form of energy". Deriving information costs energy. If the only way to provide power is by direct connections, then the need for wireless protocols is eliminated, as the cabled power link can also be used for the transmission of data. A possible solution to the problem of localized power generation is technologies that enable harvesting ambient energy to power the instrumentation [20]. While there is tremendous research into the development of energy harvesting schemes for large-scale alternative sources such as wind turbines and solar cells and that these large-scale systems have made the transition from research to commercial products, energy harvesting for embedded sensing systems is still in a development stage, and only a few prototypes exist for field-deployment.

Decentralized active sensing and processing with hybrid connection

The hybrid connection network advantageously combines the previous two networks, as illustrated in Figure 5. At the first level, several sensors are connected to a relay-based piece of hardware, which can serve as both a multiplexer and general-purpose signal router, shown as a black box. This device will manage the distributed sensing network, control the modes of sensing and actuation, and multiplex the measured signals. The device can also be expandable by means of daisy-chaining. At the next level, multiple pieces of this hardware are linked to a decentralized data control and processing station. This control station is equipped with data acquisition boards, on-board computing processors, and wireless telemetry which is similar to the architecture of current decentralized wireless sensors. This device will perform duties of a relay-based hardware control, data acquisition, local computing, and transmission of the necessary results of the computation to the central system. At the highest level, multiple data processing stations are linked to a central monitoring station that delivers a damage report back to the user. Hierarchal in nature, this sensing network can efficiently interrogate large numbers of distributed sensors and active-sensors while maintaining an excellent sensor-cost ratio because only a small number of data acquisition and telemetry units is necessary. This hierarchal sensing network is especially suitable for active-sensing SHM techniques, and is being substantially investigated by Dove et al [21]. In their study, the expandability or the sensing network was of the utmost importance for significantly larger numbers of active-sensors, as the number of channels on a de-centralized wireless sensor is limited because of the processor sharing and scheduling.

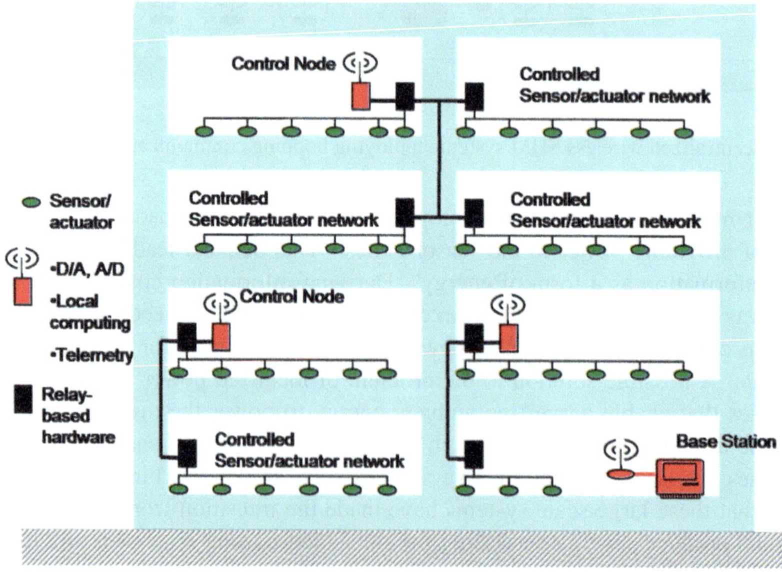

Fig. 5 Relay-based hardware with optional manual controls included

Mobile-Host Based Wireless Sensing Network

The sensing network paradigms described in the previous section have one characteristic in common. The sensing system and associated power sources are installed at the fixed locations of the structural system. The deployment of such sensing systems can be costly and the power source may not always be available.

A new and efficient future sensing network is proposed and subsequently investigated by integrating wireless energy transmission technology and remote interrogation platforms based on unmanned vehicles, such as a robot or an Unmanned Aerial Vehicle (UAV), to assess damage in structural systems [22,23,24]. This sensing network is schematically shown in Figure 6. This approach involves using an unmanned mobile host node (delivered via UAV or robot) to generate a power-providing radio-frequency (RF) signal near receiving antennas connected to the sensor nodes that have been embedded on the structure. The sensors measure the desired response at critical areas on the structure and transmit the signal back to the mobile host again via the wireless communications. This wireless communications capability draws power from the RF energy transmitted between the host and sensor node and uses it to power the sensing circuit. A recent field demonstration of this sensor network strategy is shown in Figure 7, where a remotely controlled helicopter was used to deliver power to sensor nodes mounted on a bridge structure.

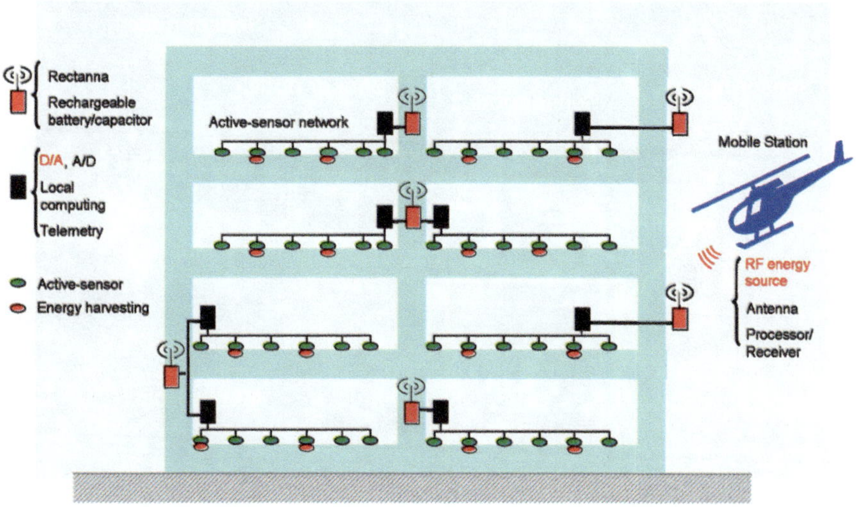

Fig. 6 A schematic of a mobile-host based sensing network that includes energy harvesting and that is interrogated by an unmanned robotic vehicle

This research takes traditional sensing networks to the next level, as the mobile hosts, that are either remotely-piloted or GPS-programmed, move to the sensor target field, identify and locate sensors, power and interrogate each sensor in turn, and perform necessary local computation to assess the system's structural health. This integrated technology will be directly applicable to rapid structural condition assessment of buildings and bridges after an earthquake as well as assessing the condition of structures where human access is limited because of safety considerations such as monitoring radioactive waste containers.

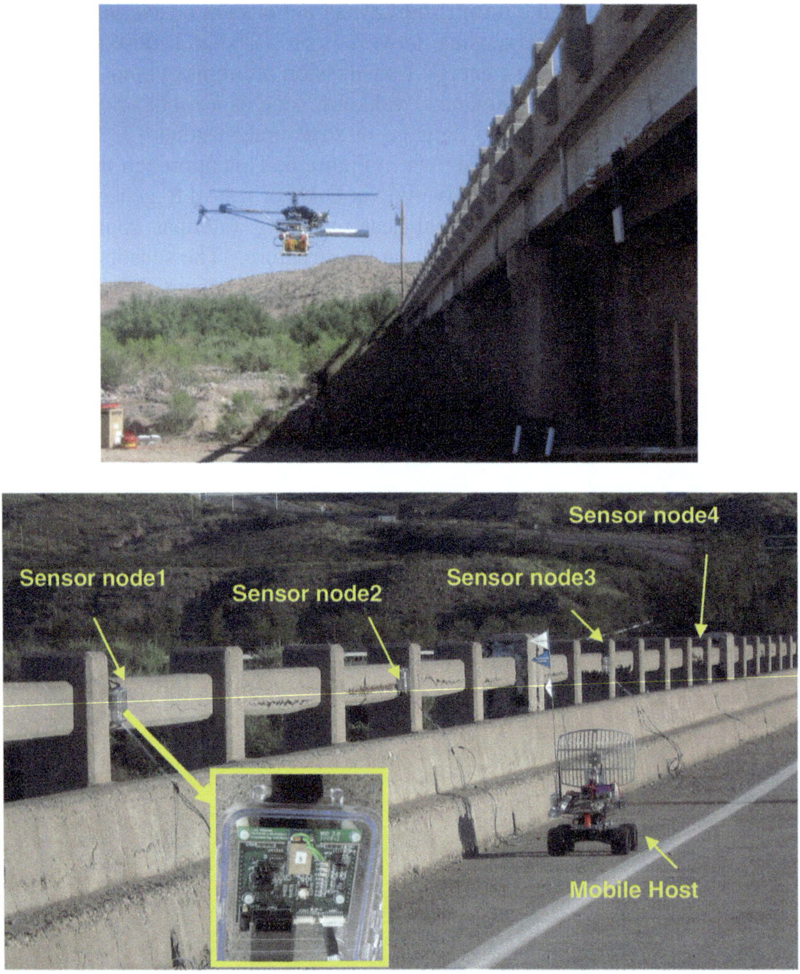

Fig. 7 Field demonstration of a mobile host based wireless sensing network for SHM on a bridge structure. UAV is used as a mobile host (top figure), while a RC controlled vehicle is used (bottom figure)

The mobile-agent paradigm also supports the use of multiple, localized sensor networks within a single structure or application. This approach would be useful in situations where the data from one network could be used by the mobile-agent to identify which network it should proceed to interrogate, following critical or catastrophic events. This would enable the mobile-agent to bypass certain networks to interrogate those which have the most pertinent data for emergency response, or security personnel, particularly in circumstances where speed of response is essential to saving human lives.

It should be emphasized that this technology can be used in a hybrid configuration where the sensor node is still equipped with energy harvesting devices and the mobile host would supply supplemental energy if the harvester is damaged or unable to provide enough power to operate the required tasks on the sensor nodes. Even if the energy harvesting device provides sufficient power, the mobile host can wirelessly trigger the sensor nodes, collect information and/or provide computational resources, significantly relaxing the power and computation demand at the sensor node level. This integrated technology will be directly applicable to rapid structural condition assessment of buildings and bridges after an earthquake. Also, this technology may be adapted and applied to damage detection in a variety of other civilian and defense-related structures such as, pipelines, naval vessels, hazardous waste disposal containers, and commercial aircraft. It should be noted however that this network paradigm is still in its infancy, some important core technologies should be further developed and integrated for full utilization of its potential.

6 Practical Implementation Issues for SHM Sensing Networks

Major concerns in the current sensing network development are the long-term reliability and sources of power. Other concerns are the abilities of the sensing systems to capture local and system level response, that is, the need to capture response on widely varying length and time scales, and to archive data in a consistent, retrievable manner for long-term analysis. These challenges are nontrivial because of the tendency for each technical discipline to work more or less in isolation. Therefore, an integrated systems engineering approach to the damage detection process and regular, well-defined routes of information dissemination are essential. The subsequent portions of this section will address specific sensing system issues associated with SHM.

Sensor Properties

One of the major challenges of defining sensor properties is that these properties need to be defined *a priori* and typically cannot be changed easily once a sensor system is in place. These properties of sensors include bandwidth, sensitivity (dynamic range), number, location, stability, reliability, cost, telemetry, etc. To address this challenge a significantly coupled analytical and experimental approach to the sensor system deployment should be used in contrast to the current *ad-hoc* procedures used for most current damage detection studies. This strategy should yield considerable improvements. First, critical failure modes of the system can be well defined and, to some extent, quantified using high-fidelity numerical simulations or from previous experiences before the sensing system is designed. The high-fidelity numerical simulations/experiences can be used to define the required bandwidth, sensitivity, sensor location and sensor number. Additional sensing requirements can also be ascertained if changing operational and environmental conditions are included in the models so as to determine how these conditions affect the damage detection process.

Another potential level of integration between modeling and sensing resides in the integration of software and hardware components. Once the actuation and sensing capability has been selected, their location has been optimized and the specification of the data acquisition system have been met, it may be advantageous to integrate model output and sensing information as much as possible. For example, surrogate models can be programmed on local DSP chips and their predictions can be compared to sensor output in real time. One obvious benefit would be to minimize the amount of communication by integrating the analysis capability with real-time sensing. In an integrated approach, features can be extracted from sensing information and numerical simulation. Test-analysis comparison and parameter estimation can then be performed locally, which would greatly increase the efficiency of damage detection.

Sensor Calibration and Ruggedness

Most sensors are calibrated at a specialized calibration facility. This type of calibration is expected to endure, but to be supplemented by self-checking and self-calibrating sensors. Calibration raises several important issues. It is not clear just what forms of calibration are essential, and what are superfluous. Some measurements are acceptable with 20% error, especially if sensor-to-sensor comparisons are accurate within a few percent. In other scenarios absolute accuracies better than 1% are required. The calibration community needs to address these issues, including both precision, for example how to calibrate a 32-bit digitizer over its entire dynamic range, and flexibility (calibration of a precise sensor vs. calibration of a coarse sensor).

Confidence and robustness in the sensors are prime considerations for SHM. If this part of the system is compromised then the overall confidence in the system performance is undermined. For sensors implemented for SHM, several durability considerations emerge:

1. The nontrivial problem of sensor selection for extreme environments, e.g. in service turbine blades;
2. Sensors being less reliable than the part. For example, reliable parts may have failure rates of 1 in 100,000 over several years time. Sensors are often small, complex assemblies, so sensors may fail more often than the part sensed. Loss of sensor signal then falsely indicates part failure, not sensor failure;
3. Sensors may fail through outright sensor destruction while the part sensed endures;

False indications of damage or damage precursors are extremely undesirable. If this occurs often the sensor is either overtly or implicitly ignored. Recently several studies are focused on issues of sensor validation [25,26,27].

Multi-Scale Sensing

Depending on the size and location of the structural damage and the loads applied to the system, the adverse effects of the damage can be either immediate or may take some time before it alters the system's performance. In terms of length scales, all damage begins at the material level and then under appropriate loading conditions progresses to component and system level damage at various rates. In terms of time scales, damage can accumulate incrementally over long periods of time such as that associated with fatigue or corrosion damage accumulation. Damage can also occur on much shorter time scales as a result of scheduled discrete events such as aircraft landings and from unscheduled discrete events such as enemy fire on a military vehicle. Therefore, the most fundamental issue that must be addressed when developing a sensing system for SHM is the need to capture the structural response on widely varying length and time scales. Sensors with a high frequency range tend to be more sensitive to local response, and therefore, to damage. This requires a sensor with a large bandwidth. Typically, as the bandwidth goes up, the sensitivity goes down. Also, it is harder to excite higher frequencies thus the excitation needs to be very local as is possible with piezoelectric actuators.

The sensing systems that is able to capture the responses over varying length and time scales has not been substantially investigated by researchers, although it is quite possible to use the same piezoelectric patches in both an active (high frequency) and passive (lower-order global) modes. When used in the passive mode, the sensors detect strain resulting from ambient loading conditions and can be used to monitor the global response of a system. In the active mode the same sensors can be used to detect and locate damage on local level using relatively higher frequency ranges.

7 Summary

In this chapter, the current research in the designing the sensing system that is used to address the data acquisition portion of the SHM problem is summarized. Several sensor systems that have been developed specifically for SHM are discussed. These sensor systems lead to the definition of several general SHM sensor network paradigms. All of these paradigms have relative advantages and disadvantages. Also, the paradigms described are not at the same level of maturity and, hence, some may require more development to obtain a field-deployable system while others are readily available with commercial off-the-shelf solutions. The chapter concludes by summarizing the practical implementation issues of the SHM sensor system in an effort to suggest a more physically rigorous approach to future SHM sensing system design.

References

[1] Farrar, C.R., Doebling, S.W., Nix, D.: Vibration-Based Structural Damage Identification Philosophical Transactions of the Royal Society: Mathematical. Physical & Engineering Sciences 359(1778), 131–149 (2001)

[2] Kulwanoski, G., Schnellinger, J.: The Principles of Piezoelectric Accelerometers. Sensors Magazine 21(2) (2004)

[3] Bernstein, J.: An Overview of MEMS Inertial Sensing. Sensors (2003), `http://www.sensormag.com` (February 1, online issue)

[4] Todd, M.D.: Optical-Based Sensing. In: Inman, D.J. (ed.) Damage Prognosis. John Wiley and Sons Inc., Chichester .(2004)

[5] Park, S.E., Shrout, T.R.: Ultrahigh Strain and Piezoelectric Behavior in Relaxor Based Ferroelectric Single Crystals. Journal of Applied Physics 82, 1804–1811 (1997)

[6] Raghavan, A., Cesnik, C.E.S.: Review of Guided –wave Structural Health Monitoring. The Shock and Vibration Digest 39, 91–114 (2007)

[7] Ihn, J.B., Chang, F.K.: Detection and monitoring of hidden fatigue crack growth using a built-in piezoelectric sensor/actuator network: II. Validation using riveted joints and repair patches. Smart Materials and Structures 13, 621–630 (2004)

[8] Kessler, S.S., Spearing, S.M., Soutis, C.: Damage Detection in Composite Materials using Lamb Wave Methods. Smart Materials and Structures 11, 269–278 (2002)

[9] Park, G., Sohn, H., Farrar, C.R., Inman, D.J.: Overview of Piezoelectric Impedance-Based Health Monitoring and Path Forward. Shock and Vibration Digest 35(6), 451–463 (2003)

[10] Chong, C.-Y., Kumar, S.P.: Sensor Networks: Evolution, Opportunities, and Challenges. Proc. of the IEEE 91(8), 1247–1256 (2003)

[11] Ni, Y.Q., Wang, B.S., Ko, J.: Simulation studies of damage location in Tsing Ma Bridge deck. In: Proc., Nondestructive Evaluation of Highways, Utilities, and Pipelines IV, pp. 312–323. SPIE, Bellingham (2001)

[12] Straser, E.G.: A Modular, Wireless Damage Monitoring System for Structures, Ph.D. Thesis, Department of Civil and Environmental Engineering, Stanford University, Stanford, CA (1998)

[13] Lynch, J.P., Sundararajan, A., Law, K.H., Kiremidjian, A.S., Kenny, T.W., Carryer, E.: Embedment of Structural Monitoring Algorithms in a Wireless Sensing Unit. Structural Engineering and Mechanics 15(3), 285–297 (2003)

[14] Tanner, N.A., Wait, J.R., Farrar, C.R., Sohn, H.: Structural Health Monitoring using Modular Wireless Sensors. Journal of Intelligent Material systems and Structures 14(1), 43–56 (2003)

[15] Spencer, B.F., Ruiz-Sandoval, M.E., Kurata, N.: Smart Sensing Technology: Opportunities and Challenges. Journal of Structural control and Health Monitoring (2004) (in press)

[16] Lynch, J.P., Loh, K.J.: A summary review of wireless sensors and sensor networks for structural health monitoring. The Shock and Vibration Digest 38(2), 91–128 (2006)

[17] Smart Structures and Systems 6(5-6) (2010)

[18] Farrar, C.R., Allen, D.W., Ball, S., Masquelier, M.P., Park, G.: Coupling Sensing Hardware with Data Interrogation Software for Structural Health Monitoring. In: Proc. of 11th International Symposium on Dynamic Problems of Mechanics, Ouro Preto, Brazil (March 2005)

[19] Lynch, J.P., Partridge, A., Law, K.H., Kenny, T.W., Kiremidjian, A.S., Carryer, E.: Design of a Piezoresistive MEMS-Based Accelerometer for Integration with a Wireless Sensing Unit for Structural Monitoring. ASCE Journal of Aerospace Engineering 16, 108–114 (2003)
[20] Park, G., Farrar, C.R., Todd, M.D., Hodgkiss, W., Rosing, T.: Energy Harvesting for Structural Health Monitoring Sensor Networks. ASCE Journal of Infrastructure Systems 14, 64–79 (2008)
[21] Dove, J.R., Park, G., Farrar, C.R.: Hardware Design of Hierarchal Active-Sensing Networks for Structural Health Monitoring. Smart Materials and Structures 15, 139–146 (2005)
[22] Mascarenas, D.M., Flynn, E.B., Todd, M.D., Park, G., Farrar, C.R.: Wireless Sensor Technologies for Monitoring Civil Structures. Sound and Vibration, 16–20 (April 2008)
[23] Mascarenas, D., Flynn, E., Farrar, C.R., Park, G., Todd, M.D.: A Mobile Host Approach for Wireless Powering and Interrogation of Structural Health Monitoring Sensor Networks. IEEE Sensors Journal 9(12), 1719–1726 (2009)
[24] Taylor, S.G., Farinholt, K.M., Flynn, E.B., Figueiredo, E., Mascarenas, D.L., Park, G., Todd, M.D., Farrar, C.R.: A Mobile-agent Based Wireless Sensing Network for Structural Monitoring Applications. Measurement Science and Technology 20(4), 45201 (2009)
[25] Park, G., Farrar, C.R., Rutherford, C.A., Robertson, A.N.: Piezoelectric Active Sensor Self-Diagnostics using Electrical Admittance Measurements. ASME Journal of Vibrations and Acoustics 128, 469–476 (2006)
[26] Kerschen, G., Boe, P.D., Golinval, J., Worden, K.: Sensor Validation using principal component analysis. Smart Materials and Structures 14(1), 36–42 (2005)
[27] Overly, T.G., Park, G., Farinholt, K.M., Farrar, C.R.: Piezoelectric Active-Sensor Diagnostics and Validation Using Instantaneous Baseline Data. IEEE Sensors Journal 9(11), 1414–1421 (2009)

Reflectometry for Structural Health Monitoring

Cynthia Furse

Department of Electrical and Computer Engineering,
University of Utah, Salt Lake City, Utah 84112
cfurse@ece.utah.edu

Abstract. Aging wiring and structural cables in buildings, aircraft and transportation systems, consumer products, industrial machinery, etc. are among the most significant potential causes of catastrophic failure and maintenance cost in these structures. Smart wire health monitoring can therefore have a substantial impact on the overall health monitoring of the system. Reflectometry is commonly used for locating faults on electric wire and cables. It can also be used for location of faults on structural cables, if they are electrically isolated. This chapter describes and compares several reflectometry methods -- time domain reflectometry (TDR), frequency domain reflectometry (FDR), mixed signal reflectometry (MSR), sequence time domain reflectometry (STDR), and spread spectrum time domain reflectometry (SSTDR) -- in terms of their accuracy, convenience, cost, size, and ease of use. Advantages and limitations of each method are outlined and evaluated for several types of aircraft cables, and the general equations that govern their performance are given. The impact of the fault location and size is also discussed.

Keywords: aging wiring, fault location, reflectometry, time domain reflectometry (TDR), frequency domain reflectometry (FDR), standing wave reflectometry (SWR), mixed signal reflectometry (MSR), spectral time domain reflectometry (STDR).

1 Introduction

Reflectometry is a method that has been used for decades to locate faults on electrical wiring, to measure the electrical properties of materials, and in some limited applications, to measure the health of non-electrical structural components as well. Reflectometry transmits a high frequency signal (electrical, optical, acoustic, etc.) down the wire or cable under test. The signal reflects (echos) off impedance changes (breaks, faults, short circuits, etc.) in the cable. This reflected signal is received at the transmitter location. The time delay of the reflection is proportional to the distance to the fault, the magnitude of the echo is proportional to the magnitude of the fault, and the nature (shape, polarity, frequency spectrum, etc.) of the reflection tells the nature of the fault. There are several kinds of reflectometry including time domain reflectometry (TDR) [9][24]-[26] which uses a fast rise time step or pulsed signal, frequency domain reflectometry (FDR) [13][14] which uses multiple sinusoidal signals, sequence TDR (STDR) which uses pseudo noise, and spread spectrum TDR (SSTDR) which uses pseudo noise modulated onto a sinusoidal carrier signal for live testing with minimal interference with low frequency

S.C. Mukhopadhyay (Ed.): New Developments in Sensing Technology for SHM, LNEE 96, pp. 159–185.
springerlink.com

signals [34]-[37]. Other methods include standing wave reflectometry (SWR), mixed signal reflectometry (MSR), and multicarrier reflectometry (MCR), all of which are related to FDR and use multiple sinusoidal signals on the wires. Noise domain reflectometry (NDR) utilizes existing noise on the wires as the effective test signal. [38] These methods are summarized in section 2. This chapter will be limited to electrical reflectometry, although other types of signals (optical and acoustic, for example), can also be used, and the theory applies in much the same way.

Reflectometry can be used in many applications. Most recently, great strides have been made in location of faults on aging electrical wiring for aircraft, and work is still very active in this area. These methods have also been applied to location of faults on anchors and metal-tensioning systems for pre-stressed concrete, with good success as long as the anchors are electrically isolated from the rest of the metallic structure (rebar, mesh grids, etc.).

Anchors for pre-stressed concrete (metal-tensioned systems) are used for construction and repair of foundations, retaining walls, and excavated and natural soil and rock slopes. At least one end of the cables is held together by a trumpet-shaped head. The other end may have a similar anchor head, or may be grouted into the cement foundation. The length of anchor cable between the two heads may be grouted (surrounded by cement) or ungrouted. Once installed, metal-tensioned systems are vulnerable to failure by corrosion of the metal elements, loss of anchorage, or both, but visual observations of the conditions at the element head assembly often do not indicate actual or potential problems, and cases of premature failure have already been documented.[1] Other methods for testing these cables include the lift off test (most common) which places a large strain on the cable (often using a crane) to see if the anchor remains intact. This method is expensive and difficult and may result in needless damage to the cable. It can also be used only for ungrouted anchors. Electrochemical tests (measurement of half-cell potential and polarization current) can be used to detect corrosion but do not give information on how much of the cable is corroded. Acoustic wave propagation methods such as impact (hammer) and ultrasound techniques have also been tested. For shorter anchors (10-20 feet), these may be useful. Attenuation and dispersion limit their use on longer cables. Electrical reflectometry has been shown to be feasible for testing anchors that are made of several steel cables, if they are electrically isolated. [2]

Location of faults on aging electrical wiring is also a key application of reflectometry in structures. Concerns over major aircraft disasters such as SwissAir 111 and TWA 800 have led to significant national commitment to find better ways to locate electrical faults before they have catastrophic consequences. [3]-[8] Over 90% of home fires are attributed to electrical faults, although it is not clear how many are due to installed wiring and how many to faulty plug-in consumer devices. [8] After the Space Shuttle Discovery disaster, the risk assessment determined that the wiring was more likely to fail than the tiles that did fail. [5][6] In addition to the safety problem, aircraft wiring systems are a maintenance burden. Wiring is pervasive in aircraft (e.g. 11 miles of wiring in an F-18C/D). One estimate is that between 1 million and 2 million man-hours are required at the operational level to troubleshoot and repair wiring system problems in the Navy alone each year. Highly trained technicians trouble shoot wiring problems using methods that are 40 years old. In fact, advances in avionics systems, such as Built-In-Test (BIT) may have hampered or even misled technicians if the fault turns out to be in the system wiring. Replacement of the complete wiring system in a typical aircraft is estimated to cost $1-7 million, depending on the aircraft [7].

Numerous federal programs have been devoted to developing methods for locating aircraft wiring faults [8]. Visual inspection, the most common traditional method, has been determined to be insufficient. Time domain reflectometry (TDR), another traditional method for locating faults, may be more accurate but is difficult to use [9]-[12]. Much of the recent work in reflectometry has been to develop better, more accurate algorithms for extracting fault information from reflectometry data as well as developing more accurate reflectometry methods. Alternatives to reflectometry are visual inspection of wiring systems (many/most faults are missed) and high voltage test systems (which can locate even small faults, but are very large and expensive and cannot be used on fueled aircraft) [9]-[12]. Methods described in this chapter are suitable for use in handheld units or small sensors built into the structure itself, and some are suitable for continual or intermittent testing even on systems carrying other live electrical signals or in very electrically noisy environments. The methods discussed in this chapter are time domain reflectometry (TDR), frequency domain reflectometry (FDR), mixed signal reflectometry (MSR), sequence time domain reflectometry (STDR), spread spectrum time domain reflectometry (SSTDR), and noise domain reflectometry [13]-[17].

2 The Basics of Reflectometry[1]

Reflectometry methods are among the most commonly used methods for testing wires. A high frequency electrical signal is sent down the wire, where it reflects from any impedance discontinuity. The reflection is received back at the transmitter, where the delay, magnitude, and nature of the reflection gives information on the location, size, and type of fault.

The reflection coefficient [19] gives a measure of how much signal is reflected from a fault or other impedance discontinuity (connectors, branches, etc.) and is given by

$$\Gamma = \frac{V_{reflected}}{V_{incident}} = \frac{Z_o - Z_L}{Z_o + Z_L} \tag{1}$$

where Zo is the characteristic impedance of the transmission line, and Z_L is the impedance of the discontinuity. The characteristic impedances for typical aircraft cables are Zo=50-200 ohms, and most other electrical cables also are in this range. [39] The characteristic impedance of anchors in concrete is typically around Z_o = 75-300 ohms. [2] The reflection coefficient for an open circuit (Z_L = infinity) on

[1] This section is adapted from [39] and reprinted with permission from TechnoPress.

any wire is 1, and the reflection coefficient for a short circuit ($Z_L = 0$) is -1. A junction of two branched wires ($Z_L = Zo / 2$) has a reflection coefficient of -1/3.

Hard faults (open and short circuits, completely broken anchors, similar high reflection coefficient faults) are readily observable by reflectometry, but soft faults (damaged insulation, corroded anchors, other low reflection coefficient faults) are much more difficult to extract from the reflectometry signature. Because of the intense desire to locate faults before they impact the electrical system (prognostic health management, condition based maintenance, etc.), the interest in locating soft faults remains intense. Fig. 1 shows the raw, roughly sampled measured spread spectrum reflectometry (SSTDR) response for load impedances ranging from 20 to 2000 ohm for RG58 coax with characteristic impedance 50 ohms. (Other reflectometry methods will have the same relative peak heights, but different shapes.) The height of the peak relative to the maximum peak height gives the reflection coefficient. Impedance discontinuities that are greater than 10% are relatively easy to identify and locate just by looking at the response, or using relatively simple algorithms to automatically detect the response of the fault. Impedance differences below 10% become progressively more difficult to identify, as

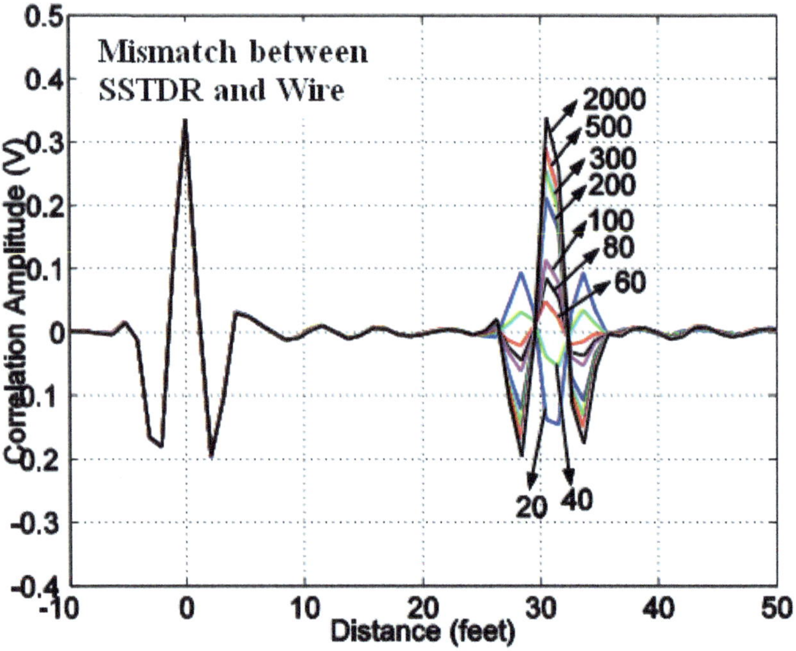

Fig. 1 Spread Spectrum Time Domain Reflectometry (SSTDR) responses for different load impedances on a 50 ohm RG58 coax that is 32 feet long. The correlation amplitude is proportion to reflection coefficient. Other reflectometry methods will have the same relative peak magnitudes, but different shapes of the pulses. From [39].

their response is much smaller, and eventually the peaks from the reflection are smaller than the measurement error and cannot be detected. Reflections for damaged insulation on electrical cables or corroded anchors imbedded in concrete are virtually invisible from the original reflectometry signature. Locating these types of faults requires use of baselines and more advanced signal processing.

The delay between the incident and reflected voltages shows up in the location of reflectometry peaks. In Fig. 1, for instance, two sets of peaks are observed. The peak at 0 feet is from the reflection from the mismatch between the wire and test circuitry. The peak at 32 feet is from the load at the end of the wire. Reflectometry measures time delay. The distance L is the velocity of propagation divided by the time delay. The velocity of propagation in typical aircraft cables ranges from 0.5 to 0. 8 times the speed of light, depending on the type of cable [13][20]. For anchors in concrete, this is slightly lower, typically 0.45-0.5 times the velocity of light. [2] It is therefore very important to know the type of wire or anchor being tested or to measure the velocity of propagation from a known length of the same cable in the same environment and configuration as you are testing. The velocity is dependent on the size and shape of the conductors, and therefore also depends on the distance between conductors. Many aircraft wires are bound together in bundles, often with several hundred wires in a bundle. The location of a specific wire within the bundle is not precisely controlled. Wires may meander through the bundle, sometimes near the center, other times near the surface, creating a change in velocity of propagation of as much as 3%. [39] Similar errors are observed if the wire is moved around between tests, even if it is closely paired with another wire (such as twisted pair or twin lead wire like lamp cord). [21]

There are several sources of error in reflectometry measurements. The error in the hardware itself (typically on the order of 1% or even less) is likely to be the least of the problems. Ambiguity in the velocity of propagation is proportional to ambiguity in the location of the fault. The inability to see small reflections can cause a fault to be missed (false negatives), or if the reflectometry is set to be too sensitive, false positives can result from normal impedance variations in the wire (proximity to other wires or metallic objects, water on the wires, connectors, bends, etc.) that can be as high or higher as the fault.[40] Another error is connection error. Since the reflectometer must be connected to a wide variety of cables or anchors, it is not generally feasible to match the impedance of the reflectometer to the wire. This means there will always be a reflection between the board and the wire being tested. The test-lead, connectors, adapters, etc. all add to this reflection in different ways. The physical connection to the wire is not always identical, particularly for handheld units. All of these types of errors can be handled by using baselines. The most accurate baselines can be expected from built in units, which can take continual baselines or baseline samples before/during/after significant changes (vibration of wires, water level changes in dams, etc.).

Another significant source of error in reflectometry methods is the so-called "blind spot". This is particularly problematic for wires or cables that are very short or when the fault is near the front of the cable. This is caused by the reflected signal overlapping the incident signal, because the time delay is so small. This makes it difficult to identify the reflected signal. Two methods can be used to reduce this problem. One is to use a longer test lead to connect the reflectometer to the wire under test. This would effectively delay the reflected signal enough that the overlap can be reduced or avoided. This may be practical for handheld applications, but it is not practical for in situ applications, where the reflectometer is actually imbedded in the system. Another method is to use a baseline identify the overlapping signals and extract the reflected response. [11][21][22]

With a basic understanding of reflectometry and the errors that are inherent in its use, the following sections describe several different types of reflectometry, each distinguished by the type of incident voltage used. Time domain reflectometry (TDR) uses a voltage step function. Frequency domain reflectometry (FDR) uses a set of stepped sine waves. Sequence time domain reflectometry (STDR) uses a pseudo noise (PN) sequence as the incident signal, and spread spectrum time domain reflectometry (SSTDR) uses a sine wave modulated PN code. Noise domain reflectometry (NDR) uses no signal at all, but rather only existing signal and its inherent noise on the wire. These methods will be compared for ease of use and interpretation, cost, size, ability to test live wires, and ability to analyze branched networks. The theoretical and practical accuracy are compared for each method.

A second class of sensors are capacitance and/or inductance sensors. The capacitance of an open circuited cable and inductance of a short circuited cable are proportional to the length of the wire. Thus, if the capacitance (for open circuited wires) or inductance (for short circuited wires) can be measured, the length can be calculated. Several such methods have been tested [18][23], and found to be very accurate for single lengths of wires. These sensors tend to be the least expensive circuits available for testing wires, however they are not able to detect faults on wire that are live, and they cannot test wires that branch into multiple arms or networks.

A. Time Domain Reflectometry (TDR)

Time domain reflectometry (TDR) uses a short rise time voltage step as the incident voltage. [9]-[12][26] For simple loads such as wiring, the reflected voltages are also step functions. As described above, the length of the cable can be calculated from the time delay between the incident and reflected voltages and the velocity of propagation (V_p) of the cable. The magnitude and polarity of reflected voltage indicate the impedance (short, open, partial opens or shorts, etc.) at the discontinuity. The TDR response of a branched wire network is shown in Fig. 2, along with responses from other reflectometry methods. Steps in the response indicate reflections returned to the test point. The source of each reflection is marked on the figure.

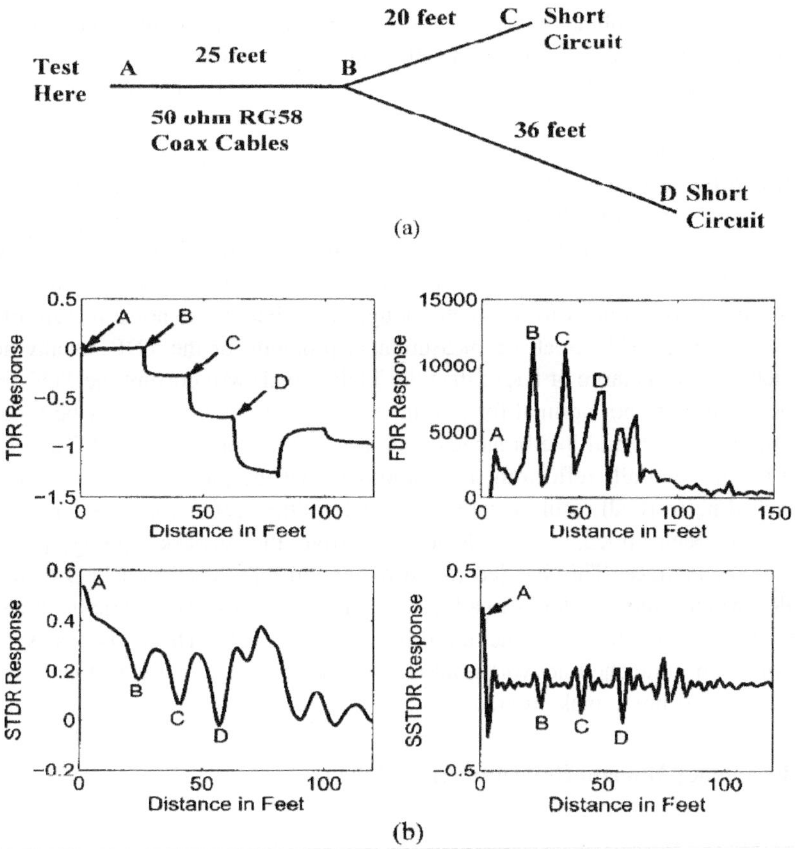

Fig. 2 (a) Network topology, (b) Reflectometry test signals of network shown (a) with TDR, FDR (MSR/SWR), STDR, SSTDR. From [39].

The accuracy of TDR is controlled by the rise time of the pulse and the sampling rate of the receiver. The TDR100 from Campbell Scientific was used in our tests. The TDR100 generates a 14 microsecond pulse and samples the reflected wave at 12.2 pico-second intervals. [26] The expected accuracy is 0.24 cm, for a typical cable with 2/3 the velocity of light. One problem that limits that accuracy of the TDR is that the voltage step contains a very broad frequency and disperses (spreads out) as it goes down the cable. It is difficult to know where to "read" this voltage step.

Due to the large bandwidth of most TDR devices, TDR has also been identified as a potential method for locating small anomalies such as frays or chafes if an extremely accurate initial baseline is available. [11][12] There are both practical and theoretical reasons that obtaining a sufficiently accurate baseline to identify small anomalies is difficult or impossible. In practice, it would be very difficult (probably impossible) to obtain a baseline test of every wire that might go bad in a fleet of aircraft. Another problem of maintaining this baseline is that if the wire is moved, even a little, the small change in impedance and velocity of propagation can easily outweigh the even smaller reflection from the fray or chafe. This issue is analyzed in detail in [12] and [40].

It is difficult to control the problem of "blind spots" with this method, except by adding a length of cable to the test lead. This method has limited application on wires that are live. If the wire is carrying a low frequency signal (400 Hz power, for instance), it may be feasible to use TDR to test the wire while it is live. The TDR signal would need to be small enough to be below the noise margin of the existing signals. This creates a measurement problem for the TDR, as any noise (which may be as large or larger than the TDR signal) will corrupt the TDR trace. TDR is therefore not optimal for testing wires that are live. TDR may be used for testing wires with multiple branches, such as the one shown in Fig. 2. The limitation of this (and all) reflectometry methods is that the junctions and ends of the branched network all result in reflections and multiple reflections that show up in the reflectometry trace, but it is difficult to extract the network topology from the reflectometry trace. This has led to the reputation that "it takes a PhD to read a TDR", which frankly extends to all reflectometry methods. Automatic methods for extracting the topology have achieved initial success [28]. Thus, TDR is as capable of testing branched networks but requires an automatic network topology extraction algorithm to make it practical.

B. Frequency Domain Reflectometry (FDR)

Frequency domain reflectometry (FDR) sends a set of stepped-frequency sine waves down the wire. There are three types of FDR that are commonly used in radar applications that are distinct in that they each measure a different sine wave property (frequency, magnitude, and phase) in order to determine distance. Related methods are also found in wire testing. These are Frequency Modulated Continuous Wave (FMCW) systems (which measure frequency shift), Phase Detection Frequency Domain Reflectometry (PD-FDR) systems (which measure phase shift) [13]-[15], and Standing Wave Reflectometry (SWR) systems (which measure amplitude or nulls of the standing wave).

1. Frequency Modulated Carrier Wave (FMCW)

Frequency Modulated Continuous Wave (FMCW) systems vary the frequency of the sine wave very quickly, generally in a linear ramp function, and measure the frequency shift between incident and reflected signals, which can be converted to time delay knowing the speed at which the frequency was ramped. This has not been implemented for wire testing, because of limitations on speed at which the frequency can be swept accurately and the accuracy at which the frequency shift can be measured [29].

2. Phase Detection Frequency Domain Reflectometry (PD-FDR)

Phase Detection Frequency Domain reflectometry (PD-FDR), shown in Fig. 3 [14], measures the phase shift between incident and reflected waves. [13][14] A voltage controlled oscillator (VCO) provides the sinusoidal signal that is stepped over a given bandwidth (f_1 through f_2) with a frequency step size Δf. A -10 dB sample of the incident sine wave is sent to the mixer, and the remainder is sent to the cable. The incident signal travels down the cable and reflects back from the load. The reflected wave is isolated from the incident wave by the second directional coupler and is sent to the mixer. The mixer multiplies the two sine waves, which gives signals at the sum and difference of the two frequencies input to the mixer. When they are at the same frequencies as they are in FDR, the difference at zero frequency (DC), and the sum is at double the original frequency. The DC voltage at the mixer output is the signal that the computer will detect and use to determine the length and load on the line. An analog-to-digital (A/D) converter used to read the mixer output effectively acts as a low-pass filter and removes the higher frequency components, The number of periods ('frequency') of the DC voltages collected over the injected frequency band is linearly dependent on the wire length. The Fast Fourier transform (FFT) of this collected waveform will give a Dirac delta function (single spike) at a location we will call *Peak*. The location of *Peak* in the FFT response is proportional to the length of the wire. The length is found from this peak index by: [14]

$$L = 2L_{Max}\left(\frac{Peak - Peak(0)}{N_{FFt} - 1}\right) = \frac{1}{2}\left(\frac{Peak - Peak(0)}{N_{FFt} - 1}\right)\left(\frac{N_F - 1}{f_2 - f_1}\right)v_p \quad (2)$$

where,

Peak = location of the Dirac delta peak in the FFT (an integer value)
v_p = velocity of propagation in the cable (m/s)
f_1 = start frequency of the FDR (Hz)
f_2 = stop frequency of the FDR (Hz)
N_F = number of frequencies in the FDR = integer[$(f_2 - f_1) / \Delta f$]
Δf = frequency step size for FDR (Hz)
L_{max} = maximum length shown below
Peak = Peak index for corresponding length in FFT
Peak(0) = Peak index for 0 length
N_{FFT}= number of points in the FFT (an integer value, generally 1024, 2048, 4096 or 8192)

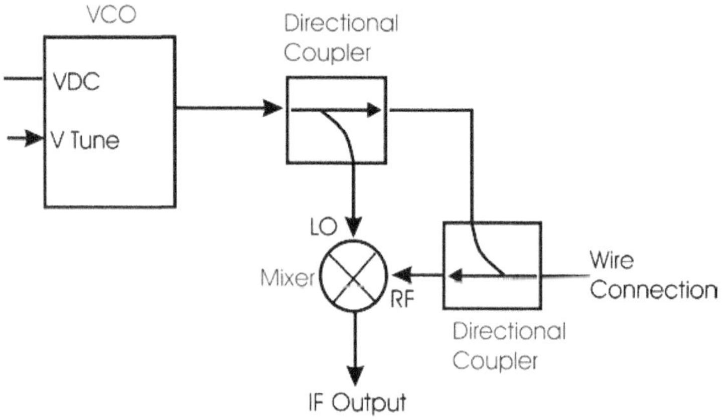

Fig. 3 PDFDR Block Diagram. © 2005 IEEE. Reprinted, with permission, from [14].

To improve the resolution of the results, the measured data can be zero padded. [30] The resolution (accuracy) of the measurements (ΔL) is given by [13][14]:

$$\Delta L = v_p / (2\, N_{FFT}\, \Delta f) \tag{3}$$

The maximum length (L_{max}) that can be measured is limited by the frequency step size and the Nyquist criterion:

$$L_{max} = \frac{v_p}{4\Delta f} \tag{4}$$

A sample set of responses of different lengths of a shielded twisted pair M27500-24SE2S23 wire is shown in Fig. 4(a), and their FFTs are shown in Fig. 4(b). The peak location in the FFT is substituted into equation (2) to find the wire length. The velocity of propagation is 0.66 times the speed of light for this wire [13][14].

Automatic analysis is quite easy with FDR methods, so they are relatively easy to use. Unlike TDR, very little frequency dispersion is seen in this method, as it is not generally as broad band as TDR, and the peak locations are clearly visible. PD-FDR is also capable of measuring branched networks of wires, where a peak in the FFT would be observed for each reflection and multiple reflections in the network, such as the response shown in Fig. 2. The same limitation that this does not directly provide the network topology exists as for TDR. FDR methods can be used on live wires, provided that the test frequencies are not within the frequency range of the existing signal on the wire, and that the FDR is below the noise margin of the signal. It is not optimal for live wires, however, as noise from the existing signal can provide significant corruption of the FDR response that may or may not be effectively filtered by the FFT. Analysis of short wires requires special treatment to remove the low frequency associated with the short connection between the PD-FDR board and the cable under test. [11][13][14][18][22] This is similar to the blind spot in TDR.

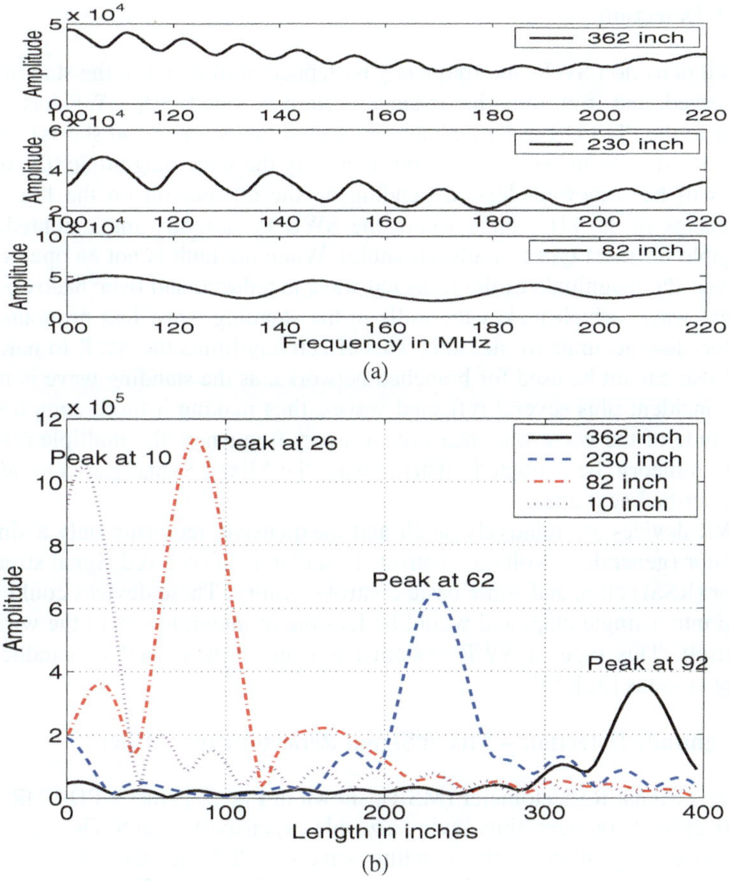

Fig. 4 PD-FDR results for open circuited RG58 50ohm coax. (a) DC output of the mixer as a function of stepped frequency, and (b) the Fourier transform of the results in (a) with N_{FFT} = 2048. The reduction in height is caused by the attenuation on the wire. © 2003 IEEE. Reprinted, with permission, from [13].

3. Standing Wave Ratio (SWR)

Standing wave ratio (SWR) systems measure the magnitude of the standing wave created by the superposition of the incident and reflected signals on the wire. The sum of these two sine waves will have a series of peaks that are caused by their constructive interference and nulls caused by destructive interference. As the frequency is swept, these nulls can be identified (as described in section 3a) or the pattern of the standing wave is proportional to the response obtained from the PDFDR (as described in section 3b). The frequency must be swept through multiple nulls, because otherwise wires that are multiples of a wavelength are indistinguishable. The two types of SWR are described below [32][33].

a. Null Detection

For null detection SWR, the frequency is stepped until a null in the standing wave is observed, and from this, the distance to fault is found [30]. SWR has accuracy similar to the PD-FDR described above for hard faults (open and shorts) where the incident and reflected signals are approximately the same magnitude (the reflected wave will be somewhat less, depending on the attenuation on the line, but for frequencies in the kHz range where the SWR is currently implemented, this is negligible for most types of aircraft cable). When the fault is not an open or short, however, the magnitude of the reflected wave is reduced and overshadowed by the incident wave, which makes the nulls in the standing wave less pronounced and therefore less accurate to measure. This effectively limits the SWR to hard faults. SWR also cannot be used for branched networks, as the standing wave is made up of the incident plus several reflected waves, thus making it more complex. If the magnitude of the wave was measured at every frequency, the multiple reflections could, in theory, be extracted. This is what the Mixed Signal Reflectometry system described next does.

SWR devices are relatively small and inexpensive, requiring only a sine wave generator (generally a voltage controlled oscillator), a received signal strength indicator (RSSI) chip, and some basic control circuitry. These devices could be integrated into a single chip, and would be feasible to integrate within the wiring system itself. This type of SWR system has been implemented in handheld wire testing systems [32][33].

b. Magnitude Detection -- Mixed Signal Reflectometry (MSR)

A Mixed Signal Reflectometer (MSR), shown in Fig. 5, is like a PD-FDR without the directional couplers (thus saving sizeable expensive) or an SWR that measures the squared magnitude of the standing wave for all frequencies (thus improving accuracy, especially for smaller reflections). Like the PDFDR, a voltage controlled oscillator (VCO) provides a sinusoidal signal that is stepped over a given bandwidth (f_1 through f_2) with a frequency step size Δf. It reflects back and is superimposed on the incident wave. The combination of the incident and reflected waves (standing wave) goes through the attenuator, which reduces the amplitude of the signal to prevent overloading the mixer. The attenuated signal feeds into both inputs of the mixer. The output of the mixer is the square of the sum of the incident and reflected signals [15]:

$$\begin{aligned}&\{B[\sin(\omega t)+\alpha\sin(\omega t+D)]\}^2\\&=B^2\{[\frac{1}{2}(1+\alpha^2)+\alpha\cos(D)]+[\frac{1}{2}\sin(2\omega t)+\alpha\cos(2\omega t+D)+\frac{1}{2}\sin(2\omega t+2D)]\}\end{aligned} \quad (5)$$

where

α : attenuation
τ : signal delay from the wire
ω : frequency of VCO output,
A : amplitude of the VCO output
B : amplitude of the sinusoidal wave after reflection and attenuation.

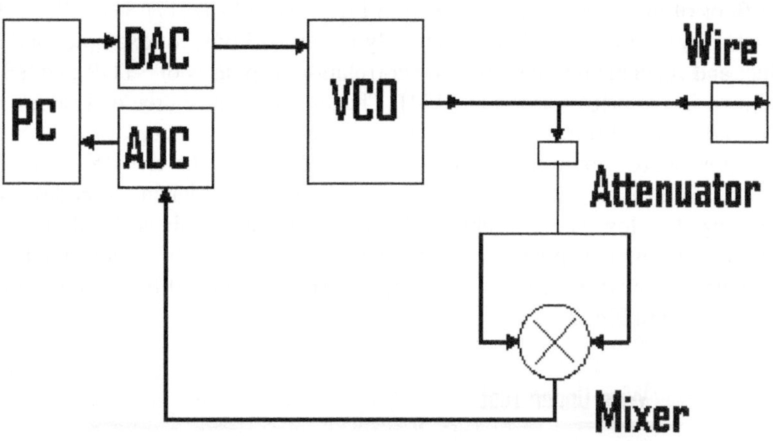

Fig. 5 MSR Circuit Diagram. © 2003 IEEE. Reprinted, with permission, from [15].

This contains the first harmonic of the sine wave and a DC value,

$$B^2[\frac{1}{2}(1+\alpha^2)+\alpha\cos(D)] \tag{6}$$

This DC value is the same as for the PD-FDR, such as shown in Fig. 4. The mixer output goes into a digital to analog converter, which automatically filters out the high frequency component. The DC values as a function of frequency are a sinusoidal wave whose frequency is linearly proportional to the wire length, virtually identical to the FDR responses shown in Fig. 4. The MSR is more accurate than the SWR for small reflections, however this advantage has not been found to have practical application, as it still cannot analyze the very small anomalies associated with frays or chafes. MSR is less expensive and smaller than PD-FDR, since it does not require the directional couplers. For branched networks, the MSR response includes the multiple reflections plus their sums and differences, which makes its response more complex to calculate than the PD-FDR branched network response. Limitations on the use of MSR for live wires and short length wires are virtually identical to those for PD-FDR.

The MSR system is less expensive than either the PD-FDR or SWR. It requires only a voltage controlled oscillator (VCO), mixer, and related control circuitry.

c. STDR/SSTDR

Block diagrams of Sequence Time Domain Reflectometry (STDR) [16][17] and Spread Spectrum Time Domain Reflectometry (SSTDR) are shown in Fig. **6** [17][34]. STDR uses a pseudo noise (PN) code as the test signal, as shown in Fig. **7**(a) [17][34]. The PN signal can be very, very small compared with the aircraft signal on the wire (-20 dB down, for instance) and is well below the allowable noise floor of the aircraft signal shown in Fig. 7(a) and (b) [17][34]. Although the PN code magnitude is small, it is relatively long (1023 bits, for example) and has a distinct and recognizable pattern. The correlation responses of STDR and SSTDR are shown in Fig. 7(c) and (d) [17][34]. The signal at the source end (a combination of incident and reflected waves) is correlated with a test copy of the PN code. Correlation delays, multiplies, and sums the signal with the test PN code. When the codes are synchronized, a high value is obtained, and when the codes are not synchronized, a low value is obtained. The correlation enables STDR to run on live wires far better than any of the other reflectometry methods described so far. The length of the wire (distance to fault) is easily determined from the correlation data, as shown in Fig. 2.

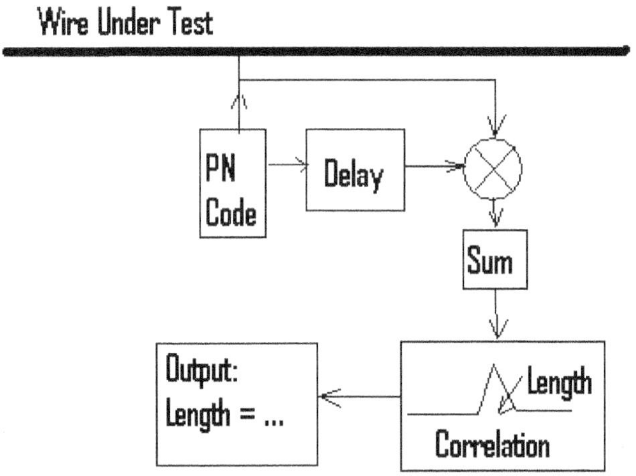

Fig. 6 Sequence (STDR) Test System. For SSTDR, the input signal is a sine wave modulated PN code. From [39].

A slight change to the STDR signal gives even better performance for live wires or for anchors requiring extremely accurate testing. Spread Spectrum Time Domain Reflectometry (SSTDR) uses a sine wave modulated PN code as the test signal, as shown in Fig. 7(b). The correlation peak obtained is sharper than the STDR peak. This method is very efficient and accurate for live wire testing, and has been shown to be accurate with the existing data signal 50 dB greater than the SSTDR signal. This is because the spectrum of the SSTDR signal is outside of the spectrum of the data signal. [34]

Height of the peaks used to determine the wire length for the S/SSTDR system relative to the noise floor depend on the speed, length, type, and integration time of the PN code [27]. The system shown here uses a PN code of length 127 with a frequency of 58 MHz. The accuracy of the S/SSTDR system is controlled by the distance between subsequent samples of the correlation peaks, which is controlled by the precision of the shifter in the correlation step. A time shift of T gives a distance error of delta L = (velocity of propagation)(T/2). If only individual chips are

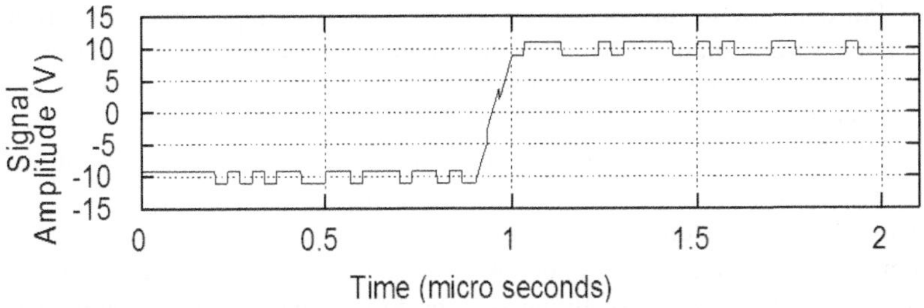

(a) STDR Signal

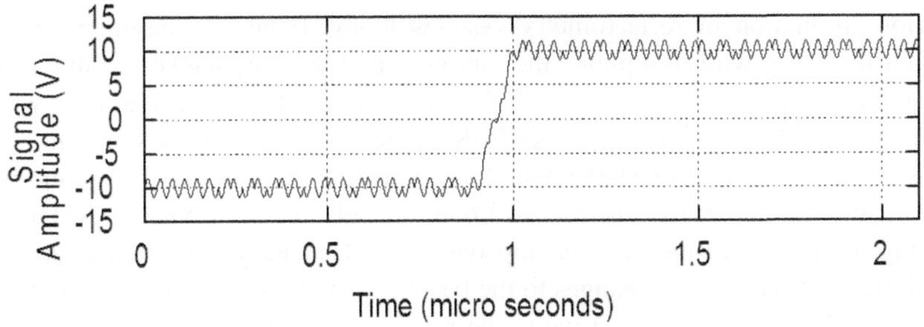

(b) SSTDR Signal

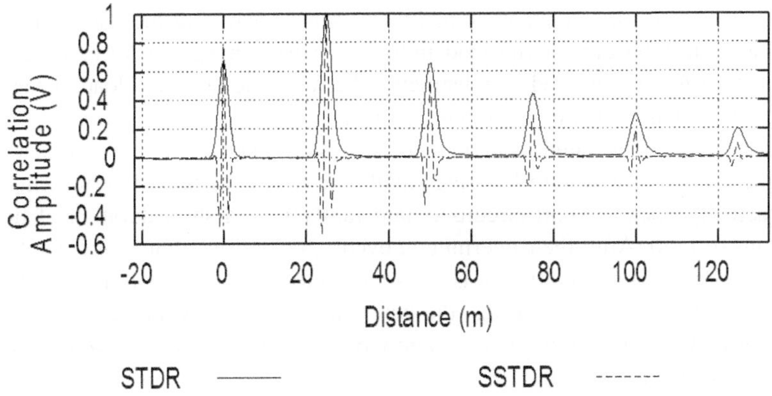

(c) Correlation response of STDR and SSTDR signals

Fig. 7 STDR and SSTDR signal added to a 10 V RMS signal at 30 MHz. The S/SSTDR signals are a Maximum Length (ML) Code 1V RMS at 58 MHz, with a 58 MHz sine wave modulation in the case of SSTDR. The magnitude of the S/SSTDR signals can be much smaller than shown here, depending on the signal on the wire. (a) STDR Signal (b) SSTDR Signal (C) Correlation response of STDR and SSTDR for a wire that is open circuited on the end. © 2005 IEEE. Reprinted, with permission, from [36].

correlated (as opposed to "subchips"), the accuracy is insufficient for this application). For our system, subchip sampling at a rate of 10 samples per chip is required to obtain a resolution of 17 cm. This error can be substantially reduced (to about 3 cm) by fitting a curve to the correlation peaks to more precisely locate peaks that are missed by sparse correlation sampling. [21] S/SSTDR has been demonstrated for location of intermittent faults that are less than 2ms in duration. Both wet and dry intermittent arcs can be located with this method.

The S/SSTDR system has several advantages over other types of reflectometry systems. First, since it can run very well on live wires, it can create and store its own dynamic baseline. Base lining is done to determine when something in the wiring system has changed. A baseline shows when the wire is "good", and the difference from the baseline shows where the fault has occurred. Base lining is a serious limitation of reflectometry systems today. Even if a baseline could be taken for every wire in a plane, the vibration and normal changes within a plane would corrupt this baseline so much that it would not be very useful later when a fault occurred, as discussed in the TDR section. The SSTDR system eliminates this problem and locates changes within a wiring system, using a dynamic baseline that it creates itself. There is still one unresolved issue about S/SSTDR base lining. Loads with time-varying impedance (such as equipment being turned on and off) will show up as changes to the baseline, and these changes need to be distinguished from real faults. It would be relatively simple to ignore all changes at the location of the load; however this would mean that a fault at the connection point to the load would be missed. Additional information would be needed to make this distinction, such as an additional sensor placed at the load, connection to the control system for the load indicating when changes were expected (and could therefore be ignored), or distinction between the fault and load change signatures (similar to an arc fault circuit breaker).

Perhaps the most significant advantage of the SSTDR system is that since it is testing while the wires are live, the small "arc faults" or other intermittent faults are actually open or short circuits ("hard faults") for a short duration of time (a few ms or less). After their intermittent event, the fault is often a "soft fault" with an impedance discontinuity that is too small to locate. The important aspect of intermittent fault location is to test the wire while the fault occurs, and the SSTDR system is the only method that we know of that can test the wire while it is live without interfering with it. [16]

Another advantage of this method is that it can be made extremely accurate by lowering the noise floor of the test system. This can be done several ways including increasing the length of the PN code or increasing the number of times it is run and averaged before a reading is confirmed. The tradeoff here is that the longer you test, the longer an intermittent fault must be in order for you to find it. The low noise floor has allowed testing of extremely long cables such as the 8500 foot long triple core, 350 MCM subsea cable shown in Fig. 8. A short circuit was located on this cable at 6900 feet with a 1.5 MHz SSTDR signal and confirmed when it was located by repair divers. [41]

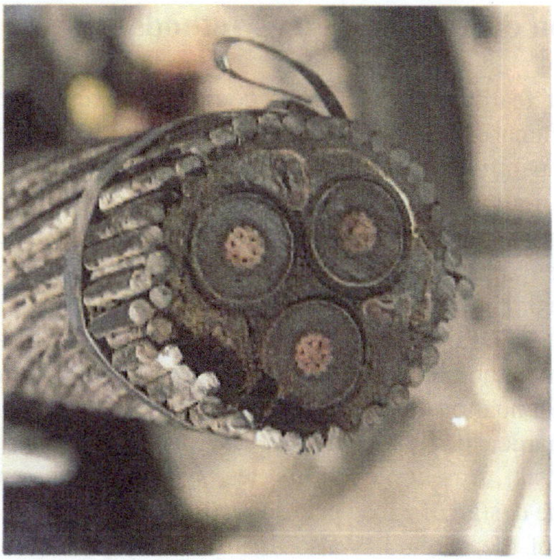

Fig. 8 3 core, 350 MCM sub sea cable

The S/SSTDR is capable of being miniaturized into a mixed signal IC, which will make it very small and likely the least expensive reflectometry system available. It is very feasible to consider imbedding this system in the wiring system. S/SSTDR is capable of analyzing branched networks, with the same limitations as FDR and TDR, that the network topology must be extracted from the multiple peaks in the reflection data.

E. Noise Domain Reflectometry (NDR)

Noise Domain Reflectometry (NDR) [38] uses existing data signals on wiring and does not need to generate any signals of its own. There are two types of NDR, type I (where incident and reflected signals are separated) and type II (where they are superimposed). NDR is totally "quiet" and passive to other signals on the media. NDR functions very similar to spread spectrum methods by utilizing correlation to determine the length of the wire. However, unlike spread spectrum methods that require a PN code as the test signal, any significant noise or high speed signal on the line can be used to passively test the wire and locate the distance to a fault. The family of Noise Domain Reflectometers (NDR) utilizes the properties of time domain autocorrelation functions and can be used to determine individual time delays or multiple reflections such as from branched networks. The advantage of using NDR over other forms of reflectometry is that there is no need to transmit a specific test signal. Instead, the existing signal or noise on the wire is used as the test signal. In other words, NDR can be totally "quiet" to other users of the media being tested. Thus, NDR may be ideal for applications where data integrity is critical such as in flight "live" wire fault location for aging aircraft wiring or applications where stealth is desired.

3 Comparison of Reflectometry Methods

There are several features on which we could compare reflectometry methods, which will be summarized here. A number of comparisons have been made, including [39], for specific applications, types of equipment, etc.

The accuracy of all reflectometry methods is controlled by their useable bandwidth. The higher the bandwidth, the greater the accuracy. The useable bandwidth is decreased (often substantially and sometimes critically) by attenuation in the system being tested. High frequencies are attenuated more than lower frequencies, so FDR, STDR, SSTDR, etc. are normally chosen to be below the range of attenuation for the type and length of cables being tested. TDR data is smoothed by high frequency attenuation (sharp rise on the front of the steps disappear), thus making it much harder to read accurately. Bandwidth is not limited by the reflectometry method itself. It is limited by the test system and the engineering choices associated with the design of each specific instrument.

The accuracy of the method is also controlled by the algorithm and methods used to extract the data. No algorithm can extract information where this is none to be extracted, so the bandwidth and frequency range must first be suitable to the application. Knowledge of the velocity of propagation, base lines that provide the expected wire system and configuration, etc. are all used to improve automatic fault location algorithms. This is an area of active research, and many new algorithms and methods are emerging.

Another major consideration when selecting a reflectometry system is its application. If you are interested in finding intermittent faults, for example, you will need to be actively testing at the instant the intermittent fault asserts itself. Systems that can be integrated into the existing electrical system or structure can provide the advantage of continually updated base lines, continual monitoring, and collection of system health information over time. This is typically more accurate than occasional testing with handheld systems. If the electrical system is live or if the environment has a lot of coupled electrical noise, the reflectometry system needs to be compatible with the existing signals so neither interferes with the other. STDR and SSTDR have been designed for location of intermittent faults on live wires, and are ideal for that application. NDR may be an option for the most sensitive applications if they have sufficiently high noise or signals already on the wires. Other methods must be specifically tailored so that they are out of the band of the existing signals, which may or may not be possible. The broader band the reflectometry test system, the more difficult that is to accomplish.

4 Testing Concrete Anchors with S/SSTDR[2]

This section describes the use of S/SSTDR for location of a partial corrosion on a multi-stranded anchor for pre-stressed concrete. In order to determine the feasibility and accuracy of this method, stranded cables were buried in trenches filled with

[2] This section is reprinted from [2] with permission. (© 2009 IEEE).

sand, deliberately damaged in a controlled fashion, and tested to determine if this damage could be detected and located. The particular challenge for this application is the attenuation of the cable, which makes the reflection from the distant end of the cable and any faults appear very small indeed by the time they return to the sending end. This was overcome using the STDR method and averaging the tests over a relatively long period of time (seconds). This significantly reduces the measurement noise of the method, thus enabling location of very small reflected signals. A baseline was taken prior to damaging the anchor. The sensor was not disconnected between tests, thus emulating the effectiveness of a built-in test system.

Fig. 8 shows the cross section of a simulated anchor used for the sand tests described in this section and the definitions of wire, strand, and anchor. It is important to note that the anchors must be electrically isolated from the surrounding metal in the dams. This depends on the construction method by which they were installed. If the anchor heads are connected into the rest of the rebar in the dam, then an isolating material is needed between the anchor head and its support.

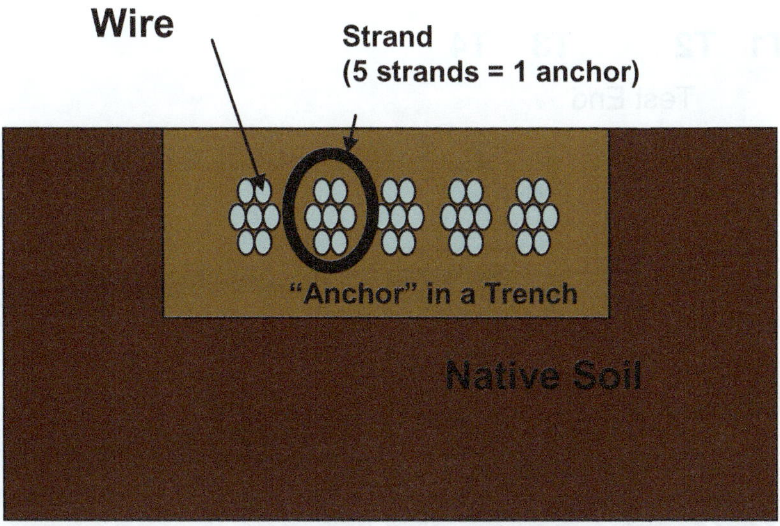

Fig. 9 Cross Section of Simulated Anchor for this Test. Another identical anchor in another trench a few feet away was used as the 'ground' reference. © 2009 IEEE. Reprinted, with permission, from [2].

A test bed was created at the Bureau of Reclamation in Denver, Colorado. The test bed consisted of four parallel 200' trenches (each 2' wide and 2' deep), as shown in Fig. 9. Each trench was filled with 1' of sand, and then five strands of 5/8" 7-wire cable were placed in parallel. Each strand was held apart by a plywood spacer to ensure that they did not touch along the length of the anchor as shown in Fig. 10.

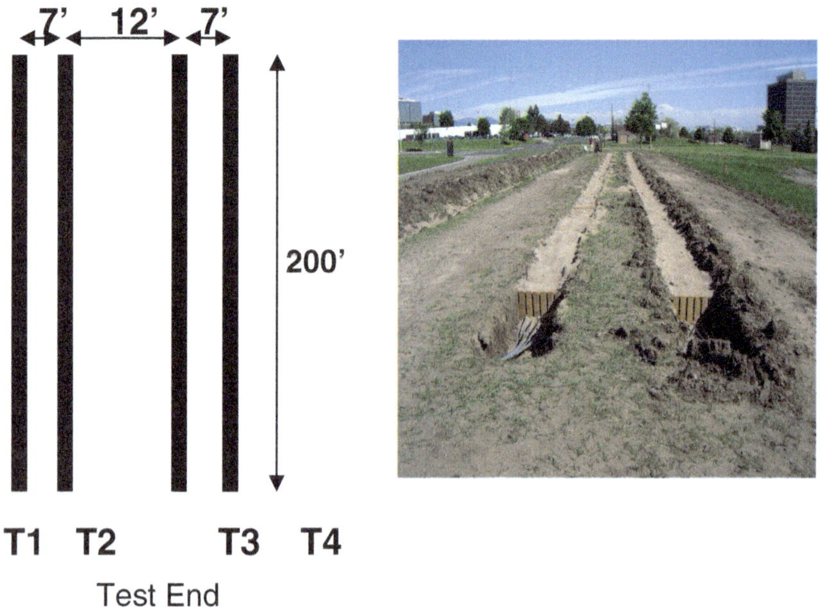

Fig. 10 Four parallel trenches were used simulate anchors in concrete. © 2009 IEEE. Reprinted, with permission, from [2]

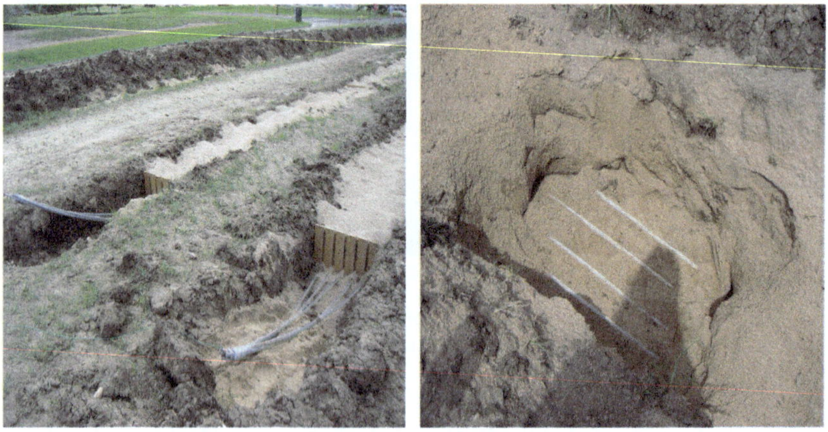

Fig. 11 (Left picture) Ends of two anchors extending from trenches 1 (left) and 2 (right), 7' apart. This shows the plywood spacers used to hold the strands approximately 4" apart in the trenches, as shown in the right photo. © 2009 IEEE. Reprinted, with permission, from [2].

In order to simulate the normal configuration where multiple strands are short circuited together at the anchor head to create a single anchor, the five strands in each trench were tightly held together with duct tape as shown in Fig. 10 (left picture). An STDR handheld test unit produce by LiveWire Test Labs was connected to the simulated anchors with approximately 10-20' of 12 gauge copper wire (available from typical home improvement centers), depending on the distance to each trench being tested. A metal pipe clamp was used to connect the 12 gauge wire to the bundle of strands representing the anchor, as shown in Fig. 10. In order to speed up collection of test data from multiple trenches, wires were run to each trench, and then connected individually to the STDR, connecting and disconnecting sequentially during each data collection. Fig. 11 shows the connection of the STDR to the simulated anchors in trenches 3 and 4. Care was taken to minimize the coils or loops in the 12 gauge (green) connection wires. (Left photo) 12 gauge wires were connected to the 90 ohm coaxial cable using a banana-to-BNC connector as shown in the right photo. Testing on subsequent days was simplified by soldering banana plugs to the 12 gauge wires, so they could be simply plugged into the banana jacks.

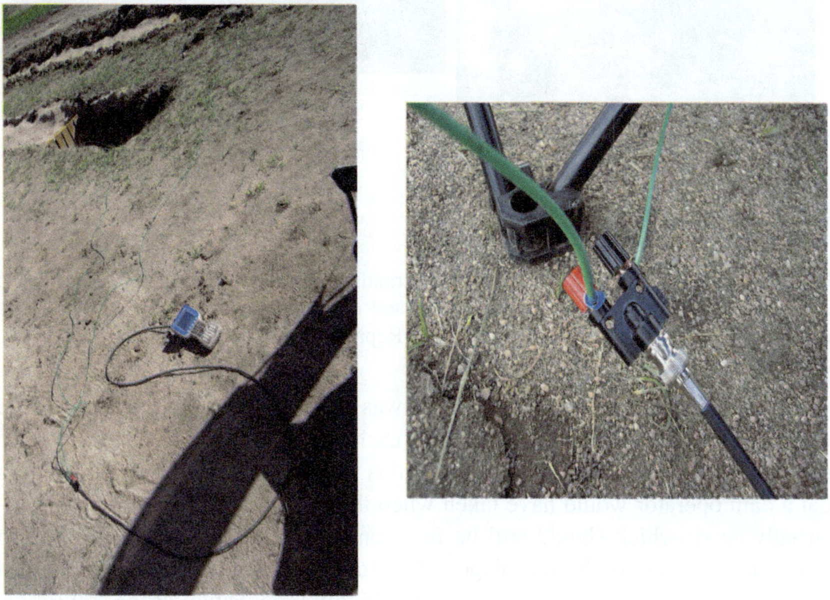

Fig. 12 Connection of STDR to simulated anchors in trenches 3 and 4. Care was taken to minimize the coils or loops in the 12 gauge (green) connection wires. (Left photo) 12 gauge wires were connected to the 90 ohm coaxial cable using a banana-to-BNC connector as shown in the right photo. Testing on subsequent days was simplified by soldering banana plugs to the 12 gauge wires, so they could be simply plugged into the banana jacks.

Damage to the anchors was simulated by cutting them with an oxygen acetylene torch. Example of these cuts are shown in Fig. 12. Fig. 12 (a) shows five strands completely cut and pulled away from each other. (b) shows strands that were cut and not pulled away from each other. Pull tests (described later) were done to determine the spacing in (b) that was detectable.

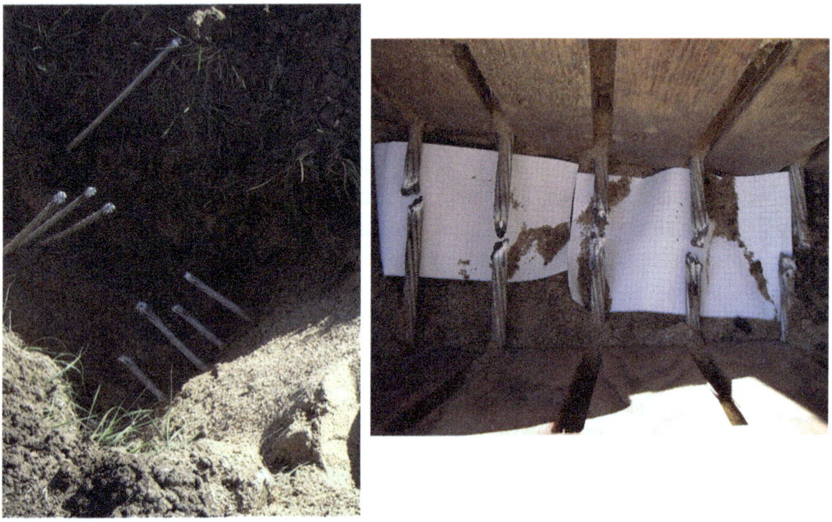

(a) (b)

Fig. 13 Simulated damage. (a) shows five strands completely cut and pulled away from each other. (b) shows strands that were cut and not pulled away from each other. Both fault types gave similar results. © 2009 IEEE. Reprinted, with permission, from [2].

For each test, an initial test (baseline) was taken when the wires were 200 feet long. This baseline, which is different for each trench, was used as the baseline for all future tests of that trench. In practice, this baseline represents the sampled data that a dam operator would have taken when the dam was new (this is optimal), or partially aged (which should still be functional). Any change from this baseline represents a change in the impedance of the anchor being measured and indicates a break or possible damage. Because of the highly lossy nature of the soil (or concrete) surrounding these anchors, the reflectometry peak that would normally be used to locate the end of the cable was not readily visible beyond a few feet. Thus, it was only possible to locate breaks on cables up to about 10' away just by examining the response (not using a baseline). Breaks beyond this distance required use of a baseline taken before the damage occurred. Also, we attempted to use one trench as a baseline for another but found that this was not functional.

There was more change between trenches than from the small changes we were seeking. Thus, the only functional method for locating breaks that were more than 10’ from the test end was to use a baseline approach that would require in situ sensors testing at continuous intervals over time.

Location of a break in the anchor was done by testing the wires when they were all 200’ long (collecting this data as a baseline), cutting one of the anchors (all 5 strands, in this case), retesting, and subtracting the new test data from the original baseline. The differences for several break locations are shown in Fig. 13 for anchors 7’ apart. For anchors that are 12’, 19’, and 26’ apart, the peaks are progressively smaller and the noise larger. Based on these tests using a baseline, a complete break in the cable can be seen for anchors that are 7’, 12’ and 19’ apart up to 160 feet and 26 feet apart up to about 140’. Breaks further away than these MAY be detectable with future improvements.

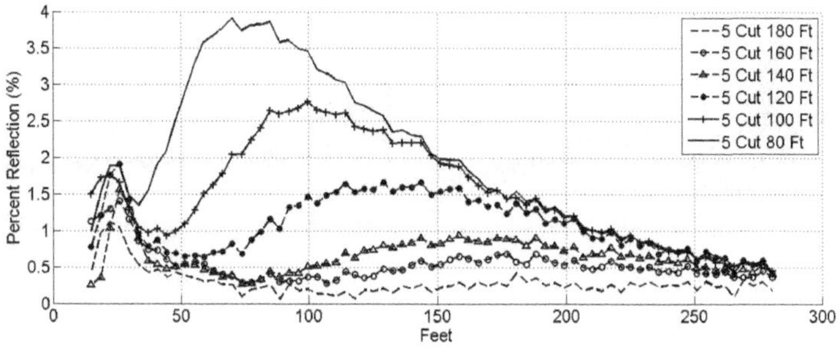

Fig. 14 Location of breaks in anchors that are separated by 7’. © 2009 IEEE. Reprinted, with permission, from [2].

In order to simulate a partially corroded (or partially broken) anchor, each of the five strands were cut one at a time and pulled physically apart from the other parts of the cable so there was no possibility of electromagnetic coupling to the other parts of the cable. Smaller breaks were also tested, and found to be virtually identical to those that were pulled well apart. Partially damaged anchors showing effect of cutting 1,2,3,4 or 5 strands are shown in Fig. 14 for anchors 7’ apart. For cuts up to 160’ it appears that partial damage to the anchor can be identified. As for anchors that are fully cut, increasing the separation between anchors reduces the sensitivity of the method. It should also be noted that the strands in these tests were separated by wooden spacers, representing the configuration where multiple strands are separated in space. Other types of anchors have all of the strands touching or bundled together. These types of anchors were found to have reflectometry responses that were significantly less sensitive to partial damage.

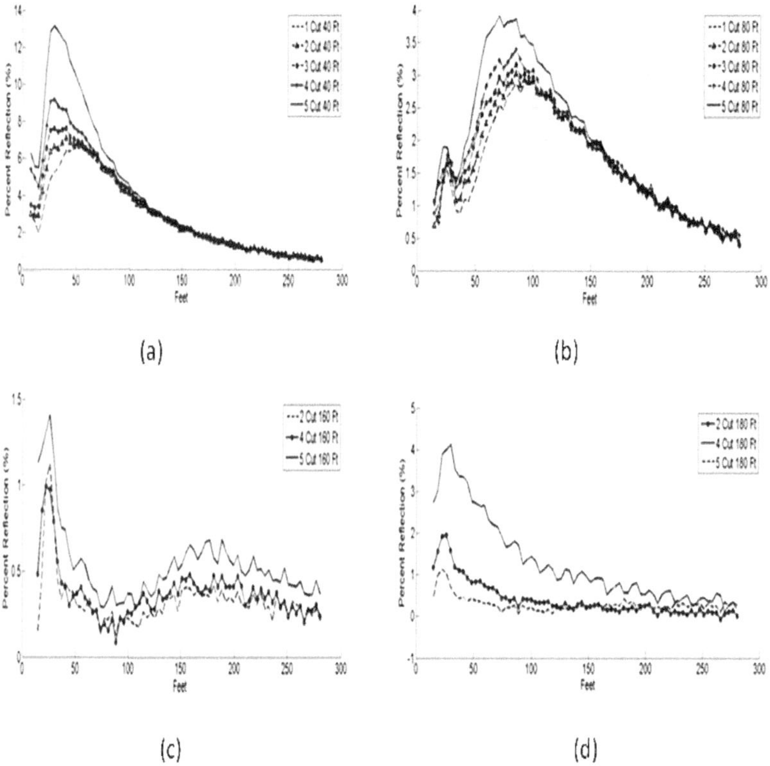

Fig. 15 Partially Damaged Anchors showing effect of cutting 1,2,3,4 or 5 strands. (a) Cuts at 40', (b) cuts at 80', (c) cuts at 160', (d) cuts at 180'. All data is compared to a baseline at 200'. All anchors are in trenches 7' apart. For cuts up to 160' it appears that partial damage to the anchor can be identified. © 2009 IEEE. Reprinted, with permission, from [2].

6 Discussion

This chapter compared several types of reflectometry methods for structural health monitoring. Reflectometry methods transmit high frequency signals on a wire or structural metallic element (an anchor used for pre-stressed concrete, for example). These signals reflect off impedance discontinuities on the wire or cable, and are received at the transmitter location. The time delay, magnitude, and nature of the reflections tell the distance to the fault, the magnitude of the fault, and the type of the fault, respectively. There are numerous types of reflectometry methods, each using a different type of transmitted signal. This chapter described electrical reflectometry methods, but many of the same principles apply when using optical or acoustic reflectometry systems.

Smart imbedded test systems for wiring hold the promise of revolutionizing the way large wiring systems are designed and maintained and may also be used for structural health monitoring. The ability to precisely identify and locate faults on wires and cables remotely enables monitoring, diagnosis, control, and potentially even prognosis of degrading systems. Critical elements including sensors that are small enough to be imbedded, that are capable of locating faults on live or noisy systems, and that can be used on branched networks are all rapidly emerging and are showing excellent results.

Aging wiring and cable systems have plagued us for decades, and the proliferation of electronic systems within our society is further propagating that problem. Test methods to locate faults, or to locate early intermittent predecessors to catastrophic faults, can dramatically decrease the maintenance cost and time burdens as well as improve safety. Handheld systems are rapidly emerging, and systems that can be used on live wires are following close behind. These new methods promise a dramatic shift in electrical maintenance and open up opportunities for robust and inexpensive imbedded structural sensors that have not previously existing.

References

1. Withiam, J., Fishman, K., Gaus, M.: Recommended Practice for Evaluation of Metal-Tensioned Systems in Geotechnical Applications, National Research Council Transportation Research Board, National Highway Coorperative Research Report #477, National Academy Press, Wash DC (2002)
2. Furse, C., Smith, P., Diamond, M.: Feasibility of Reflectometry for Non-destructive Evaluation of Prestressed Concrete Anchors. IEEE Journal of Sensors 9(11), 1322–1329 (2009)
3. Furse, C., Haupt, R.: Down to the Wire: The Hidden Hazard of Aging Air Craft Wiring. IEEE Spectrum, 35–39 (February 2001)
4. NASA (2000), Wiring Integrity Research (WIRE) Pilot Study A0SP-001-XB1 (August 2000)
5. Lloyd, R.: 64 Cases of Wiring Problems found on Shuttle Fleet, CNN Reports (September 3, 1999),
`http://www.cnn.com/TECH/space/9909/03/shuttle.repairs/`
6. Lloyd, R.: NASA Delays Shuttle Launch to Inspect Wiring, CNN Reports (August 13, 1999), `http://www.cnn.com/TECH/space/9908/13/shuttle.update/`
7. Conley, T.: The Relationship among Component Age, Usage (Reliability) and Cost of Naval Aviation Repairables. In: Aging Aircraft Conference 2003, New Orleans (September 2003)
8. NSTC Review of Federal Programs for Wire System Safety, White House Report (November 2000)
9. Steiner, J., Weeks, W.: Time-Domain Reflectometry for Monitoring Cable Changes: Feasibility Study, EPRI GS-6642 (February 1990)
10. Waddoups, B.: Analysis of Reflectometry for Detection of Chafed Aircraft Wiring Insulation, MS Thesis, Utah State University, Logan, Utah (2001) (all theses and dissertations in this paper can be obtained from `http://www.lib.umi.com`
11. Schmidt, M.: Use of TDR for Cable Testing, MS Thesis, Utah State University, Logan,Utah (2002)
12. Jani, N.: Location of Small Frays using TDR, MS Thesis, Utah State University, Logan,Utah (2003)

13. Furse, C., Chung, Y., Dangol, R., Nielsen, M., Mabey, G., Woodward, R.: Frequency Domain Reflectometry for On Board Testing of Aging Aircraft Wiring. IEEE Trans. Electromagnetic Compatibility, 306–315 (2003)
14. Chung, Y., Furse, C., Pruitt, J.: Application of Phase Detection Frequency Domain Reflectometry for Locating Faults in an F-18 Flight Control Harness. IEEE Trans. EMC 47(2), 327–334 (2005)
15. Tsai, P., Lo, C., Chung, Y., Furse, C.: Mixed Signal Reflectometer for Location of Faults on Aging Wiring. IEEE Sensors Journal 5(6), 1479–1482 (2005)
16. Furse, C., Smith, P., Safavi, M.: Feasibility of Spread Spectrum Reflectometry for Location of Arcs on Live Wires. IEEE Sensors Journal 5(6), 1469–1478 (2005)
17. Furse, C., Lo, C., Chung, Y., Pendayala, P., Nagoti, K.: Spread Spectrum Sensors for Critical Fault Location on Live Wire Network Structures. Journal of Structural Control and Health Monitoring 12, 257–267 (2005)
18. Chung, Y., Amarnath, N., Furse, C.: Capacitance and Inductance Sensors for Open and Short Ends Circuit Wire Faults Detection. IEEE Trans. Instrument and Measurement 58(8), 2495–2502 (2009)
19. Iskander, M.: Electromagnetic Fields and Waves. Prentice Hall, Englewood Cliffs (1992)
20. White, E.: Personal Communication (April 13, 2004)
21. Pendayala, P.: Development of Algorithms for Accurate Wire Fault Location Using Spread Spectrum Reflectometry, MS Thesis, University of Utah (2004)
22. Basava, S.: Detection and Location of Cable Faults Using Reflectometry Methods, MS Thesis, Utah State University (2004)
23. Amarnath, N.: Capacitance and Inductance Sensors for the Location of Faults in Wires, MS Thesis, University of Utah (2004)
24. Mackay, N., Penstone, S.: High-Sensitivity Narrow-Band Time-Domain Reflectometer. IEEE Trans. Instrumentation and Measurement 23(2), 155–158 (1974)
25. Chen, C., Roemer, L., Grumbach, R.: Cable Diagnostics for Power Cables. In: IEEE Annual Conference of Electrical Eng. Problems in Rubber and Plastic Industries, 20–22 (April 1978)
26. Campbell Scientific, TDR100 Instruction Manual, `ftp://ftp.campbellsci.com/pub/outgoing/manuals/tdr100.pdf`
27. Arcade Electronics, Psiber CT50 CableTool Multifunction Cable Meter, `http://www.arcade-electronics.com/psiber/psiber_ct50_cabletool.html`
28. Mahoney, A., Lo, C., Chung, Y., Furse, C.: Use of Genetic Algorithms and Reflectometry for Identification of Network Topologies. Personal Communication
29. Furse, C., Kamdar, N.: An Inexpensive Distance Measuring System for Navigation of Robotic Vehicle. Microwave and Optical Tech. Letters 33(2), 84–97 (2002)
30. Oppenheim, V.: Digital Signal Processing. Prentice-Hall, Englewood Cliffs (1975)
31. Chung, Y.: Non-Destructive Fault Location on Aging Aircraft Wiring Net-works Part 1 – Cost-Optimized Solutions. IEEE APS and USNC/URSI National Radio Science Digest, Columbus Ohio (2003)
32. Eclypse Co. SWR meter, `http://www.eclypse.org/Home.htm`
33. Medelius, P., Simson, H.: Non-intrusive Impedance-Based Cable Tester, US Patent 5977773 (November 1999)
34. Smith, P.: Spread Spectrum Time Domain Reflectometry, Ph.D. Dissertation, Utah State University (2003)

35. Smith, P., Furse, C., Gunther, J.: Fault Location on Aircraft Wiring Using Spread Spectrum Time Domain Reflectometry. IEEE Sensors Journal 5(6), 1469–1478 (2005)
36. Furse, C., Smith, P., Safavi, M., Lo, C.: Feasibility of Spread Spectrum Reflectometry for Location of Arcs on Live Wires. IEEE Journal of Sensors 5(6), 1445–1450 (2005)
37. Furse, C., Lo, C., Chung, Y., Smith, P., Pendayala, P., Nagoti, K.: Spread Spectrum Sensors for Critical Fault Location on Live Wire Networks. Journal of Structural Control and Health Monitoring 12, 257–267 (2005)
38. Lo, C., Furse, C.: Noise Domain Reflectometry for Wire Fault Location. IEEE Trans. EMC 47(1), 97–104 (2005)
39. Furse, C., Chung, Y., Lo, C., Pendayala, P.: A Critical Comparison of Reflectometry Methods for Location of Wiring Faults. Smart Structures and Systems 2(1), 25–46 (2006)
40. Griffiths, L., Parakh, R., Furse, C., Baker, B.: The Invisible Fray: A Critical Analysis of the Use of Reflectometry for Fray Location. IEEE Journal of Sensors 6(3), 697–670 (2006)
41. LiveWire Test Labs Personal Communication from M. Mason, Dubai Petroleum (2010), http://livewiretest.com

Sensor Fusion in Transportation Infrastructure Systems Using Belief Functions

Stephen Mensah, Nii O. Attoh-Okine, and Ardeshir Faghri

Department of Civil and Environmental Engineering
University of Delaware, Newark Delaware 19716
{samensah,okine,faghri}@udel.edu

Abstract. Civil infrastructure systems such as bridges, buildings, highways and dams play a crucial role in today's socio-economic development. Constructing these exacts a heavy financial toll and even more important is maintaining them at an acceptable level of performance over the design period. Several methods are employed today in infrastructure health monitoring from simple visual inspection to complex image analysis in order to detect flaws in a timely manner and take appropriate steps to mitigate any adverse effects. The present era of microelectromechanical systems (MEMS) and nanotechnology have the potential to greatly impact infrastructure monitoring even revolutionizing the whole process. Tiny microsensors with remote telemetry capability can be embedded in a structure to monitor its health and performance in real-time or quasi real-time. One of the issues to grapple with is that doing so will generate abundant data from different sources with inherent problems like data conflict, data incompleteness, or other forms of uncertainty which need to be addressed appropriately. The objective of this research is to expound sensors and sensor networks and their impacts on civil infrastructure systems; highlight the strengths of the Belief Function method and its application in sensor fusion for transportation infrastructure systems. This work shows how sensors for monitoring infrastructure can be described in a graphical model framework with the individual sensors representing the nodes. The resulting graphical model is then solved using the Belief Function approach.

1 Introduction

Civil infrastructure such as buildings, highways, bridges, dams and the like have become the backbone of modern societies and the vehicles for development and other socio-economic activities. Through use, aging and the effects of the elements -such as ice, snow, wind loading, tectonic events, thermal cycles- these infrastructures begin to deteriorate and over time have to be maintained and eventually replaced since their failure can lead to adverse consequences: damage to property and worse still loss of human life. Such failures and their consequences have been well documented. In our quest to reduce the risk posed we seek ways to improve monitoring of these infrastructures in order to take timely action to preempt unfavorable consequences. Also since it costs money to provide these infrastructures and maintain them for safe public use, the constraints on our scarce resources compels us to seek better ways to improve infrastructure health monitoring.

S.C. Mukhopadhyay (Ed.): New Developments in Sensing Technology for SHM, LNEE 96, pp. 187–203.
springerlink.com

This paper will illustrate how sensor networks can be used for transportation infrastructure monitoring with potential benefits such as superior damage detection and evaluation. Also with a real-time monitoring capability, sensor network affords asset managers the ability to make timely decisions to protect the infrastructure as well as the general public. Rapid renewal with little disruption of service is very vital. The microsensors can measure intrinsic properties that can be used to evaluate the failure modes of an infrastructure while in service. With this kind of capability maintenance can even be predicted and scheduled to a very high fidelity. This will be an invaluable tool to asset managers who will no longer be left guessing but will have adequate time to successfully tackle any anticipated challenges. Also there is the potential to positively impact the design process making it safer and more cost effective.

In addition this work also gives further impetus to exploit the sensor networks technology in the civil infrastructure systems community making use of belief networks. The Belief Function method of reasoning is gaining more appeal for its application in decision modeling. This method enables a more general development of the uncertainty problems compared to other methods such as the Bayesian method. Under some special conditions it reduces to the Bayesian method of reasoning. Thus the belief function method has the advantage of modeling more challenging decision scenarios that cannot be handled under the Bayesian approach. This paper however will focus on the discrete form of discernment with the belief function framework.

This whole process can be done in a seamless way since sensor information can be combined with experience accrued over time from individuals thus making its implementation more appealing. A successful implementation of the new methodology is intimately linked to how it is perceived by stakeholders. Since to some extent experience plays a role in the way infrastructure is managed today, the loss of experienced personnel could seriously cripple the process. A sensor network based approach will preempt this problem and furthermore provide a basis for a more scientific approach to a procedure otherwise steeped in individual biases.

2 Health Monitoring

The primary goal of health monitoring of civil infrastructure is to determine, by a measured parameter, the location and severity of damage in the structure [1]. There are several methods for infrastructure health monitoring ranging from simple visual inspections to complex image analysis. While each has its merits and demerits, the general consensus among engineers and infrastructure managers is that the state-of-the-art methods of health monitoring do not give sufficiently accurate information to localize and determine the extent of damage [1]. Ideally it will be great to have a system which can monitor infrastructure in real time and quantify and locate any damage that occurs. There is no doubt that technological advancements will continue to open up new frontiers and spawn a new genre of sensors with signal processing capabilities that take infrastructure monitoring closer to this goal. Current researches lend credence to this.

Nonetheless with the available monitoring techniques, a lot can still be achieved if we tap into innovative tools and procedures that will help mitigate some of the challenges we have to wrestle with. As mentioned earlier the uncertainty associated with the current methods of monitoring can begin to be contained when for instance statistical tools are brought to bear, and in fact they have been used. Another methodology that can be successfully applied in infrastructure monitoring is the use of microsensors and sensor fusion.

3 Sensor Fusion and Health Monitoring

Sensor fusion has been described as the process for combining information gathered from multiple sources to estimate or predict entity states [2]. Klein [3] indicated that this process is a multilevel, multifaceted process dealing with the automatic detection, association, correlation, estimation, and combination of data and information from single and multiple sources. There are other terminologies used that essentially refer to the same process such as data fusion or information integration. Sensor fusion or data fusion happens all around us especially in biological organisms. Just as ubiquitous as data fusion is, so there are terminologies for describing similar processes, and repetitive research [2]. A common thread that runs through is that data from different sources are combined to make the best inference. Figure 1 illustrates a data or sensor fusion system.

Distributed sensor networks is a collection of a large number of heterogenous intelligent sensors distributed logically, spatially and geographically over an environment and connected through a high-speed network. The main components of a sensor network are sensor nodes capable of sensing, processing data and communicating. These sensors may be cooperative, competitive or independent depending on how they are configured to collect data. The data from different sensors collecting information from different aspects of the domain is then combined to give better insight into the domain. For instance if the sensors are measuring the concentration of a gas in the environment, it is almost impossible to tell if the reading is flawed due to any biases or malfunction on the part of just one sensor in place. However if information from all the sensors monitoring the same gas in the environment is pooled together, it helps to construct a domain that is globally consistent. Data fusion is the methodology through which the information gathered can be processed in order to determine the state of the domain. This can be achieved by several different topologies which can be employed for distributed sensor networks. Sensor networks have seen several applications in the robotics industry or target tracking. In the case of target tracking where an objected has to be classified, multiple sensors can be used to observe the object in motion either simultaneously or not. The observed data will then be used to determine out of say N possible classes which particular class the target belongs to. The decision process devolves to selecting a single hypothesis from a given set of hypotheses [4]. In the context of infrastructure systems, sensors can be embedded in a structure to monitor the deleterious effects of say ASR, cracking, strains etc. and all this pooled together to evaluate the health and serviceability of the structure. Technology advancement in wireless communication and electronics has enabled the development of low-cost, low-power multifunctional sensor nodes, that are small in size and communicate untethered in short distances [5] and have broader application. Figure 1 below is a schematic diagram to show how information from individual sensors distributed throughout a domain can be used collect useful information and processed for decision making.

Sensor networks are versatile and can lend themselves to many varied applications. Sensor networks can be used to monitor the environment as well as objects and their interaction with the environment. Some examples are environmental and habitat monitoring; structural monitoring and condition based equipment maintenance; disaster management and emergency response [6].

Data fusion may improve the inference that can be made from one single sensor. This is due to the statistical advantage gained by combining same-source data (redundant observations). While one school of thought believes that the use of multiple types of sensors may increase the accuracy with which a quantity can be observed and characterized, another asserts that that may not always be true. There is the fear that fusion will not always yield good results. This is because fusion may actually produce worse results than could be obtained by tasking the most appropriate sensor in the sensor suite.

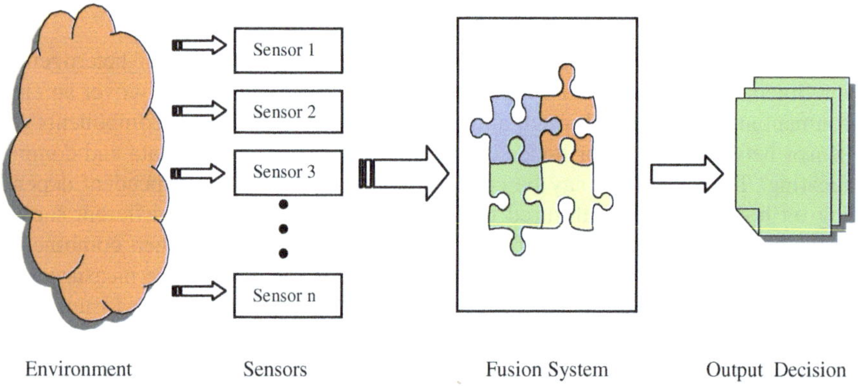

Fig. 1 Schematic for sensor fusion

This is caused by the attempt to combine good or accurate data with inaccurate or biased data especially if the variances are unknown [7]. The challenge of data or information fusion is thus made apparent here-obtaining reliable information from sources that are not fail-safe. This brings into sharp focus the need to properly deploy sensors and to have a mechanism for assessing and quantifying associated uncertainty. Herein lies the strength of the Dempster-Shafer approach to the fusion process which will be discussed presently. Figure 2 is a schematic adapted from [7] to show the various ways in which data can be fused.

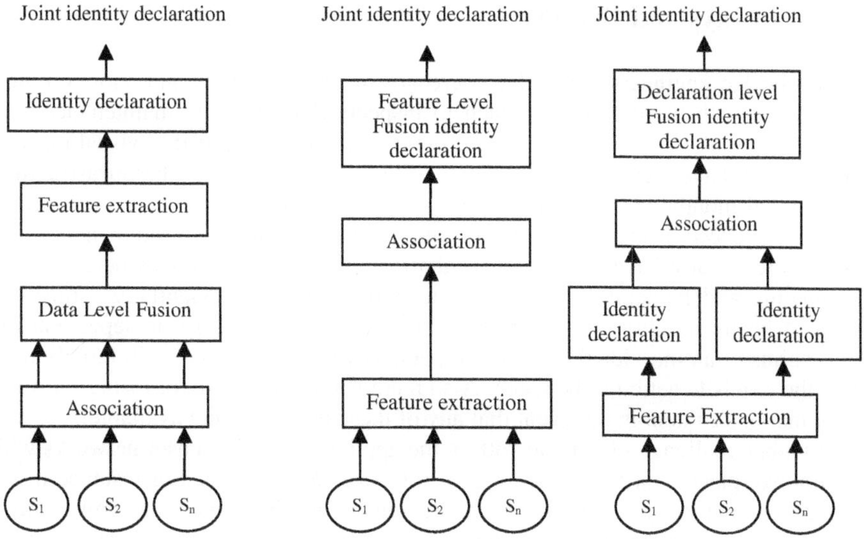

Fig. 2 Variaous methods for fusing data. Adapted from [7]

4 Application in Transportation Infrastructure Systems

The importance of structural health monitoring or damage detection techniques for maintenance of civil infrastructure cannot be overemphasized. Wireless sensor networks can make a significant impact in this area in many ways. First, by collecting data from both the physical structure and its environment in a timely unbiased manner. There is the potential to achieve complete monitoring by employing a dense network of sensors in the structure as well as the environment the structure is located. Furthermore remote inaccessible areas can benefit from wireless sensor networks especially in cases where sensors are designed with systems on board to harness energy from the environment. Second, MEMS and nanotechnology have the potential to enable us measure intrinsic material properties as well as the effects of processes. Visual inspection can only reveal so much to the human eye and many deleterious conditions can go unnoticed. What these microsensors will help us do is to be able to monitor and predict material characteristics under different environmental conditions. This has a great potential in changing our design protocol to enhance safety and ensure more cost-effective designs. A dense network of sensors with signal processing and communication capabilities can process data and extract important information from any structural system in real-time. The benefits here include an automated system that can gather information that will be either global or localized through distributed micro sensing. Third, there is the concept of self-healing structures where for instance cracking can rapture and release an adhesive from an embedded microdevice to immediately start healing of the crack. While conceptually these advantages should be achievable, there are no doubt challenges that must be surmounted to realize this. The following section will highlight one specific area of application in civil infrastructure systems.

5 Highways and Bridges

Many bridge engineers agree that there are many limitations and shortcomings associated with the current approach to inspection, evaluation, maintenance and construction of existing bridges. The current methods are steeped in visual inspections which have significant costs and can restrict operations of the infrastructure for several months [8]. Also, much as these inspections are conducted by trained and experienced bridge engineers or inspectors according to well-standardized procedures, many have argued the limitations and shortcomings associated with evaluating and managing bridges on the basis of what is essentially subjective data. A health monitoring system leaves much to be desired if it is dependent on the whims of an individual or group of persons whose experience will largely dictate the requisite action to be taken. Also there is the probability of losing relevant information or talent in the event that any of these persons is not available.

Another challenge to grapple with in the application of the sensor networks will be optimal placement of sensors in civil infrastructure systems. For instance in an extensive highway project, where should sensors be distributed and how many? The placement of sensors has to be done in a way that does not interfere much with the current methods of construction used by contractors. Even more critical is that an optimal configuration can minimize the number of sensors required, increase accuracy and provide a robust system [9]. Also optimal sensor placement is important in cases where the properties of a system, described in terms of continuous functions, need to be identified using discrete sensor information. Structures like highways may permit uniform distribution of sensors in an array as shown in the Figure 3 below. In other situations where there is no control over the distribution of sensors it is still possible to use sensors in monitoring if the appropriate sensor network is designed such as is the case in ad hoc sensor networks.

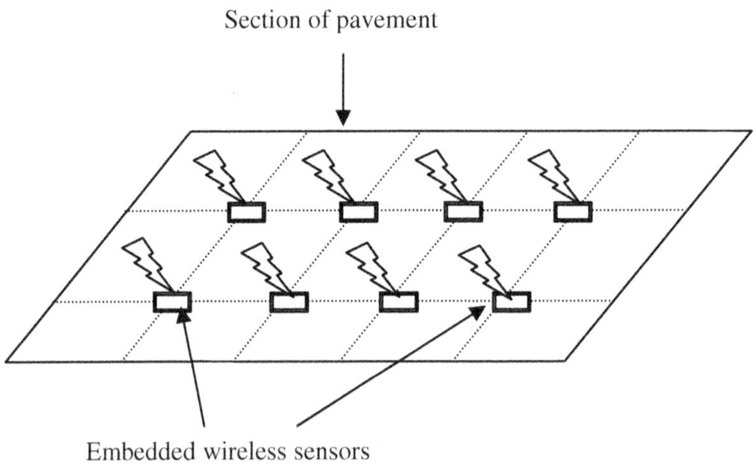

Fig. 3 Distribution of sensors in a domain

6 Graph Theory and Sensor Networks

Graphical belief models are both mathematical structure which specifies which variables are directly connected, and a picture that provides an intuitive description of the model. Graphical models are very useful because they can translate very complex problems into easily understood forms. A highly complex system can have only secondary or indirect interactions between certain components or subsystem through other subsystems. Using independence assumptions we can take advantage of the structure of the problem to provide computationally tractable model [10]. A potentially complex problem can be transformed into an easily understood form. Such an explicit representation of a problem allows one to validate the model and revise it when it does not behave well [11]. In a nutshell, a graphical model is used to capture the structure of the problem. This model graph has a twofold advantage [10]: first, the model graph is both a mathematical structure that specifies which variables are directly connected and second, a picture that provides an intuitive description of the model. A potentially complex problem can be transformed into an easily understood form. Such an explicit representation of a problem allows one to validate the model and revise it when it does not behave well. Several applications of graphical models are cited in the literature [10]. Some examples are counting of evolutionary trees in biology, the intractability of optimizing phylogenies, problems in chemistry and physics, operations research, electrical engineering, industrial engineering, science and civil engineering. Graphical models are a versatile tool for analyzing complex systems.

The universal applicability of graphs can be attributed to the following inherent properties especially in the area of statistics [12]: graphs can visually represent the scientific content of a given model and facilitate communication between researcher and statistician; models are naturally modular so that complex problems can be described and handled by careful combination of simple elements; graphs are natural data structures for modern digital computers. Due to uncertainties good decision making requires building models to assess risk of critical events. The model may stem from information that is incomplete or imprecise. In either case it is necessary to pay careful attention to how the uncertainty is represented [11].

Graphical models can play a crucial role in handling uncertainties and its effect on a system. A complex system with several components will have even more variables describing component and subsystem states. Graphical models help to specify and manipulate such a large system with techniques that take advantage of structure in the problem. Graphical models have proven to be very powerful tools in various applications. Graphical models are well suited for system level reliability which is critical to system design improvement. It can provide a mechanism to identify systems and components which could potentially create problems and study the effects of proposed changes [11].

Figure 4 is an illustration of an infrastructure with embedded sensors for measuring some parameters of interest. The sensors can be designed so all measure the same parameter or different parameters. The infrastructure can be pavement, bridges, buildings etc. In pavements, these sensors could be measuring moisture, temperature and deformation. In bridges the sensors could monitor corrosion or strain; in buildings they can monitor temperature humidity and other gases that might be present in the air. Our goal here is to use the embedded sensors to collect enough information to enable an estimate of the state of health of the infrastructure. Figure 4 thus gives us a schematic diagram of how the sensors can be used to monitor any infrastructure.

The performance requirements of the infrastructure will have a bearing on the topology of the sensor networks that will be used to monitor it. The appropriate sensors to monitor parameters of interest will be deployed from a sensor suite. These sensors with the appropriate algorithm will be able to form a sensor network to collect and process information. The information collected can then be fused using the belief function approach and the output used in the decision making process. The question to ask is which method of fusion will be most appropriate? How does the task at hand affect the chosen fusion approach? A review of the literature shows that a belief function approach will be an invaluable tool. Beynon et al. [13] discussed some cogent reasons to support this claim.

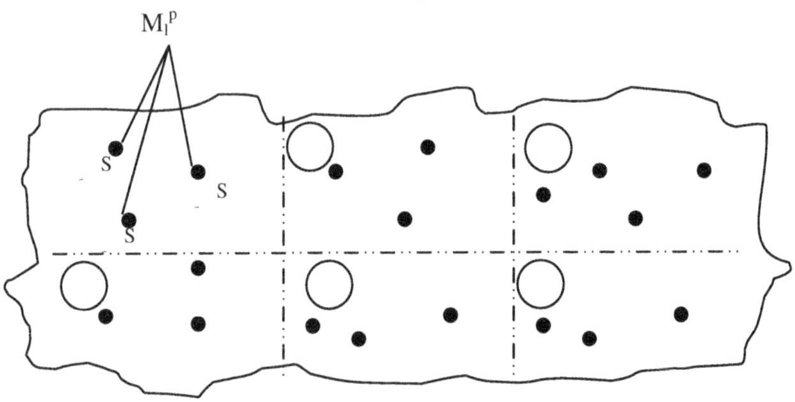

Fig. 4 Aggregation of sensor information

7 Inference Based on Belief Functions

The basic belief mass function (m-values) is similar in notion to the probability function. The concept is best explained with an example and reference is made to the following papers [14] and [15]. If we consider a decision scenario with n possible elements or states of nature that are mutually exclusive and exhaustive, then the set of all these possible outcomes is referred to as the frame of discernment. In other words

$$\Theta=\{ a_1,a_2,a_3,...a_n\}$$

In classical probability theory each of these states is assigned a probability, a number in the interval [0,1] and these probabilities must add up to 1. Shafer [16] discusses the formalism where propositions are represented as subsets of a given set. When interested in the true value of some quantity where its possible values form the set, then the propositions of interest can be declared precisely of the form the true values of Θ is in A where A is a subset of Θ. The set of all propositions of interest corresponds to the set of all subsets of Θ, which is denoted by the symbol 2^{Θ}. Thus for a situation where n=3

$$2^{\Theta} = \{ \emptyset, a_1, a_2, a_3, \{a_1,a_2\}, \{a_2,a_3\}, \{a_1,a_3\}, \{a_1,a_2,a_3\}\}$$

Under the belief function framework, basic belief masses or m-values are assigned not only to each state of nature but also to all possible combinations of these states. That is m-values will be assigned to all the single elements, to all subsets containing two elements, three elements and so on and also to the entire frame of reference. The m-values must sum up to 1 just like the case in classical probability theory. The basic belief assignment can therefore be expressed mathematically as a function m from 2^{Θ} to [0,1] satisfying the following where A represents all the subset of the frame:

$$0 \leq m(a_n) \leq 1$$
$$\sum m(A)=1$$
$$m(2)=0$$

The basic belief mass m(A) represents the part of belief exactly committed to the subset of A of a given piece of evidence, or equivalently to the fact that all we know is that A holds. The belief function over a frame , is denoted by Bel(A), and it corresponds to every proper subset A_i of A ($A_i \subset A$) and is a sum of all basic probability assignments committed to every subset A_i.This can be represented mathematically as follows:

$$Bel(\{A,B,C\})=m(\{A,B,C\})+m(\{A,B\})+m(\{A,C\})+m(\{B,C\})+m(\{A\})+m(\{B\})+m(\{C\})$$

Therefore Bel(A) is a measure of the total amount of belief committed to all possibilities(combinations) implied by A, and not exclusively to A, as expressed by m(A) [17]. The properties of belief functions are given below:

$$Bel(\Theta)=1 \quad \text{as } \sum m(A_1)$$
$$Bel(A)=0 \text{ if } A \surd \Theta$$
$$0<Bel(A) \quad \text{if } A \subseteq \Theta \text{ and } A \neq \Theta$$

$$Bel(A)=m(A) \quad \text{for each } A \subseteq \Theta \text{ containing only one element}$$

$$Bel(A)+Bel(\sim A) \leq 1$$

The plausibility of an element or a set of elements, say A, of a frame, Θ ,is defined to be the maximum possible belief that could be assigned to A if all future evidence were in support of A [14]. A proposition is plausible in the light of the evidence to the extent that the evidence does not support its negation. The degree of plausibility is a number in the interval [0,1] with zero representing evidence refutes a hypothesis and one indicating there is no evidence against the hypothesis at all [16].Belief in the hypothesis is considered the lower probability (degree of belief) based on evidence, while plausibility is the upper probability (degree of belief) based on evidence [17]. For instance the plausibility of a hypothesis A is given as follows

$$Pl(A)=1-Bel(\sim A)$$

The ambiguity in a state A is defined as the difference between the plausibility of A and the belief in A. This can be represented as follows: Ambiguity in A=Pl(A)-Bel(A) or it can also be described by the expression below:

$$Pl(A)=\sum m(B)$$

8 Rules for Combination of Evidence

Uncertainty arises from information that is incomplete, imprecise, contradictory, vague, unreliable, fragmentary or deficient in one way or the other [18]. In the context of sensor networks, it may be the result of sensors that are faulty, broken down or unreliable and for whatever reason which cannot be isolated. A method of combination is required to fuse all the information gathered to facilitate the decision making process. Dempsters rule strongly emphasizes the agreement between multiple sources and ignores all the conflicting evidence through a normalization factor [19]. The normalization factor is necessary to preserve the basic properties of the belief functions [20]. This approach sometimes leads to counterintuitive conclusions and some modifications of the combination method have been developed to rectify this problem. The issues with "counterintuitive" results are a hotly debated subject as some researchers see the problem arising only because of incorrect or incomplete modelisation [21]. It appears different combination rules have to be understood in the context in which they are applied in order to do so appropriately [19].

The Dempster Shafer theory also provides a method for combining measure of evidence from different independent sources using Dempster's rule of combination. This rule reflects fusion of evidence. It must be pointed out that the belief functions to be combined must be based entirely on distinct bodies of evidence - mutually exclusive sources of data [17]. If m_1 and m_2 are the bpa's associated with Bel_1 and Bel_2 respectively and Bel_1}and Bel_2 are independent, then a function $m_1 \oplus m_2 : 2^{\Theta} \rightarrow [0,1]$ defined by

$$m_{12}(A)=K^{-1}\sum m_1(B_1)m_2(B_2)$$

where $m_{12}(A)$ is the resultant m-value for the subset of the frame , and K is the renormalization constant given as

$$K=1-\sum m_1(B_1)m_2(B_2)$$

The significance of k is that it forces the sum $m_1 \oplus m_2$ to take the value of 0 when the subset $A=B_1 \cap B_2$ is the empty set. Also k is a measure of the degree of conflict between two belief functions. Shafer [16] describes a renormalizing constant K, described as follows:

$$K=(1/(1-k))$$

which is seen to increase with k and can therefore serve as a measure of the extent of the conflict. Even more useful is the quantity

$$\log K=\log(1/(1-k))=-\log(1-k)$$

which Shafer [16] called the weight of conflict. It is a weight function because it may take any value from zero to infinity whereas K only takes values greater than or equal to one. However worthy of note is the fact that when k=1 we cannot apply Dempster's rule of combination [22]. The above operation is the orthogonal sum. It can be shown that the operation of orthogonal sum of belief structures satisfies the following properties [22]:

1.commutativity

$$m_1 \oplus m_2=m_2 \oplus m_1$$

2.associativity

$$(m_1 \oplus m_2)\oplus m_3=m_1 \oplus (m_2 \oplus m_3)$$

These two properties according to [22] allow the combination of multiple belief structures or fusion of information by repeated application of Dempster's rule. Thus for instance if we have n pieces of evidence, their combination is

$$m=m_1 \oplus m_2 \oplus \ldots \oplus m_n$$

9 Numerical Example

As discussed in the outset of this paper, the goal is to apply the Dempster-Shafer method in the sensor fusion problem for infrastructure health monitoring and evaluation. Infrastructure through use and being exposed to the elements begins to deteriorate. As the deterioration or damage progresses, the serviceability of the infrastructure gradually begins to be compromised. There are several states of damage for any infrastructure. For instance for a concrete structure which is susceptible to cracking among other distresses, cracking may range from minor cracks which may not warrant an immediate intervention to severe cracks that pose a real threat of imminent failure. It behooves asset managers to know the state of the infrastructure and its needs to keep it serviceable and safe. Generally, these different states can be thought of as hypotheses given by $H=\{\Omega_1,\Omega_2...\Omega_n\}$ which represent all possible states and a single hypothesis from the n possible hypotheses has to be chosen. The challenge here is to be able to successfully do the classification task using multisensor data fusion.

Assume a sensor network is employed to collect the following data as part of a pavement management system-transverse cracking, alligator cracking, rutting and alkali-silica reactivity (ASR). Based on these parameters a decision is made on the condition of the pavement and the requisite maintenance action to take. We can envision a decision scenario of the following possibilities which for the purpose of the work here will be assumed to be mutually exclusive and exhaustive: {rehabilitation required[X1]; routine maintenance required [X2] ; more tests required [X3]; pavement condition OK ie do nothing [X4]}. Again assume we have been able to deduce our belief in the required course of action based on the information reported from the sensor network. We can use this hypothetical situation to illustrate the belief function approach. The belief masses deduced be represented as shown below:

Fusion Process

Sensor Cluster p:

$$M_p[X1,X2]=0.4$$
$$M_p[X2,X4]=0.1$$
$$M_p[X3]=0.3$$
$$M_p[B]=0.2$$

Sensor Cluster r:

$$M_r[X1,X4]=0.2$$
$$M_r[X3]=0.3$$
$$M_r[X1,X2]=0.15$$
$$M_r[X1,X2,X3]=0.25$$
$$M_r[B]=0.1$$

Based on the above information, we can calculate the belief and plausibility values for the sensor cluster labeled p and r:

Belief and plausibility values (Cluster p):

$$Bel([X1,X2])=0.4$$
$$Bel([X2,X4])=0.1$$
$$Bel([X3])=0.3$$
$$Pl([X1,X2])=0.4+0.1+0.2=0.7$$
$$Pl([X2,X4])=0.1+0.4+0.2=0.7$$
$$Pl([X3])=0.3+0.2=0.5$$

Similarly for the sensor cluster labeled r the following belief and plausibility values can be calculated.

Belief and plausibility values (Cluster r):

$$\mathrm{Bel}([X1,X4])=0.2$$
$$\mathrm{Bel}([X3])=0.3$$
$$\mathrm{Bel}([X1,X2])=0.15$$
$$\mathrm{Bel}([X1,X2,X3])=0.25$$
$$\mathrm{Pl}([X1,X4])=0.2+0.15+0.1=0.45$$
$$\mathrm{Pl}([X3])=0.3+0.25+0.1=0.65$$
$$\mathrm{Pl}([X1,X2])=0.15+0.2+0.25+0.1=1$$
$$\mathrm{Pl}([X1,X2,X3])=0.25+0.2+0.3+0.15+0.1=1$$

In order to combine the evidences from these two sources to obtain the fused belief we can compute the k-values and the combined beliefs as shown below.

Computation of K-values:

$$K_{rp}=0.4x0.3+0.1x0.3+0.3x0.2+0.3x0.15=0.255$$

The combined evidences become

$$M_{rp}[X1,X2])=(0.4x0.15+0.4x0.25+0.4x0.1)/(1-0.255)=0.268$$

Similarly

$$M_{rp}[X2,X4]=0.013$$
$$M_{rp}[X3]=0.262$$
$$M_{rp}[X1,X4]=0.054$$
$$M_{rp}[X1,X2,X3]=0.067$$
$$M_{rp}[B]=0.040$$

10 Inference

Ambiguity and uncertainty are inherent characteristics in all disciplines. Ambiguity deals with situations of uncertainty where we are unable to quantify a judgment about a chance of each outcome occurring. Uncertainty deals with scenarios where one is not sure about the outcome of an event [14]. It is obvious that the concepts of ignorance are accounted for in the example given above which is represented as $M_{rp}[B]=0.040$. The good thing about the belief functions is that it allows you to represent partial or total ignorance whereas in for instance the Bayesian framework one is forced to exactly specify probability distributions which are not known. Under the belief function the $M_{rp}[B]$ is the undeclared quantity is left for subjective reasoning. The belief function approach therefore has the ability to handle uncertainty and also ambiguity.

11 Network of Infrastructures

The description above can be applied to two bridges in an entire network of bridges. Figure 5 and Figure 6 below show respectively a schematic of the bridges in the network and the associated graphical model showing the fusion process. This process need not be limited to the same kinds of infrastructure but sensors and the sensor fusion methodology can be deployed to monitor entire network of critical infrastructure especially in times of emergency for optimal performance. This is shown in Figure 6 below.

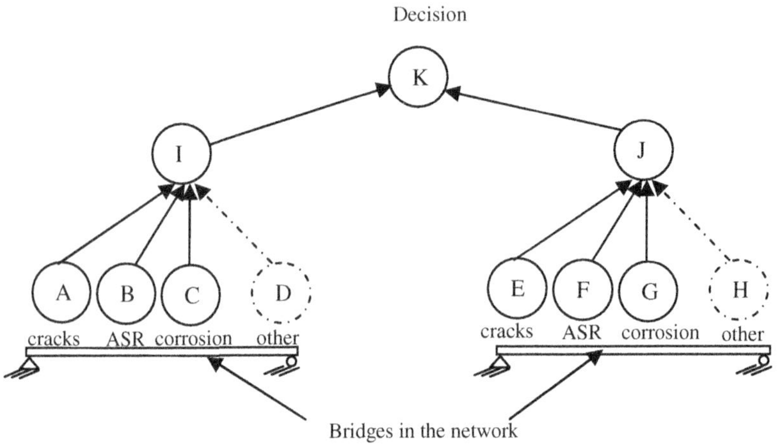

Fig. 5 Network showing two bridges and how distress data is collected and passed on for further processing

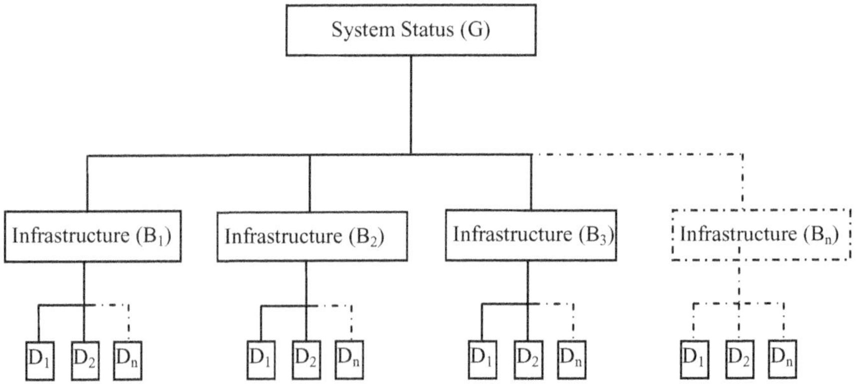

Fig. 6 Network of multiple infrastructures. D_k is a distress variables such as corrosion, cracking, ASR, vibration, rutting, etc which is used to assess the status of each infrastructure and furthermore the whole system status

The importance of the information on the fused beliefs is that it forms the basis for setting policy for rehabilitation and maintenance. From decision node K in Figure 5, network level decisions will be made which will in turn devolve into program level decision (that is the planning and allocating budget for network optimization); project selection which will rank projects within the constraints of the available budget and set objectives; and finally project level decision which will encompass the rehabilitation or maintenance details for implementing the individual projects.

This procedure could be used for more bridges than this example has demonstrated. Also many more variables can be included in this analysis depending on the availability. The attractive thing about a graphical model based approach is that it allows easy modifications to the model with varying degrees of detail when a modular approach is used.

12 Conclusion

Infrastructures today are very important assets that need to be protected. The demands placed on infrastructure from our activities in a modern society compels all stakeholders - owners, consultants, contractors- to look for innovative ways of managing the infrastructure in order to reduce disruption of service to the general public. It is a known fact that the current approach used in structural health monitoring leaves much to be desired and there is a need for an approach that addresses some of the issues faced. This paper has expounded a paradigm shift that will not just facilitate the process, but provide superior damage detection and evaluation. Embeddable micro sensors and sensor networks have a great potential in giving the necessary breakthrough. However in order for this approach to be successful it has to be implemented in tandem with an appropriate technique that helps us to process information with a higher level of abstraction. This is achieved with a sensor fusion methodology based on the Dempster-Shafer theory.

This research has provided some impetus for using high-level monitoring for civil infrastructure systems. It has delved into the state-of-the-art of sensors and sensor networks and proposed a new way to exploit the technology. It has also highlighted a highly marketable but dormant area of microsensor research and development for civil infrastructure systems. Also a foundation has been laid for using graphical models and sensor networks as well as a sensor fusion methodology that can address some of the innate problems of civil infrastructure systems. Also the use of sensor networks affords asset managers the possibility of real-time monitoring of infrastructure which means problems can be detected almost immediately and the appropriate action taken in order to minimize the overall cost of maintenance. In the light of the above, it is envisaged that bridge owners, consultants and contractors will take advantage of innovative paradigms that have the potential to save money and provide an objective scientific approach to infrastructure health monitoring.

Furthermore, the Dempster-Shafer approach to sensor fusion requires the use of independent sources of evidence. This implies the current approach in structural health monitoring, which is not very sophisticated as is the case with visual inspection, can be included in the fusion process along with information gathered from hightech or sophisticated systems such as sensor networks. This has a significant advantage in the sense that the current methodology can be used or included in the process while a progressive shift is made to a more sophisticated approach based on sensor networks. In other words the objective information from sensors can be combined with subjective human estimates acquired through experience. Also the gradual shift means it will not be viewed as too drastic and intimidating and stakeholders are more prone to embrace it. A successful implementation of the new methodology is intimately woven with how stakeholders perceive it. Since to some extent experience plays a role in the way infrastructure is managed today, the loss of experienced personnel could seriously cripple the process. A sensor network based approach will preempt this problem and furthermore provide a basis for a more scientific approach to a procedure otherwise steeped in individual biases. Moreover, reliability based maintenance can begin to take on real meaning. The microsensors can measure intrinsic properties that can be used to evaluate the failure modes of any infrastructure while in service. With this kind of capability maintenance can even be predicted to a very high fidelity. This will be an invaluable tool to asset managers who will no longer be left guessing but will have adequate time to schedule maintenance. Also there is the potential to positively impact the design process making it safer and more cost effective.

Although the methodology discussed in this work is promising for infrastructure management, there is a whole lot of research that needs to be done in key areas to ensure its success. Firstly, in new construction it is much easier for microsensors to be embedded to form sensor networks. However existing infrastructure may not afford us the opportunity or ease of embedding the microsensors. Secondly, sensors may not have lifetimes commensurate with some infrastructure. They may stop functioning after a while. How to replace faulty sensors embedded in an infrastructure can be a real challenge. While it is true that sensor networks can reconfigure and recalibrate based on which sensor nodes are alive, in time these sensors will run out their design life and not be able to collect and transmit data. Future work should focus on addressing some of these issues and developing sensors and a scheme that will enable such high level monitoring with sensor lifetimes commensurate with the lifetime of the infrastructure in order to reap the benefits of using sensor networks at discussed in this paper.

References

1. Chang, P.C., Flatau, A., Liu, S.C.: Review Paper: Health Monitoring of Civil Infrastructure. Structural Health Monitoring 2(3)
2. Steinberg, A.N.: Data Fusion System Engineering. IEEE AESS Systems Magazine (June 2001)
3. Klien, L.A.: Sensor and Data Fusion Concepts and Applications, vol. 14. SPIE Opt. Engineering Press, Tutorial Texts (1993)
4. Braun, J.: Dempster-Shafer theory and Bayesian reasoning in multisensor data fusion. Proceedings of IEEE Communication Magazine 40(2) (August 2002)

5. Akyildiz, I.F., Su, W., Sankarasubramaniam, Y., Cayirci, E.: Survey on Sensor Networks. IEEE Communication Magazine 40(2) (August 2002)
6. Martinez, K., Hart, J.K., Ong, R.: Environmental Sensor Networks. IEEE Computer Society, Los Alamitos (2004)
7. Hall, D.L., Llinas, J.: An introduction to multisensor data fusion, vol. 85(1). IEEE, Los Alamitos (January 1997)
8. Emin Aktan, A., Necati Catbas, F., Grimmelsman, K.A., Pervizpour, M.: Development of a Model Health Monitoring Guide For Major Bridges. Report submitted to Federal Highway Administration Research and Development for Contract/Order No. DTFH61-01-P-00347
9. Meo, M., Zumpano, G.: On the optimal sensor placement techniques for a bridge structure. Engineering Structures 27, 1488–1497 (2005)
10. Foulds, L.R.: Graph theory applications. Springer, New York (1992)
11. Almond, R.G.: Graphical Belief Modeling. Chapman and Hall, Boca Raton (1995)
12. Lauritzen, S.: Graphical Models. Oxford University Press Inc., NY (1996)
13. Beynon, M., Curry, B., Morgan, P.: The Dempster-Shafer theory of evidence: an alternative approach to multicriteria decision modeling. Omega 28, 37–50 (2000)
14. Srivastava, R.P., Mock, T.J.: Belief functions in accounting behavioral research. Advances in Accounting Behavioral Research 3, 225–242
15. Elouedi, Z., Mellouli, K., Smets, P.: Assessing sensor reliability for multisensor data fusion within transferable belief model. IEEE Transactions on systems, man and cybernetics-Part B: Cybernetics 34(1) (February 2004)
16. Shafer, G.: A mathematical theory of evidence. Princeton University Press, Princeton (1976)
17. Mertikas, P., Zervakis, M.E.: Exemplifying the theory of evidence in remote sensing image classification. International Journal on Remote Sensing 22(6), 1081–1095 (2001)
18. Klir, G.: Measures of Uncertainty in the Dempster-Shafer Theory of Evidence
19. Sentz, K., Ferson, S.: Combination of Evidence in Dempster-Shafer Theory. SANDIA Report SAND2002-0835
20. Lefevre, E., Colot, O., Vannoorenberghe, P.: Are alternatives to Dempster's rule of combination real alternatives? Comments on About the Belief function combination and conflict management problem - Lefevre et al. Information Fusion 3, 149–162 (2002)
21. Haenni, R.: Are alternatives to Dempster's rule of combination real alternatives? Comments on About the Belief function combination and conflict management problem. Information Fusion 3, 237–239 (2002)
22. Yager, R.R.: On the Dempster-Shafer framework and new combination rules. Information Sciences 41, 93–137 (1987)

Pulsed Eddy Current Thermography and Applications

G.Y. Tian[1], J. Wilson[1], L. Cheng[1], D.P. Almond[2], E. Kostson[2], and B. Weekes[2]

[1] School of Electrical, Electronic and Computer Engineering, Newcastle University, UK
[2] RCNDE, Department of Mechanical Engineering, University of Bath, UK

Abstract. In this chapter we report on the application of the pulsed eddy current thermography inspection technique to the detection and quantification of defects in a variety of materials. After introducing the appropriate modelling and simulation techniques an overview of a typical PEC thermography system setup is provided. Applications of the system for defect detection in nickel alloys, composite materials and ferritic materials including multiple complex cracking in rail-tracks are discussed.

Keywords: Induction heating, pulsed eddy current thermography, defects, NDT & E.

1 Introduction

The use of thermography for non-destructive (NDE) defect detection predates the development of the infrared camera by several decades. Early thermographic defect detection techniques date back to the 1960s, but it was the development of the infrared camera in the late 1970s which made it possible to directly detect the temperature contrast over large inspection areas. The continuing development of infrared (IR) cameral technology has led to increases in spatial resolution, frame rate and temperature sensitivity. These improvements have allowed thermography to develop from a qualitative overall inspection technique which needs to be supplemented by other NDE inspection techniques to a stand-alone technique able to supply quantitative information through the acquisition and analysis of image sequences.

The major advantages of thermography over other techniques are the ability to inspect a relatively large inspection area within a short time and the capacity to provide real time imaging of any defects which may be present in the inspection area. However, there is a trade-off between detectable defect size and inspection area. Thermography is also capable of inspecting a wide range of materials with proper selection of the optimal excitation technique for the chosen application. Although excitation through heat deposited on the surface using flash lamps [1,2,3], etc. is still dominant, newer techniques such as eddy current [4], laser thermography [2], optical lock-in thermography [5], or sonic excitation [6] are gaining in popularity. In pulsed eddy current (PEC) thermography (also known as induction thermography) a short burst of electromagnetic excitation is applied to the material under inspection, inducing eddy currents to flow in the material. Fig 1a shows the basic configuration of a PEC thermography system; a coil powered by an

S.C. Mukhopadhyay (Ed.): New Developments in Sensing Technology for SHM, LNEE 96, pp. 205–231.
springerlink.com

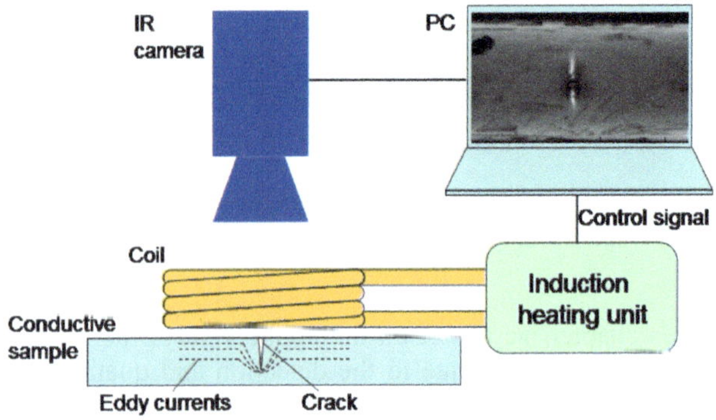

(a)

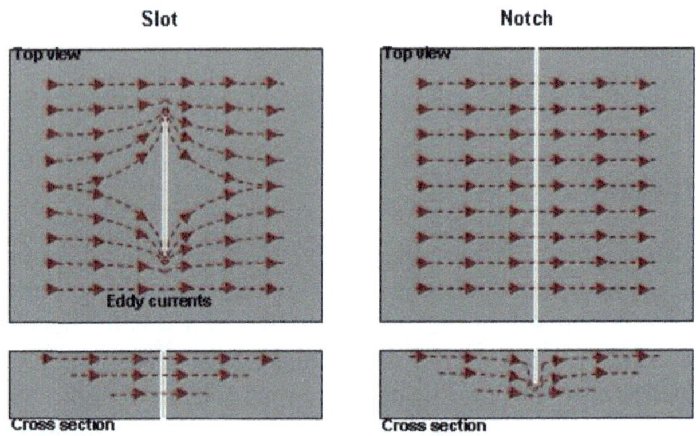

(b)

Fig. 1 a) Basic configuration of pulsed eddy current thermography system, b) Principle of PEC thermography crack detection for two different types of defect

induction heating unit is used to induce eddy currents in the sample under inspection, while a thermal imaging camera is used to record the temperature change in the sample over time. Where these eddy currents encounter a discontinuity, they are forced to divert, leading to areas of increased and decreased eddy current density. Areas where eddy current density is increased experience higher levels of Joule (Ohmic) heating, thus the defect can be identified from the IR image sequence, both during the heating period and during cooling. An alternating current (see Fig. 1b) flowing through a coil or wire (inductor) induces a current in an electrically conducting material placed nearby. If a crack in the sample blocks the current it has to flow around the crack leading to an increased current density at the crack tip. Therefore, after the heat has diffused to the surface, it can be detected with an IR camera [7,8].

The temperature history for any pixel which corresponds to a section of the sample under inspection which has experienced a level of heating can be split into two sections; heating and cooling (see Fig. 2b). The change in temperature in the heating section of the curve is due to a combination of direct eddy current (Joule) heating, which is proportional to the eddy current density, and diffused heat. The change in temperature in the cooling period is entirely due to heat diffusion in the sample. Consequently, analysis and comparison of the two parts of the signal yields different information about any defect which may be present in the material under inspection. Greater heat retention in the cooling period indicates a strong contribution from diffused heat, and has been found to correlate to subsurface heat sources, such as subsurface defects and heat generated at the bottom and sides of surface breaking defects.

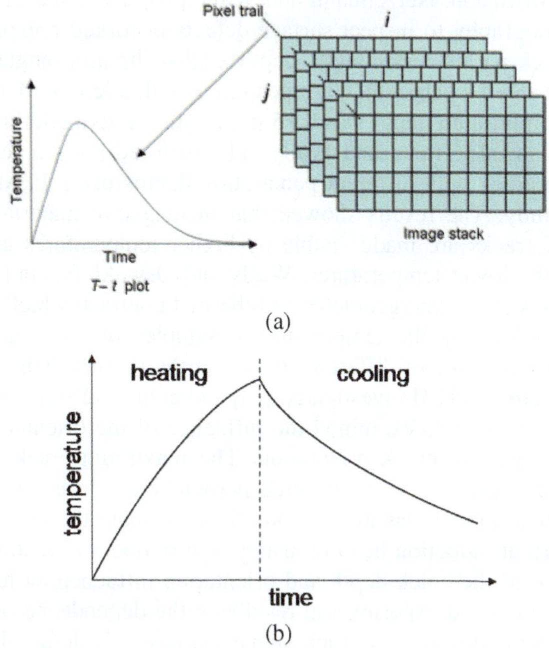

Fig. 2 a) Extraction of temperature history from image stack, b) Heating and cooling sections of the temperature history plot

In contrast to flash lamp heating, in PEC thermography there is a direct interaction between the heating mechanism and the defect. This can result in a much greater change in heating around defects, especially for vertical, surface breaking defects. However, as with traditional eddy current inspection, the orientation of a particular defect with respect to induced currents has a strong impact, sensitivity decreases with defect depth and the technique is only applicable to samples with a minimum level of conductivity (ferromagnetics, paramagnetics and conductive non-metals, i.e. carbon fibre).

Eddy current stimulated thermography is increasingly receiving attention from academic researchers. Zenzinger et al. [9] simulated inductive heating by using finite element method (FEM) models and investigated the detection limits with experiments. In order to gain fundamental knowledge about the induced current density distribution in the component under test, Vrana et al. [7] presented an analytical model for the calculation of the current density distribution in a finite body. Mechanisms and models for detection of open and closed cracks were also examined and the effects of cracks on the current density distribution were investigated with FEM and experimental methods. The results showed that the heating process depends on the type of crack. Cracks can be detected mainly by a direct observation of the heating process due to an increased current density or because of the pattern of heat diffusion. Netzelmann and Walle [10] discussed the application of induction thermography to inspect surface defects in forged components. The effects of the crack parameters, length, depth, and inclination angle, were investigated. In ferrite steel, a perpendicular open crack with a length of 7.5 mm was detected when its minimum depth was 0.15 mm, with the induction frequency set at 100–200 kHz. Oswald-Tranta and Wally [11] explored the temperature distribution around the crack with different penetration depths using FEM modeling and experimental study. The results showed that in magnetic materials after a short heating period, cracks are made visible by higher temperatures and in nonmagnetic materials by lower temperatures. Wally and Oswald-Tranta [12] studied the influence of crack shape and geometry and thermal contrast, which is the temperature at crack divided by the temperature at sample surface, was introduced to demonstrate the influence of different shapes on the thermal behaviour of cracks. Walle and Netzelmann [13] investigated perpendicular and slanted surface cracks in ferric steel. The authors examined the influence of the orientation of the eddy currents with respect to crack orientation. The maximum crack signal was observed when eddy currents were oriented perpendicular to crack length orientation. An analytical model was also proposed to calculate the temperature signals due to eddy current induction heating, using high frequency excitation. Zenzinger et al [14] discussed the crack depth and orientation influence on temperature signals. The theoretical and experimental results on the dependence of the crack signal on crack depth showed that crack signal increases as defect depth increases, with the best performance from defects perpendicular to induced eddy currents in the material.

2 PEC Thermography Systems

2.1 Modeling and Simulation of PEC Thermography Systems

2.1.1 Theoretical Considerations

In this section an analytical model is established for the eddy current (electromagnetic) and heat diffusion phenomena. Consider the change in temperature in a conductive material caused by resistive heating from eddy currents flowing through that material. The generated resistive heat Q is proportional to the square of the eddy current density J_s or electric field intensity E. The relationship between Q, J_s and E is governed by following equation.

$$Q = \frac{1}{\sigma}|J_s|^2 = \frac{1}{\sigma}|\sigma E|^2 \tag{1}$$

The electrical conductivity σ in Eq. (1) is dependent on temperature and governed by Eq. (2), but σ is seen as temperature independent in numerical simulations to simplify calculations.

$$\sigma = \frac{\sigma_0}{1+\alpha_T(T-T_0)} \tag{2}$$

where σ_0 is the conductivity at the reference temperature T_0 and α_T is the temperature coefficient.

According to Maxwell's equations, the magnetic vector potential A can be calculated from Eq. (3).

$$\frac{1}{\mu}\nabla^2 A - \sigma\frac{\partial A}{\partial t} = -J_s \tag{3}$$

Subsequently, the electric field intensity vector E and the eddy current density J_s can be derived via Eqs. (4) and (1).

$$E = -\partial A/\partial t \tag{4}$$

The heat conduction equation of a specimen caused by Joule heating source Q is governed by

$$\rho C_p \frac{\partial T}{\partial t} - \nabla \cdot (k \cdot \nabla T) = Q \tag{5}$$

where ρ, C_p, k are density, heat capacity and thermal conductivity respectively.

2.1.2 Simulation Set-Up

In order to model the PEC thermography response to the presence of defects in a variety of materials, the models shown in Fig. 3 and Fig. 4 have been created. The excitation frequency and current are set at 256 kHz and 380 A_{rms} respectively to match the experimental results presented later in the this paper. Separate models have been created to represent the rectangular coil and Helmholtz coils used in experimental studies. The rectangular coil is constructed from 6.35 mm hollow high-conductivity copper tube and is used to induce parallel eddy currents, perpendicular to any defects which may be present. For tests on CFRP, which has directional conductivity, the sample is aligned so that the eddy current direction coincides with the direction of highest conductivity. The eddy currents are induced dominantly by the coil edge which is close to the sample. Thus, only one edge of the rectangular coil is simulated, drawn as a cylindrical wire in Fig. 3. For the Helmholtz coil, the coil is modelled with a thickness of 5mm, diameter of 60mm and a distance of 30mm between the two halves of the coil, as shown in Fig. 4.

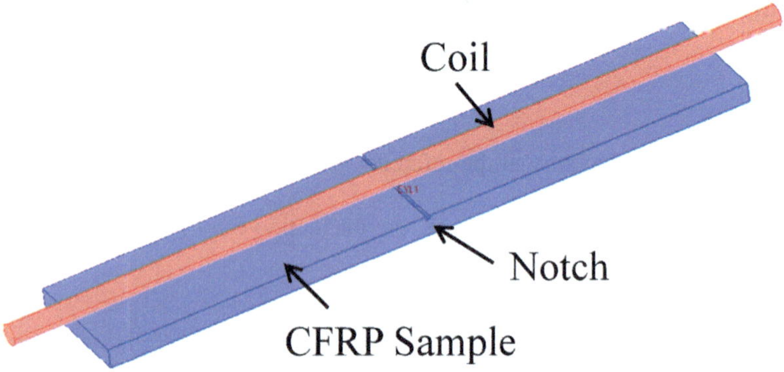

Fig. 3 The simplification of rectangular coil with sample modelled in 3D in COMSOL

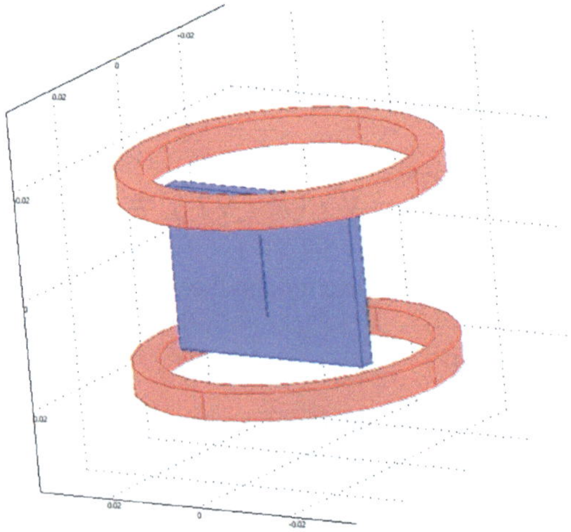

Fig. 4 The Helmholtz coil with sample modelled in 3D in COMSOL

2.2 PEC Thermography System Configuration

Fig. 5 shows the PEC thermography system used in the tests reported in this paper. The excitation sub-system is based around a commercial induction heating system, the Easyheat 224 from Cheltenham Induction Heating. The Easyheat has a maximum excitation power of 2.4 kW, a maximum current of 400 ARMS and an excitation frequency range of 150 kHz - 400 kHz. The system has a quoted rise time (from the start of the heating period to full power) of 5 ms, which was verified experimentally. As the material under inspection is to be heated for a relatively short period (>=20 ms), this was an important factor in system selection.

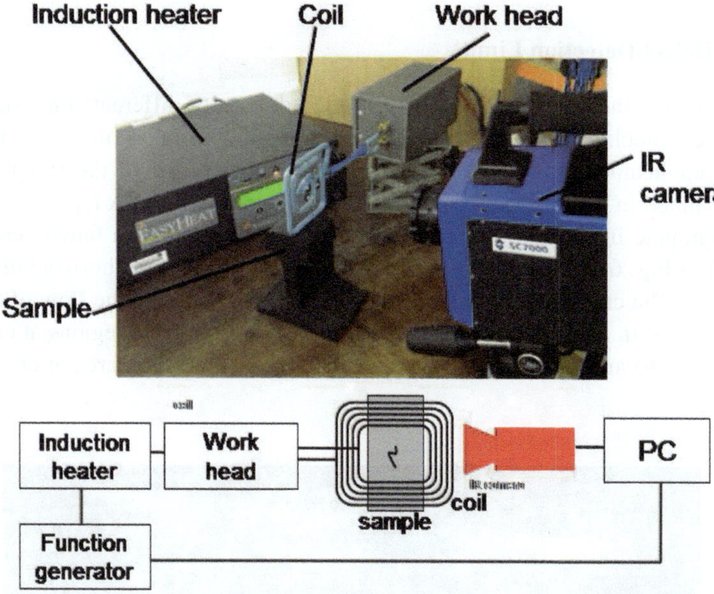

Fig. 5 System design

The Easyheat consists of the main induction heating control box which supplies power to the work head. The work head contains a transformer-coupled resonant circuit, including two capacitors and the excitation coil itself. The excitation frequency is dictated by the value of the capacitors, the inductance of the coil and the load on the circuit, *ie*. the material, volume and proximity of the sample under inspection.

Preliminary tests with a variety of cameras showed that many of the interesting features of the measured temperature change in a material under inspection are within the first few tens of milliseconds of the heating period and, after numerous tests, it was decided that the minimum heating period would be set at 20 ms. Hence a fast frame rate was identified as a critical factor in camera selection, along with excellent thermal sensitivity. After auditioning several cameras for the system, the FLIR SC7500 was chosen for the work. The SC7500 is a Stirling cooled camera with a 320 x 256 array of 1.5 - 5 µm InSb detectors. The camera has a sensitivity of <20 mK and a maximum full frame rate of 383 Hz. The 383 Hz frame rate provides 1 frame every 2.6 ms, thus nearly eight frames are generated within our minimum test period, with the option to increase the frame rate with windowing of the image.

3 PEC Thermography Applications

3.1 Quantification of Defect Detections Limits and the Effects of Defect Orientation

3.1.1 Defect Detection Limit

In this section the sensitivity of this method to defects of different crack size is investigated. Steel, titanium and nickel-based superalloy samples often found in aero engine applications are used in this preliminary study. All of the samples were spray-painted in black acrylic paint to increase the emissivity. A typical dark field thermographic image from a metallic (nickel alloy) part with a fatigue crack can be seen in Fig. 6. In this case, the induced currents are flowing horizontally in the test piece. The crack in the center of the specimen is blocking the flow of the current resulting in an increase in heating at the crack tips (white regions at crack location, Fig. 6) and a decrease at the center of the defect (dark area at crack location, Fig. 6).

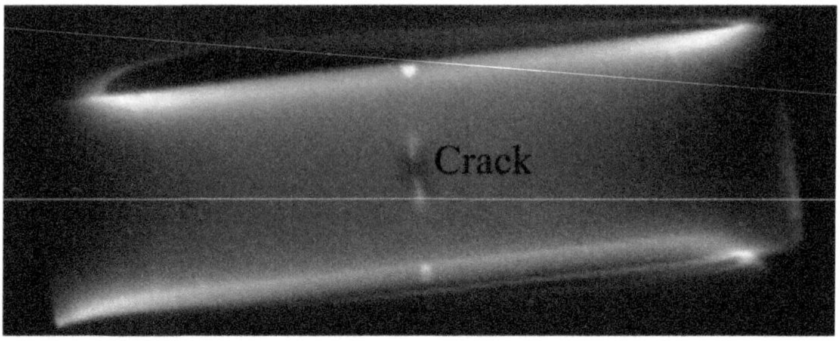

Fig. 6 Thermographic image of a nickel alloy sample with a 6 mm long crack visible at the centre of the specimen; line shows the measured region

Fig. 7a shows an image of a steel sample with a 0.34 mm long fatigue crack present. The defect is hardly visible in the center of this image. In this steel sample only a cold region is visible, compared to the larger defect shown in Fig. 6 where a hot region is also seen. A similar investigation was performed on a steel sample with as slightly larger crack (~ 0.5 mm long). The defect is clearly visible in

Fig. 7b, with a stronger crack signature than in the previous specimen. In this case quite a significant amount of extra heat is observed at the crack tips, while a cold region can be seen at the center of the defect. Again the cold region is more predominant than the hot region. For the last steel sample which was investigated in this set of experiments the defect is clearly visible with a typical crack signature (Fig. 7c). The defect was about 1 mm long generating significant heat at the edge of the defect. The two hot regions at the crack tips and the cold region in the center of the specimen can clearly be seen. Figure 7d shows the image of a titanium alloy sample with the presence of a 0.8 mm long fatigue crack. The crack in that sample is in this case clearly visible. To conclude, the results presented here show that the cold region at the centre of the crack is more indicative of the presence of a defect can than the hot region at the crack tips for small defects.

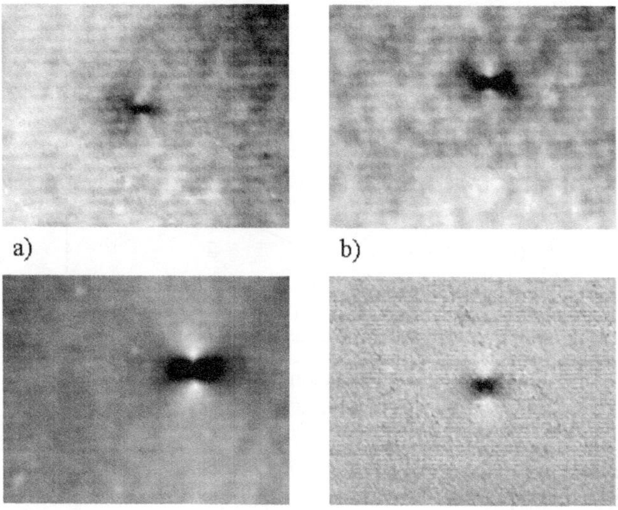

a) b) c) d)

Fig. 7 Thermographic images of steel and titanium samples with fatigue cracks; a) steel sample with 0.34 mm long crack; b) steel with 0.5 mm long crack; c) steel with 1 mm long crack; d) titanium with 0.8 mm long crack

Fatigue cracks in 37 nickel-based superalloy (Waspaloy), 43 titanium 6246 and 25 steel samples were trialed for detectability. Crack lengths ranged from 0.27-5.3 mm in Waspaloy, 0.05-4.2 mm in titanium and 0.23-3.9 mm in steel. The nominal crack lengths were determined optically at 500x magnification for steel, whilst for Waspaloy and titanium the machined surface finish necessitated sizing by dye penetrant inspection (level 4 ultra-high sensitivity post-emulsified fluorescent penetrant to RPS702). Three non-consecutive tests were performed on each test-piece. For Waspaloy and titanium, a frame immediately after the excitation was turned off was considered. Processing was then limited to subtraction of an

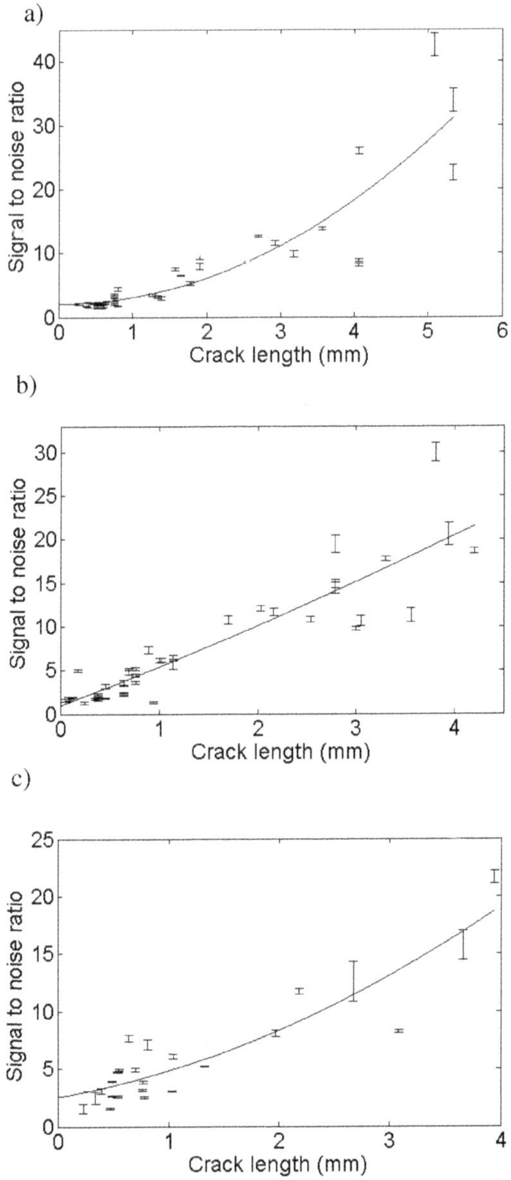

Fig. 8 Measured signal to noise ratios for a range of fatigue cracks in a) nickel superalloy, b) titanium 6246 and c) ferromagnetic steel alloy

average of the pre-excitation frames to form a dark-field image, and spatial median filtering (3x3 kernel). For the steel samples, it was found that a better dark-field image was obtained by subtracting a frame just after the excitation was turned off from a frame of a similar bulk temperature just prior to excitation-off. These frames are only separated by a single frame (e.g., frames 30 and 32, acquisition at 60 Hz) and the defect is only detected in the former (excitation-on) frame. This is because the significant temperature gradient between the neighbouring hot and cold spots of the detection signature (observed to be up to ~11°C), together with the high thermal conductivity of steel causes the detection signature to 'blink' out of existence between frames. Each crack was manually bound within a region of interest box, and the signal taken as the mean of the 10 pixels in the region of interest which deviate furthest from the bulk temperature rise (i.e., hotter or colder than the bulk temperature, response-rectified).

The noise was taken as the standard deviation of a reference area adjacent to the bound area of the crack. The results of these studies are shown in Fig. 8. The smallest manually discernible cracks were ~0.6-0.7 mm in Waspaloy, ~0.4-0.6 mm in titanium and 0.23-0.27 mm in steel. Whilst the temperature rise in steel was significantly higher than that in Waspaloy and titanium, the SNR remained comparable. This was likely in-part due to the finishing quality of the paint applied to the extremely shiny surface of the steel samples. Further, use of frames with the excitation on caused additional noise due to electromagnetic interference with the focal plane array. Repeat tests showed minimal variation in all cases. Some vertical scatter from the best-fit is observed to be a function of the specific detection characteristic, i.e., cracks with point-contacts cause localized hot-spots along the crack-length. Cracks with these additional hot-spots are less strongly detected since the contiguous areas of the hot and cold spots are smaller, supporting lesser deviation from the bulk temperature. Significant horizontal error for Waspaloy and titanium is a consequence of defect sizing by dye-penetrant inspection.

3.1.2 Influence of Crack Orientation

In this section the influence of the crack orientation on the crack signal is reported. A non-ferromagnetic nickel alloy and a ferromagnetic steel sample were used in these investigations. The samples were cut so they could be rotated inside the center of the coil. A 4 mm and an 8 mm long fatigue crack was present in the steel sample and in the nickel alloy sample respectively. In Fig. 9 results are shown for these two samples for various crack angles. Fig. 9a shows an image of the non-ferromagnetic sample with the crack oriented parallel to the induced currents. In this case it is not possible to see the crack. As the angle increases (Fig. 9b, ~45 °) the crack becomes more visible. At an angle of 90 ° (Fig. 9c) where the induced currents flow perpendicular to the crack orientation the crack signature is the strongest.

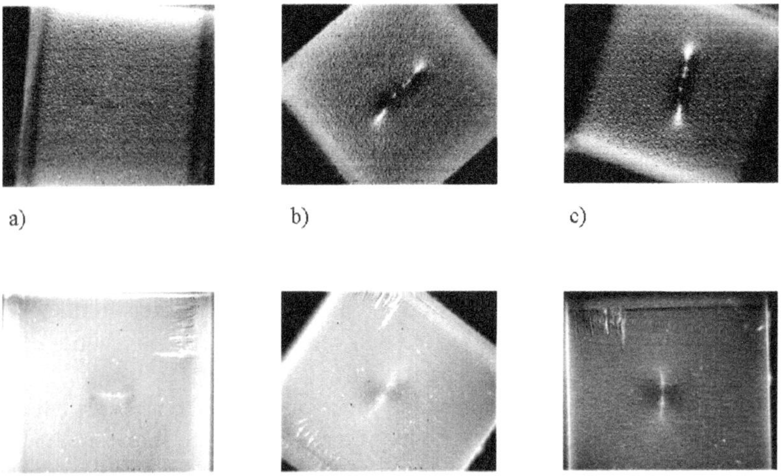

a) b) c)

d) e) f)

Fig. 9 Comparison of thermographic images for non-ferromagnetic and ferromagnetic specimen with defects present (8 mm and 4 mm long crack resp.) at different angles relative induced currents; non-ferromagnetic: a) 0 °; b) ~ 45 °; c) 90 °; ferromagnetic: d) 0 °; e) ~ 45°; f) 90 °

In contrast to the non-ferromagnetic sample, the crack is clearly visible for currents parallel to the crack orientation in the ferromagnetic material (Fig. 9d). This is due to the added heating effect caused by magnetic flux leakage at the crack boundary. The heating pattern at the crack is slightly different from a typical crack signature (Fig. 6), with observed heating along the whole boundary of the crack. As the angle increases (Fig. 9e) the crack signature becomes slightly stronger, its shape changes with a cold region in the center of the crack and line heating along the ends of the crack. For the case when the crack is perpendicular to the induced currents the crack can be seen clearly (Fig. 9f). The SNR was calculated for different crack angles (0-90 °) for these two samples. Results from these calculations can be seen in the Figure 10. Figure 10a shows the SNR as a function of the crack angle in the non-ferromagnetic nickel alloy sample. An angle of 90 ° corresponds to a crack which is perpendicular to the induced currents and 0 ° for a crack parallel to the induced currents. It can be seen that for 0 ° the SNR is very low, showing no heating (Fig. 9a). This suggests that a crack with this orientation cannot be detected in non-ferromagnetic material. From the SNR value it can be seen that a crack with an orientation of about 30° would most probably be detected with the current setup. As the crack angle increases even more the SNR value increases until about 70 ° where its value (~16) stays almost constant.

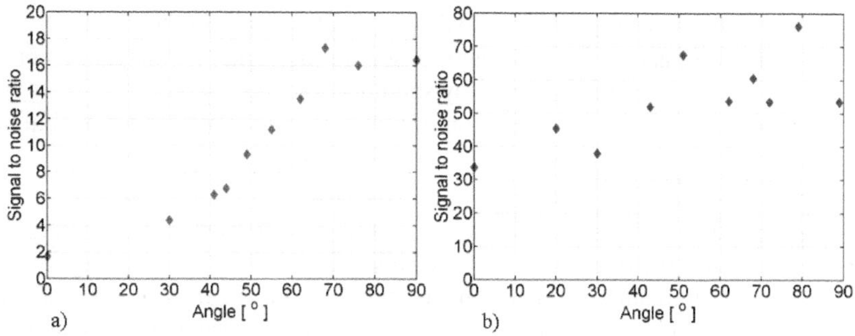

Fig. 10 Measured signal to noise ratios for a) non-ferromagnetic nickel alloy sample and b) ferromagnetic steel alloy sample

Fig. 10b shows the results for a similar investigation performed on the ferromagnetic steel sample. It can be seen that there is quite a variation in the measurements. This was most probably caused by the experimental variation in the different measurements. The SNR value for a crack parallel to the induced currents is about 50 % of its value at about 90°. This is in quite good agreement with results presented by Walle et al. [13] for a similar study. To conclude, a crack parallel to the induced currents can be detected in ferromagnetic material (Fig. 9d), but not in non-ferromagnetic material (Fig. 9a). As discussed in [15], For ferrous metals like iron and some types of steel, there is an additional heating mechanism that takes place at the same time as the eddy currents mentioned above. The intense alternating magnetic field inside the work coil repeatedly magnetises and demagnetises the iron crystals. This rapid flipping of the magnetic domains causes considerable friction and heating inside the material. Heating due to this mechanism is known as Hysteresis loss, and is greatest for materials that have a large area inside their B-H curve. This can be a large contributing factor to the heat generated during induction heating, but only takes place inside ferrous materials.

3.2 Detection of Multiple Complex Cracks in Rail Track

3.2.1 Rolling Contact Fatigue (RCF) Cracks

Since the introduction of the steel rail to rail transport systems around 150 years ago, much work has been carried out to perfect manufacturing processes to minimise defects introduced during fabrication and to aid the detection of in-service defects. The dominant mode of failure in early steel rails was transverse defects initiating from internal fissures caused by uneven cooling after hot rolling, but the introduction of retarded cooling processes has minimised the occurrence of these types of defects [16]. Faults found in modern rails can be classified in three groups:

- Faults originating from manufacturing defects. Such as tache oval or kidney defects originating from hydrogen shatter cracks in the rail head.
- Faults originating from damage caused during handling, installation or use, i.e. wheelburn defects caused by spinning wheels.
- Faults caused by the exhaustion of the steel's resistance to fatigue damage, i.e. gauge corner cracking initiated from rolling contact fatigue.

During the last two decades the incidences of failure from defects initiating from surface cracks on the running surface of rails due to rolling contact fatigue (RCF) has increased dramatically [17]. The reason for this is mainly due increased stresses on rails due to high speed trains, more frequent usage and increased axle load for goods vehicles (in Australia axle loads of 37t have been reported [16]). But the improved resistance to wear of modern steels has also contributed to the increase in surface defects; in the past the wear on rails was so great that surface defects were effectively removed through normal usage, but modern steels are so resistant to abrasion that material wear is no longer sufficient to prevent the growth of cracks in the rail surface [18]. Surface defects can to some extent be addressed by surface grinding [19], but in order to carry out an effective programme of maintenance, an effective and sufficiently frequent programme of surface condition assessment must be carried out [20].

The most high profile incident of rail failure due to RCF in the UK was the Hatfield train derailment on Tuesday 17 October 2000, where four passengers were killed and over seventy people were injured. The Hatfield derailment occurred when an outer rail in a 1500m radius curve shattered over a length of tens of metres under a passenger train travelling at about 185 km/h [21]. A 2006 report by Health and Safety carried out under the supervision of an independent Investigation Board [21], found that the "fracture and fragmentation of the rail was due primarily to extensive fatigue cracking", due to RCF, "initiated at or near the surface of the rail head due to high contact stresses at the wheel/rail interface". The report found that "in many cases, these surface initiated fatigue cracks developed into deep transverse (downward) cracks, which severely weakened the rail." It was also found that "grain boundary ferrite in the surface layer of the rail running surface probably acted as initiation sites for rolling contact fatigue cracks." [22] Despite the section of rail being ground at some point between its manufacture in 1995 and the derailment in 2000, over 300 cracks were found at the site, leading to an extensive programme of rail inspection in the UK, and consequently much disruption to the UK train service.

Previous work [4] has shown that angular defects such as those found in RCF constitute a very specific set of circumstances as far as PEC thermography is concerned. Fig. 11 illustrates the phenomena; the angle of the defect causes a modification of the eddy current distribution in the sample, leading to a buildup of eddy currents in the corner of the slot (see area marked as heat source in Fig. 11a). This area experiences increased levels of Joule heating, much greater than would typically be found around a straight defect in the same sample. Because the area is bounded by the defect, the heat is trapped between the slot and the surface and propagates through this bounded area over time (see simulation result in Fig. 11b).

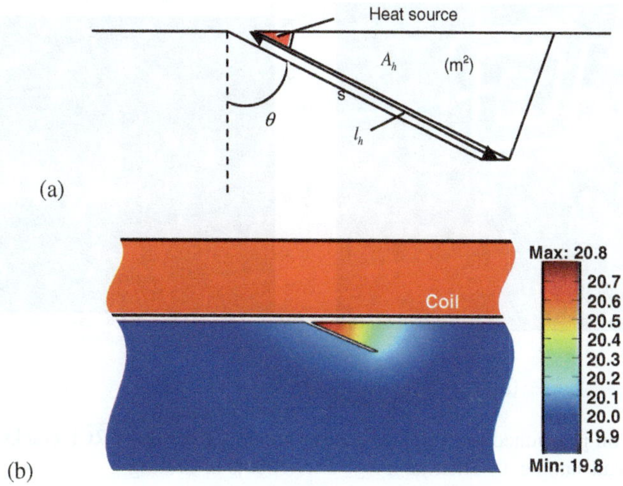

Fig. 11 a) Illustration of an angular slot inside a sample, where θ is the slot angle, b) Simulated heat distribution after 100ms of heating from cross section view for a 67.5° angular slot.

The result of this process is a characteristic heat distribution at the surface which changes over time. It starts with an intense level of heating at the corner of the defect in the early stages, which manifests itself as a thin line of heating conforming to the shape of the defect opening. At this stage, shallow and deep defects of a similar angle present a very similar surface heat distribution and multiple defects can be identified. As the heating time continues, the heat spreads out into the area bounded by the defect, leading to a spreading of the heat at the surface in the defect angle direction. At this point, deeper defects begin to dominate. After the cessation of heating, the material starts to cool; heat is retained in the areas bounded by the defect, with larger defects retaining more heat. For multiple defects, this has the effect that after a short time only larger defects are evident.

3.2.2 Multiple Defect Mapping

In the experiment shown in Fig. 12, a square coil is positioned normal to the sample surface, near the edge of the rail head (Fig. 12a), where the RCF induced cracking is known to be concentrated. This configuration mimics a line inductor, with localised heating in the area under the coil. Fig. 12b shows the thermal image captured by the IR camera after 100ms of heating which discloses the presence of defects at the edge of the rail head. The presence of the cracks is made visible through the increase in temperature at the crack edges, resulting from the diversion of the induced eddy currents which conforms to the shape of the cracks to complete it path. This shows the effectiveness of the PEC thermography technique in detecting the presence of multiple defects through the visualisation and mapping of the resulting temperature distribution from the eddy current interaction with defects.

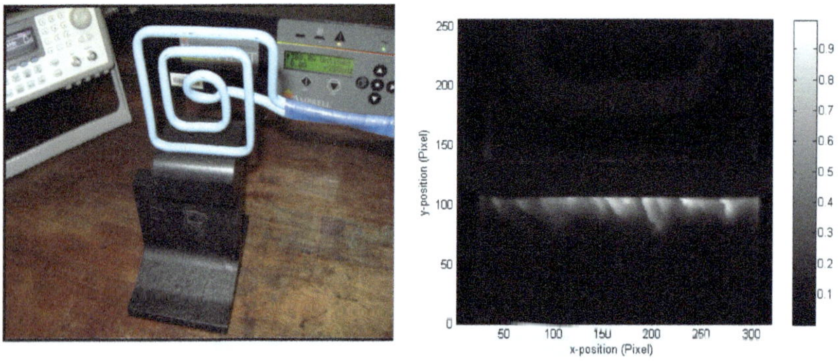

(a) (b)

Fig. 12 a) Coil positioned for localised heating for the detection of RCF cracks at the edge of the rail head sample, b) Thermal image after 100ms of heating

Fig. 13 illustrate the change in the type of defect that become evident at different times in the heating cycle. It can be seen from the figure that the change in heat distribution with time follows this pattern:

- Early stage heating: Fine network of cracks visible with similar amplitude for shallow and deep cracks
- Late stage heating: Deeper (and more acute angle) cracks result in greater heating at surface. The result is that the deeper cracks dominate the heat distribution, though the heat generated from the shallower cracks is still evident and is superimposed on the larger heating gradients caused by deeper cracks.
- Cooling stage: Only very deep/acute cracks evident.

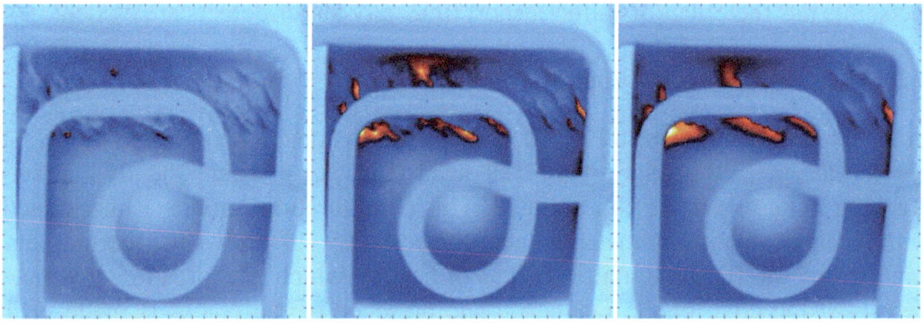

(a) (b) (c)

Fig. 13 Change in heat distribution with time; a) Early stage heating, b) Late stage heating, c) Cooling

3.2.2 Transient Analysis for Defect Quantification

Fig. 14 shows the transient temperature change in two positions on the sample surface:

- Pos 1: Over a deep defect, with a large temperature change.
- Pos 2: Over a shallower defect with a smaller temperature change.

It can be seen from Fig. 14b that the transient temperature change supports the observations in the previous section; in the early stages of heating, both defects cause a similar change in temperature at the surface, but as heating continues the rate of change of temperature for the shallower defect decreases, whereas the rate of change in temperature for the deeper defect stays roughly the same. A similar thing can be observed in the cooling period, where the shallower defect cools much more quickly than the deeper one.

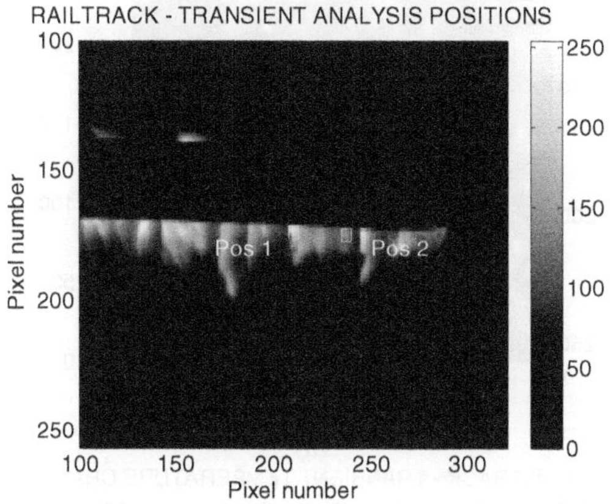

(a)

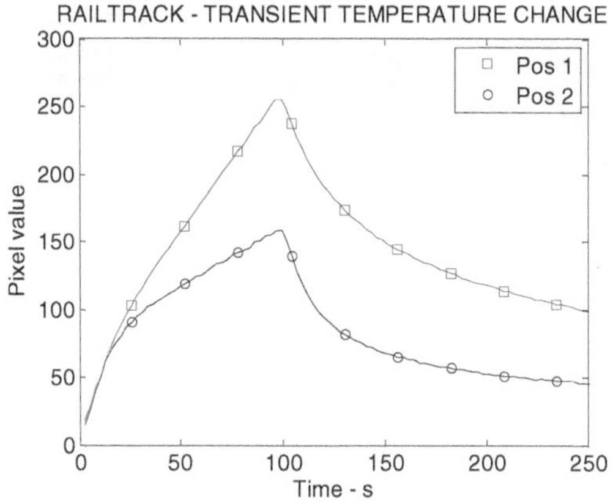

(b)

Fig. 14 a) Transient analysis positions, b) Transient temperature change with time in selected positions

Fig. 15 shows the transient temperature change in four positions moving away from the opening of a large angular defect in the rail head. As might be expected, as we move away from the opening of the crack, the surface heats up less quickly and consequently reaches a lower maximum temperature. However, it can be seen from the plot that areas away from the opening of the crack retain more heat in the cooling period. If we relate this back to the explanation pertaining to figure 5, in the cooling period, the areas away from the crack opening are kept warm by heat propagating from the area of increased eddy current density in the corner of the crack.

By comparison of Fig. 14and Fig. 15, it is clear that although a shallow defect and an area some distance from a deep, acutely angled defect can result in a similar overall level of heating, the transient change in temperature follows a very

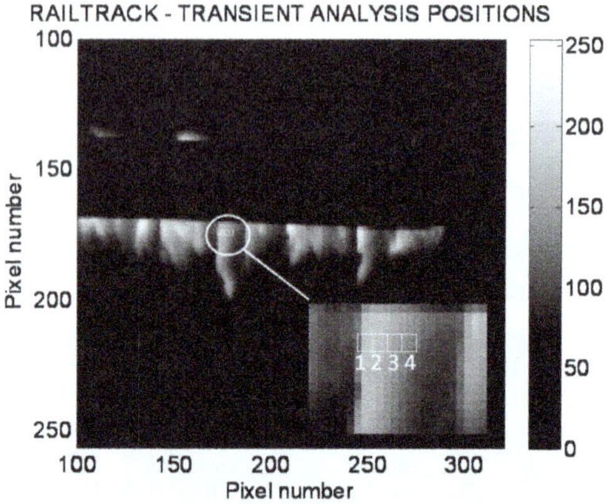

(a)

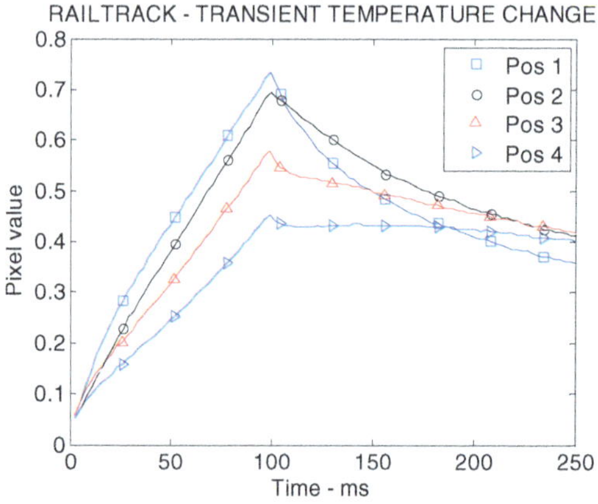

(b)

Fig. 15 Difference in transient temperature change moving away from a deep defect (Pos. 1 is closest to the crack and Pos. 4 is furthest away); a) Transient analysis positions, b) Transient temperature change with time in selected positions

different course. These different characteristics of the transient temperature change clearly have the potential to provide a solution to the inverse problem and allow defect geometry to be determined to some extent.

3.3 Composite Materials

In this section, the results of a set of tests carried out on samples made from carbon fibre reinforced plastic (CFRP) provided by Exel Composites are presented. The size of the CFRP samples is approximately 350 mm × 38 mm × 6 mm. The sample used in these tests contains a number of machined notches with varying depth, introduced to simulate the presence of surface breaking cracks. PEC thermography is proposed as a new inspection technique, allowing the users to observe the eddy current distribution in a structure using infrared imaging,

The sample was inspected using the system previously described and shown in Fig. 5, A heating period of 200ms was chosen empirically, as the shortest heating time which provides sufficient thermal contrast to perform a thorough analysis of the transient temperature change in the material. The rectangular coil shown in Fig. 12a was supplied with and excitation waveform with a frequency of 256 kHz and current of 380 A_{rms}. Images were acquired for a total of 500 ms (200 ms heating followed by 300 ms cooling) at the maximum frame rate of 383 fps.

3.3.1 Directional Conductivity Experiment

As CFRP exhibits directional conductivity, dependent on the fiber orientation in the composite, coil orientation has a large impact on experimental results. Thus before inspecting the sample for defects, the directional conductivity is first ascertained. This allows optimisation of excitation direction and notch direction to achieve the best temperature contrast between defected regions and healthy regions.

Two coil orientations with respect to the sample surface; horizontal (Fig. 16a) and vertical (Fig. 16b), are investigated. For horizontal coil orientation, the eddy currents are flowing in a horizontal direction, hence, the conductivity of Exel sample in horizontal direction is investigated in this case. For vertical coil direction, the conductivity of Exel sample in vertical direction is tested.

Fig. 16a and Fig. 16b show the thermal image in terms of digital level (DL) at 2 second heating using horizontal and vertical coil directions respectively. From the comparison of these two excitation directions, it can be seen that the increase in temperature at the sample surface with the coil orientated vertically is much greater than when the coil is orientated horizontally. According to Eq. (1), it can be concluded that the conductivity in the vertical direction is much larger than that in horizontal direction, thus it can be ascertained that the fibre orientation is in the vertical direction, since conductivity is greater along the fibre orientation. With awareness of the fibre orientation, the coil orientation is fixed in the vertical direction in the following experiments.

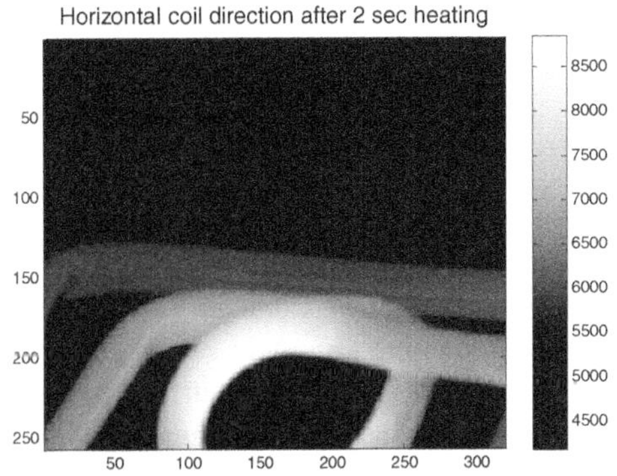

(a)

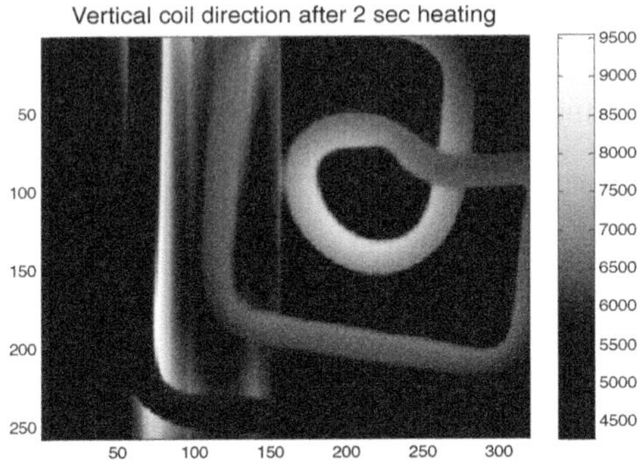

(b)

Fig. 16 Thermal image of sample at maximum heating for: (a) horizontal current excitation; (b) vertical current excitation

3.3.2 Influence of Notch Depth

Notches with differing depths were inspected while retaining the same positional relationship between notch and coil. As an example the thermal image at the maximum heating time for a 2mm deep notch is shown in Fig. 17. The transient temperature change at the same point at the notch bottom and close to the coil is investigated. The simulation and experimental thermal responses for varied notch depths are shown in and Fig. 18 and Fig. 19. From the comparison of the thermal responses at the investigated point for the three notches shown in Fig. 18 and Fig. 19, it can be ascertained that the deeper the notch is, the higher the increase in temperature, when notch depth is smaller than skin depth, as is the case here. The relationship between notch depth and transient temperature change from experimental results has agreement with that from simulation results illustrated in Fig. 18. From Fig. 18b and Fig. 19b, we can find the amplitude of temperature rise for the deeper notch is the larger due to the highest eddy current density at the notch bottom. From the comparison of the normalised transient temperature behaviours

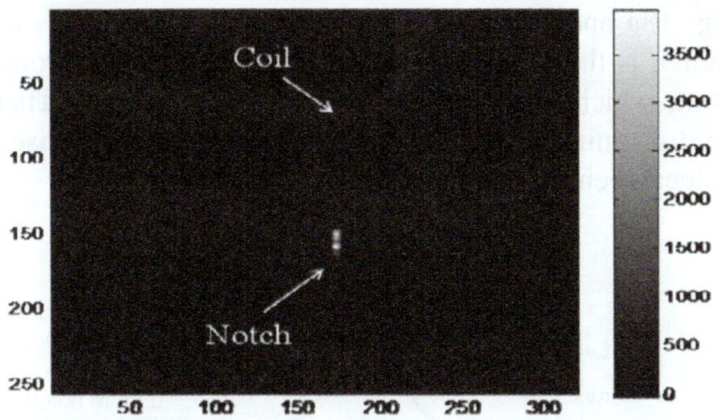

Fig. 17 Experimental results for 2mm deep and 1mm wide notch; thermal image at the maximum heating time of 200ms, unit: digital level

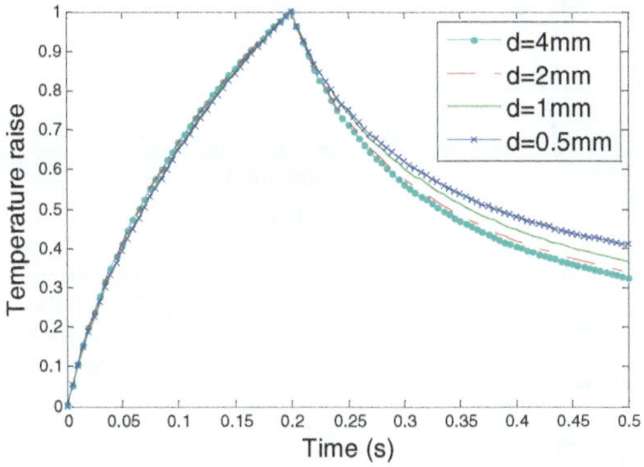

(a)

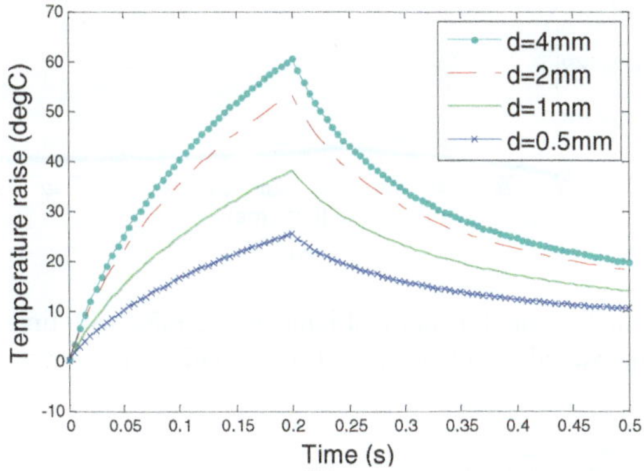

(b)

Fig. 18 Simulation results for transient temperature with time at notch bottom for varied notch depth at notch width *w*=1mm: (a) normalised responses; (b) non-normalised (raw) responses

shown in Fig. 18a and Fig. 19a, we can see that temperature decay rate for the 2mm deep notch is the largest due to the smallest distance from notch bottom to sample bottom, which leads to a faster temperature decay. Therefore, the notch depth can be discriminated by the amplitude of temperature rise and the transient temperature decay behaviour.

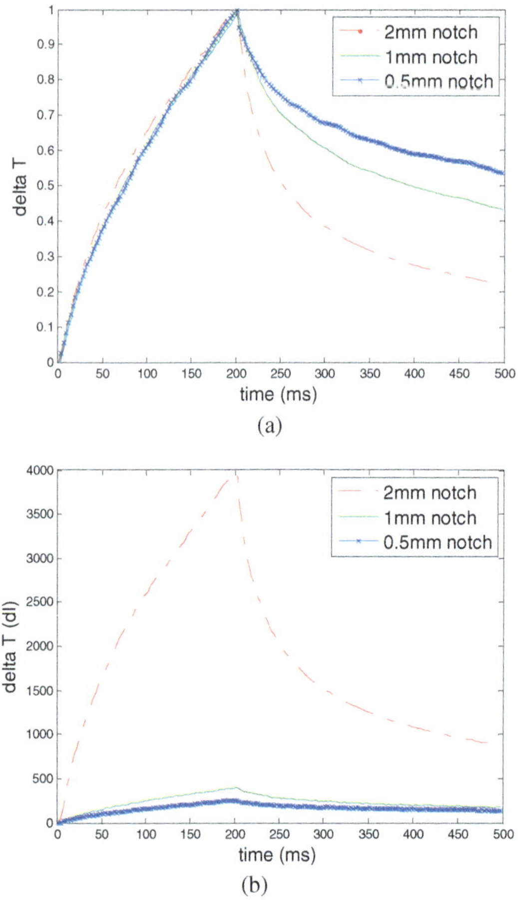

Fig. 19. Experimental results for transient temperature raise with time at notch bottom for width w=1mm and varied depth notches: (a) normalised responses; (b) non-normalised (raw) responses

3.3.4. Influence of Notch Width

As the simulation results presented in the previous section closely agree with the experimental results, it is feasible to use simulation to predict the impact of notch width on thermal response. The relationship between transient temperature change and notch width w is shown in Fig. 20b, where the figure indicates that the maximum amplitude of the temperature change increases as notch width w becomes smaller. It implies that the narrower notch will force eddy currents to divert around a narrower area at the notch bottom. Thus a narrower notch leads to larger temperature rise (seen in Fig. 20b), as well as a greater rate of change in temperature in the early stages of the heating phase (see Fig. 20a). In addition, it is clear that investigation after normalisation of the temperature curve, shown in Fig. 20a has some advantages in the analysis of the signal. The results also indicate that a narrower notch has a faster temperature decay in the cooling phase.

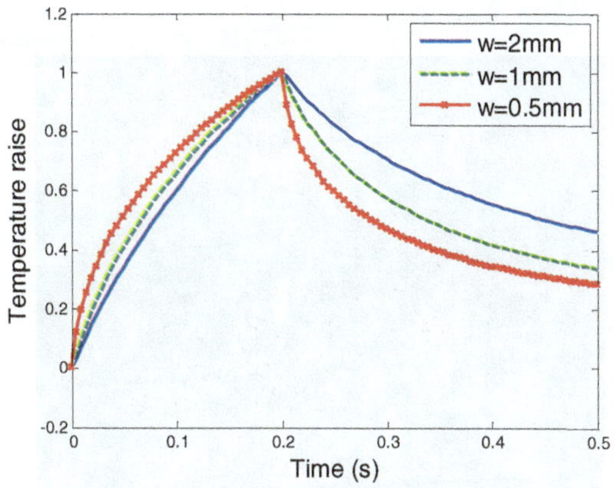

(a)

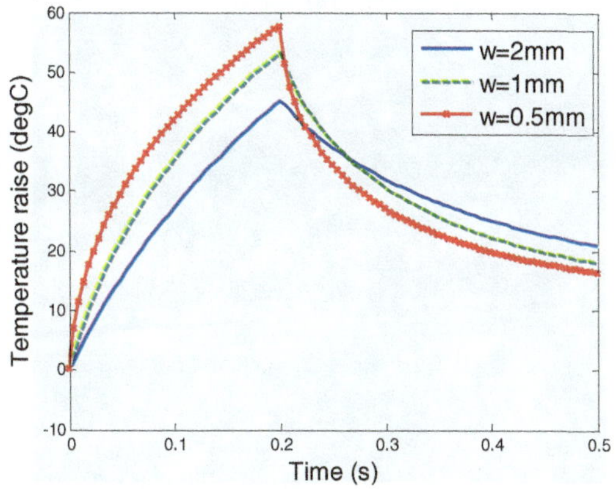

(b)

Fig. 20 Simulation results for transient temperature with time at notch bottom for varied notch width at notch depth d=2mm: (a) normalised responses; (b) non-nomalised (raw) responses

3.3.5 Notch Position Invariants along Fibre Orientation

The variation in thermal response when the notch position with respect to the coil along the fibre orientation is increased is investigated in this section. As the fibre orientation is identified in section 3.3.1, in this experiment, the notch is moved only horizontally along the fibre orientation, shown in Fig. 21. Thermal videos are captured at different notch positions with respect to the coil. A 1 mm wide and 2 mm deep notch is tested in this experiment. When the distance between the coil and 2mm notch is increased to 8cm, the heating on the notch can still be seen, but the temperature rise is less than one third for the 2cm coil-notch distance, shown in Figs. 21a and 21b. To compare the influence of notch location, 0 cm, 2 cm and 8 cm coil-notch distances are tested. The normalised and non-normalised thermal responses at the notch bottom are shown in Fig. 22.

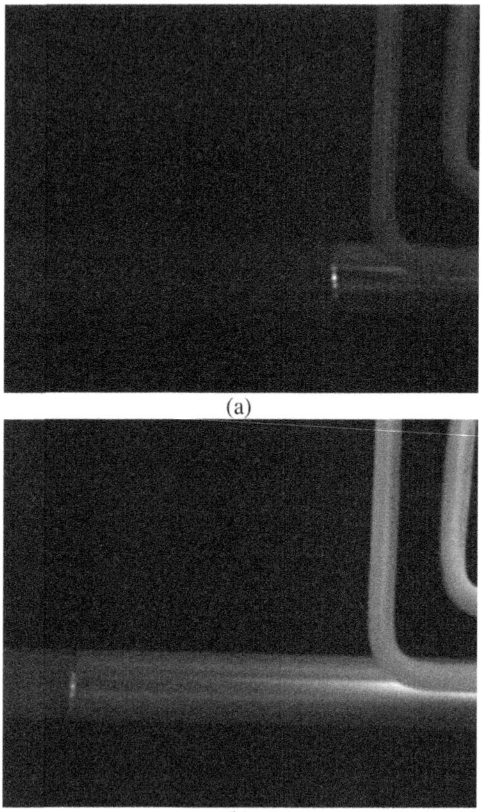

(a)

(b)

Fig. 21 Varied distance between the coil and 2mm deep notch: excitation current in length direction: (a) 2cm coil-notch distance; (b) 8cm coil-notch distance.

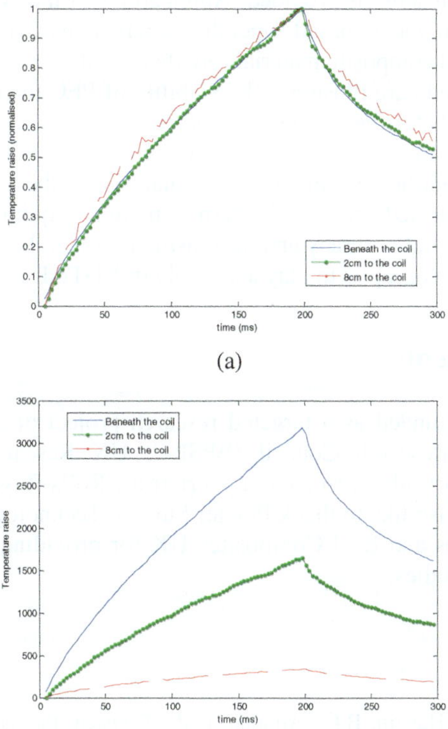

(a)

(b)

Fig. 22 Thermal response at notch bottom versus distance between coil and notch: (a) Normalised responses; (b) non-normalised (raw) responses.

From the results, the location of notch only influences the maximum amplitude of the temperature rise in the heating phase, seen in Fig. 22b. The temperature rise and decay rate after the normalisation is not affected shown in Fig. 22a, because the notch shape and dimensions are not changed. Therefore, the transient temperature change with time at varied notch positions during both heating and cooling is not changed.

Unfortunately, the time delay of thermal or eddy current propagation from the region beneath the coil to the notch cannot be observed in thermal videos, because the propagation velocities of the thermal wave and eddy currents are in the order of 10^3 and 10^8 m/s respectively. The time delay of either thermal wave or eddy current is much shorter than the minimum detectable time interval from the thermal camera (2.6 ms).

4 Conclusions

In this paper, the design, development and application of a pulsed eddy current thermography system is reported. The introduction of modelling, simulation and experimental system setup is provided. Applications of the systems for defect detections for titanium, nickel based superalloys, ferritic material and rail-track with multiple defects and composite materials are discussed.

The work reported here illustrates the viability of PEC thermography to inspect a variety of materials for the presence of defects such as cracks and delaminations. The technique is an attractive one, as it offers real time imaging of defects coupled with scope for quantitative work through analysis of the transient temperature change over the affected area. With thermal imaging equipment simultaneously increasing in speed and accuracy and decreasing in price, the authors of this chapter expect PEC thermography to play a key role in NDT&E in the future.

Acknowledgements

This research was funded as a targeted research project of the Engineering and Physical Science Research Council (EPSRC) UK Research Centre in NDE (RCNDE). The work also received support from Rolls-Royce plc. and Alstom Power. We would also like to thank Praxair Surface Technologies, Inc. for coating nickel alloy samples and Exel Composites UK for providing the CFRP samples for experimental studies.

References

1. Avdelidis, N.P., Hawtin, B.C., Almond, D.P.: Transient thermography in the assessment of defects of aircraft composites. NDT&E International 36(6), 433–439 (2003)
2. Hung, Y.Y., Chen, Y.S., Ng, S.P., Liu, L., Huang, Y.H., Luk, B.L., Ip, R.W.L., Wu, C.M.L., Chung, P.S.: Review and comparison of shearography and active thermography for nondestructive evaluation. Materials Science and Engineering: R: Reports 64(5-6), 73–112 (2009)
3. Nino, G.F., Ahmed, T.J., Bersee, H.E.N., Beukers, A.: Thermal NDI of resistance welded composite structures. Composites Part B: Engineering 40(3), 237–248 (2009)
4. Abidin, I.Z., Tian, G.Y., Wilson, J., Yang, S., Almond, D.: Quantitative evaluation of angular defects by pulsed eddy current thermography. NDT & E International 43(7), 537–546 (2010)
5. Zöcke, C.M.: Quantitative analysis of defects in composite material by means of optical lockin thermography, Dr. Ing. Dissertation, Saarbrucker Reihe Materialwissenschaft Und Werkstofftechnik (December 2009)
6. Morbidini, M., Cawley, P.: The detectability of cracks using sonic IR. Journal of Applied Physics 105(9), 093530–93530-9 (2009)
7. Vrana, J., Goldammer, M., Baumann, J., Rothenfusser, M., Arnold, W.: Mechanisms and models for crack detection with induction thermography. In: 34th Annual Review of Progress in Quantitative Nondestructive Evaluation. AIP Conference Proceedings, vol. 975, pp. 475–482 (2008)
8. Wilson, J., Tian, G.Y., Abidin, I.Z., Yang, S., Almond, D.: Modelling and evaluation of eddy current stimulated thermography. Nondestructive Testing and Evaluation 25(3), 205–218 (2010)

9. Zenzinger, G., Bamberg, J., Dumm, M., Nutz, P.: Crack Detection Using Eddytherm. In: Thompson, D.O., Chimenti, D.E. (eds.) CP760, Review of Quantitative Nondestructive Evaluation, vol. 760, pp. 1646–1653. American Institute of Physics, New York (2005)
10. Netzelmann, U., Walle, G.: Induction Thermography as a Tool for Reliable Detection of Surface Defects in Forged Components. In: 17th World Conference on Nondestructive Testing, Shanghai, China, October 25–28 (2008)
11. Oswald-Tranta, B., Wally, G.: Thermo-inductive surface crack detection in metallic materials. In: ECNDT 2006, Berlin, Paper Number We.3.8.3 (2006)
12. Wally, G., Oswald-Tranta, B.: The Influence of Crack Shapes and Geometries on the Results of the Thermo-Inductive Crack Detection. In: Proc. SPIE, vol. 6541, p. 11 (2007)
13. Walle, G., Netzelmann, U.: Thermographic Crack Detection in Ferritic Steel Components Using Inductive Heating. In: ECNDT 2006, Berlin, Paper No. Tu.4.8.5 (2006)
14. Zenzinger, G., Bamberg, J., Satzger, W., Carl, V.: Thermographic Crack Detection in Ferritic Steel Components Using Inductive Heating. In: ECNDT 2006 Tu.4.8.5 (2006)
15. `http://www.richieburnett.co.uk/indheat.html`
16. Cannon, D.F., Edel, K.O., Grassie, S.L., Sawley, K.: Rail defects: an overview. Fatigue & Fracture of Engineering Materials & Structures 26(10), 865–886 (2003)
17. Hesse, D., Cawley, P.: Excitation of Surface Wave Modes in Rails and their Application for Defect Detection. In: AIP Conf. Proc., vol. 820, pp. 1593–1600 (March 2006)
18. Pohl, R., Erhard, A., Montag, H.-J., Thomas, H.-M., Wüstenberg, H.: NDT techniques for railroad wheel and gauge corner inspection. NDT & E International 37(2), 89–94 (2004)
19. Wang, W.J., Guo, J., Liu, Q.Y., Zhu, M.H., Zhou, Z.R.: Study on relationship between oblique fatigue crack and rail wear in curve track and prevention. Wear 267(1-4), 540–544 (2009)
20. Grassie, S.L.: Rolling contact fatigue on the British railway system: treatment. Wear 258(7-8), 1310–1318 (2005)
21. Office of Rail Regulation, Train Derailment at Hatfield: A final Report by the Independent Investigation Board (July 2006), `http://www.rail-reg.gov.uk/upload/pdf/297.pdf` (accessed October 2010)
22. Garnham, J.E., Davis, C.L.: Very Early Stage Rolling Contact Fatigue Crack Growth in Pearlitic Rail Steels 27(1-2), 100–112 (2011)

The Use of Optical Fibre Sensors in Dam Monitoring

Ian Platt, Michael Hagedorn, and Ian Woodhead

Lincoln Ventures Limited
platti@lvl.co.nz

1 Introduction

The building and maintenance of dams can require considerable investment for any country, organization or individual. Depending upon its size and use, dam failure may result in significant damage to the environment and economy or in the case of unexpected catastrophic failure the loss of life. These issues have been well understood for thousands of years over which design has evolved with the advent of new materials and the increased water demand that push dams to become larger and more numerous. While various forms of monitoring have been in place for as long as dams have been built, the development of mechanical and electronic sensors enables an increasingly more thorough and accurate measurement of dam parameters, such as strain (e.g. for structural members), water level, water pressure and temperature.

Such devices however are still point monitoring sensors that often require specialized housing and communication paths, limiting their deployment and thus overall effectiveness. With the development of optical fibre technology, sensors either embedded into the line of the fibre or as branches to it allow the possibility of deploying a large number of sensor points on a single fibre. The advantages of optical fibre sensing are many [10] [18] including, 1) inertness to extraneous environmental factors (e.g. moisture, most naturally occurring chemicals, electromagnetic fields etc.), 2) potentially small cross section (minimal interference to structural integrity), 3) low signal attenuation over large distances together with high bandwidth enable large numbers of sensors to be multiplexed over distances of, potentially many kilometres, 4) the low cost of the fibre itself. The cost of the associated monitoring equipment, while relatively expensive in the past, is rapidly reducing as the technology becomes more prolific and 5) much of the progress in optical fibre sensing technology is due to advances from the highly funded field of communications technology.

As with the development of most technology in the field of Structural Health Monitoring (SHM) it is the current disadvantages that impede mass uptake into industry. While these disadvantages continue to be diminished with ongoing research and development some of the most important ones include 1) sensitivity to many different parameters. This sensitivity to everything can often make it difficult to extract signal relating to the required observable. For example the spectral shift observed from Bragg gratings is

S.C. Mukhopadhyay (Ed.): New Developments in Sensing Technology for SHM, LNEE 96, pp. 233–251.
springerlink.com

the same for both strain and temperature changes on the grating, 2) placement of the sensor so that it measures the required parameter. For example to measure strain on a structural component the strain must be transferred to the fibre directly and not lost in the fixing material. As a consequence the fixing method invariably increases the size of the sensor and much of its small cross sectional advantage is lost. This is of course a problem with most other sensors measuring similar parameters, and 3) cost of the monitoring equipment. Though the cost of equipment is diminishing rapidly there is still a significant outlay for many of the types of optical sensors proposed for SHM.

This work discusses the types of Optical Fibre Sensors (OFS) most commonly available and their use in monitoring some aspects of dam structure integrity. Sections 2 and 3 begin by a brief review of both the operating principles behind some OFS used in SHM and the types of dams in which they may be employed. Section 4 looks at existing OFS dam monitoring systems and those under development, while Section 5 introduces the Finite Difference Time Domain (FDTD) technique for modelling the expected performance of several new Bragg fibre configurations.

2 Optical Fibre Sensors

A detailed description behind the physics of guided light propagation is beyond the scope of the text and for the interested reader works by either [14] or [10] provide an excellent technical introduction. There are many different types of optical sensors and only those that are commonly used for the types of measurands specific to the SHM of dams are discussed here. A basic picture of the main types of fibre sensors available for this application and their major detection parameter is given in Table 1. In this table the distributable ability of the sensors is described as follows. Distributive sensing is defined as the ability to extract measurements of the required parameter anywhere along the fibre. In these cases the whole fibre itself is the sensor and no special attachments are required. The methods used here are the material scattering modes, which either involve scattering from inhomogeneity within the fibre material (Rayleigh scattering) or result from the light field interaction at a molecular or atomic level of the fibre material (Raman and Brillouin scattering). In either case some of the incident signal is scattered backward or forward from which the required parameter is inferred. On the other end of the scale, point sensors are those defined as usually being at the end of some path along which the signal is carried to the interrogation equipment. Such sensors have one sensor per fibre. Quasi-distributive sensors are really many point sensors along the one fibre and are usually interrogated by isolating their position by time of flight of the light pulse (Optical Time Domain Reflectometry – OTDR) or in the case of Bragg Grating frequency encoding.

A considerable amount of OFS work has been directed towards the health monitoring of structural systems where a rigid structural member is used (e.g. bridges, buildings, [5] [9]) and concrete dams have benefited from some of this

Table 1 OFS types and their properties. Note that only the major measurands influencing the fibre are represented. For example, Bragg, interferometer and Brillouin devices can be arranged to measure pressure by altering the mechanical design. The * indicates that it is relatively straightforward to adapt the sensor for this measurement.

Sensor Type	Bragg Grating	Interferometer Interferometer	Rayleigh Scattering	Raman Scattering	Brillouin Scattering
	Quasi Distributive	Point	Distributive	Distributive	Distributive
Internal (Intrinsic)	Intrinsic/Extrinsic	Intrinsic/Extrinsic	Intrinsic	Intrinsic	Intrinsic
Strain	y	y	y		y
Temperature	y	*	y	y	y
Pressure	*	*			
Displacement	*	y			

structural, or strain, monitoring development. Surprisingly little research has been conducted in the geotechnical area however, where monitoring different types of movement and seepage in rock or compact soil are important. A look at the next section will show that while strain in rigid structural members is important for dams, equally important (certainly in the case of embankment dams) is the monitoring of strain in fill material and seepage of water flow through and under the dam. Measuring strain in non-rigid structures requires a different approach to those in structural members and seepage can best be monitored via water pressure or temperature changes within the wall.

The two measurands that are naturally measured by most fibre sensors are temperature and strain (Table 1). In fact one of the most common problems in both Bragg, some interferometers and Brillouin based sensors is the difficulty in uncoupling the two. While Bragg grating sensors have received the most attention over the years in developing the ability of OFS to monitor these two parameters, they are still point sensors that usually require considerable modification to the fibre line. As the optical fibre technology advances researchers can realize the benefits of fully distributive sensing where the unmodified fibre itself is the sensor. Thus there is a growing trend towards development of fully distributed sensors and while there are still difficulties to be overcome, particularly in spatial resolution and temperature/strain coupling when deployed in real structures, it is growing more likely that they will be the long term future of optical fibre sensing.

In the remainder of this section the operation of the main type of fibre sensors that have been used (or show potential to be used) in dam structures is discussed. While there are many variants in both construction and fibre composition the underlying physical principles remain similar for the mechanical and temperature type optical sensors used for this type of civil engineering structure.

2.1 Fibre Bragg Gratings (FBG)

The operation of a typical short period grating can be described by reference to figure 1.

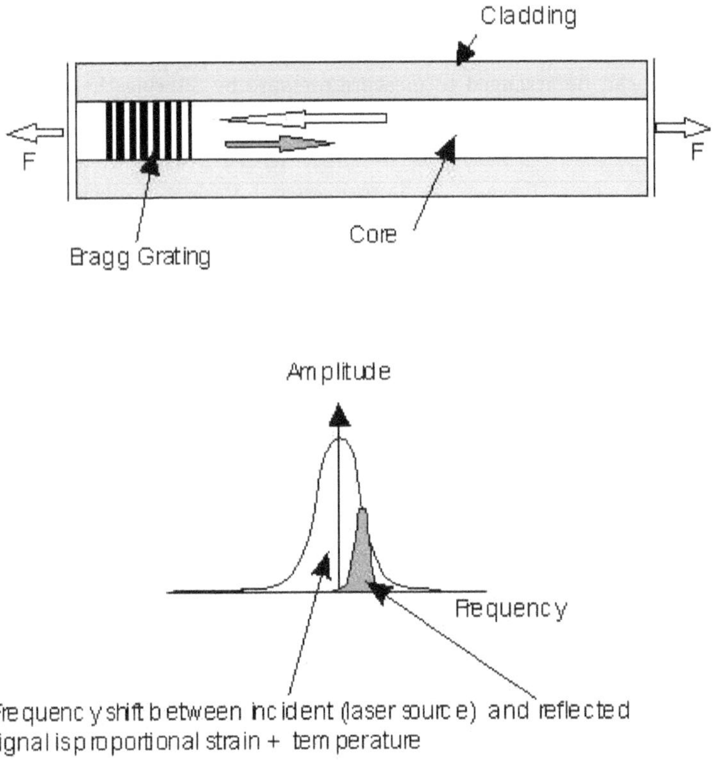

Fig. 1 Bragg grating sensor

When force is applied to either end of the fibre containing the Bragg grating, the spacing between the Bragg lines is increased resulting in a slight frequency shift of the reflected signal. The spacing between the Bragg lines given in terms of wavelength λ_G is related to the backscattered wavelength λ_B by:

$$\lambda_B = 2n\lambda_G \tag{1}$$

Where n is the refractive index of the fibre core. The change in the backscattered wavelength due to both strain and temperature can be given by [10] as:

$$\delta\lambda_B = 2n\lambda_G[(1 - \frac{n^2}{2}(P_{12} - v(P_{11} + P_{12})))\delta\epsilon + (\alpha + \frac{1}{n}\frac{dn}{dT})\delta T] \tag{2}$$

Where P_{11} and P_{12} are components of the fibre strain tensor, $\delta\epsilon$ is the applied longitudinal strain, v is Poisson's ratio, α is the coefficient of thermal expansion of the fibre and T is the temperature.

Equation 2 shows that the reflected spectral shift is dependent upon both strain and temperature and in practice it can be difficult to resolve the effect of the two. The most common method to overcome this with FBG's is to provide a dual grating system where one is a reference sensor under no strain and the other is the collocated sensor under strain. The reference sensor can then be used to compensate for the temperature in the combined system. Other methods for resolving the two components include using the different response from two gratings at different wavelengths or gratings etched into fibre regions with different characteristics such as refractive index and diameter (e.g. [7][16]).

Variations in the Bragg grating geometry can also be used to enhance specific propagation characteristics. For example the Long Period Grating (LPG) where $\lambda_{source} << \lambda_G$ may be used to convert forward propagating bound modes to forward propagating cladding modes for use in sensors that rely on some interaction with this part of the fibre. Other grating configurations included, chirped, tilted, tapered and combinations of these.

2.2 Interferometer Type Sensors

All OFS interferometers use the principle of detecting the phase difference between two or more optical paths by analysing the interference pattern caused by their sum. In the dual path interferometers the interference pattern describing the change in the measurand results from two separately propagating beams. The most commonly used of these for civil engineering has been the Michelson interferometer or some variant of its principle.

Early on in OFS development the Michelson interferometer technique (figure 2) was used to perform long gauge measurements of displacement between two points (strain). Two fibres with mirrored ends are used, one fixed to the structure being measured (test fibre) and one remaining unfixed (reference fibre). The resulting interference between the two is used to determine the displacement of the test fibre to within a micron or so. The most commonly used form of this sensor in civil engineering structures is the Long Gauge OFS (LGFOS) where the distributed strain is measured over a long length of the fibre (up to tens of metres). The SOFO (Surveillance d´Ouvrages par Fibres Optiques) long gauge sensor of this type was initially developed by the Swiss Federal Institute of Technology (EPFL) and has been installed in many civil engineering structures [6]. Other common two path interferometers include the Mach-Zehnder and Sagnac configurations.

Another interferometer sensor gaining some commercial exposure is the Fabry-Perot sensor (see for example [12]). This low coherence interferometer is capable of high resolution and can be configured to measure all of the parameters described in Table 1. Two mirrors on the ends of a small cavity reflect the signal back and forth within the cavity to produce a highly sensitive interference pattern (figure 3). The amount of signal emerging from the cavity to be analysed depends upon the reflectivity of the mirrored ends and the sensitivity to changes in the cavity length (or refractive index of cavity material) depend of the number on reflections inside it. Thus the more light

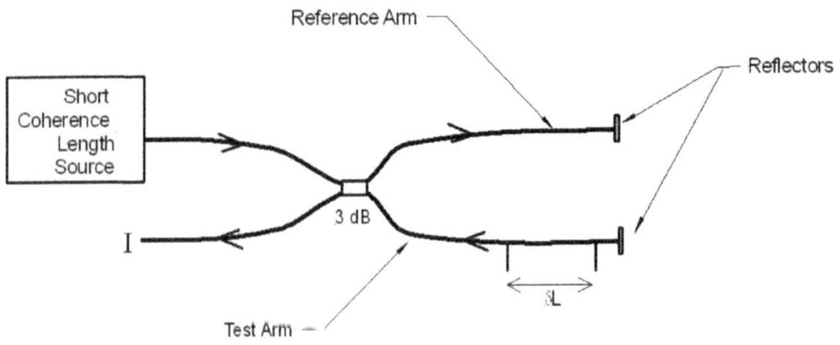

Fig. 2 The Michelson interferometer. A low coherence light source directs light into two fibres, each with mirrored ends. The Test arm is bonded to the structure and undergoes movement due to stress while the reference arm is free (i.e. not bonded). The interference pattern between the two is an indication of the change in length due to strain, or δL.

that escapes from the cavity the less number of significant reflections inside it and so there is a trade off between resolving the phase difference at the measurement end of the fibre and sensitivity to the measurand.

2.3 Distributed Sensors

The three most commonly researched forms of distributive measurements in optical fibres are the Rayleigh, Raman and Brillouin scattering modes. Optical Time Domain Reflectometry (OTDR) or Optical Frequency Domain Reflectometry (OFDR) may be used to isolate the position of the portion of scattering being observed at a resolution and distance dependent upon the scattering mode and any modifications to the fibre. OTDR measures the propagation time of the pulse from the scatterer and can provide a resolution of around 1 m, depending upon the system, over many tens of kilometres. OFDR on the other hand, while more accurately fixing the scattering position, is only reliable up to around hundred metres.

Rayleigh scattering results from scattering off micro inhomogeneity regions of refractive index (most commonly silica impurities) within the fibre core or cladding. Some scattering is always present and changes in its intensity can be related to a modification of the fibre by either mechanical means or some form of measurand coupling to the cladding. The mechanical change to the core of the fibre is often induced by a device (e.g. microbend wedges, wire coil etc.) wrapped around the fibre while chemical interaction with special cladding material is commonly used to measure the composition or presence of various liquids. Because both of these uses require special attachment or modification to the fibre at point locations these types of configurations of the Rayleigh scatter become more quasi-distributive than fully distributive. This, together with their large amplitude losses makes Rayleigh scattering

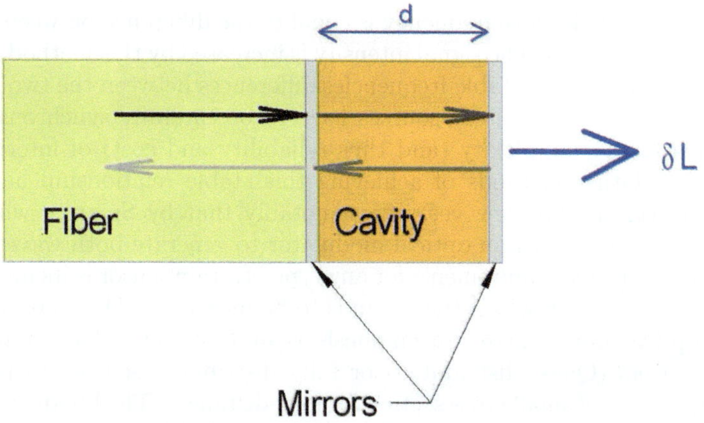

Fig. 3 The Fabry Perot interferometer is a point sensor that can be either all in fibre (as depicted here) or housed in an external structure from the fibre. The basic principle is the same where a number of reflections between the partially mirrors causes constructive and destructive interference within the cavity. The magnitude of the interference is dependant upon the wavelength and cavity length, d.

for these configurations less attractive than the other scattering type sensors for measuring strain and temperature.

Fibre systems that measure the Raman scattering components are used in truly distributive sensing to measure temperature over longs distance (up 20 – 30 km). In Raman scattering the light is absorbed by the fibre and re-emitted at a wavelength (or energy) dependent upon the temperature and composition of the fibre. The change in wavelength takes two values either side of the incident signal at the Stokes and anti Stokes positions. The amplitude of the anti Stokes shift relative to the Stokes shift is particularly sensitive to the temperature and this can be measured to provide a very accurate ($< 1°C$) value for the temperature. Raman type sensors can only be used for temperature measurements.

Brillouin scatter sensors are sensitive to both strain and temperature. The scatter arises due to the interaction of the light with acoustic waves set up by thermal excitation. These waves, or acoustic phonons, introduce periodic variation along the fibre whose phase velocity, v_b is dependent upon both strain, ϵ and temperature, T, [11]:

$$\delta v_b = C_T \delta T + C_\epsilon \delta \epsilon \tag{3}$$

Where C_T and C_ϵ depend upon the type of fibre. Notice again the coupling between temperature and strain.

The signal intensity of this spontaneous Brillouin scatter is small however and thus difficult to measure. Stimulated Brillouin amplification can be used to increase the phonon response by injecting two waves, one from either end of the fibre. The interaction between these two waves is at a maximum when the stimulated acoustic wave frequency is equal to the difference between the two injected light sources. The signal intensity is increased by this method, but the requirement for highly stable frequencies differences between the two injected light waves means that laser sources have to be carefully synchronised and this adds to the complexity (and thus reliability and cost) of interrogation equipment. Other methods of achieving this stable relationship have been explored over the last few years most notably that by Smartec who use a single laser source with an optical modulator to generate both waves.

One of the prime requirements for any type of strain sensor is its interaction with the structure in which the strain is to be measured. This is particularly so for optical fibre where the emphasis is upon either a large number of points sensors (Quasi distributed) or fully distributed sensors to maintain their advantage of small cross section for long distances. The bonding must be accomplished so that the structure's strain is coupled directly to the sensitive part of the fibre and not lost in any of the fittings or adhesives.

While there are still a number of technical issues to be fully resolved before the widespread use of optical fibre sensors become common there are at least two other, more general factors, that inhibit the wide spread use of OFS in Structural Health Monitoring. Firstly, more conventional sensors such as strain gauges and extensometers are well understood and their performance variations usually predictable. Physical size and communication requirements make their placement (i.e. position and number) limited and this has always been the case. With the advent of optical fibre sensors expectations of increased placement ability and performance introduce another dimension of complexity by requiring strong coupling to the material to be measured over long distances with little disruption to its structural integrity. Not surprisingly establishing the best approach to meet these deployment requirements for different projects is ongoing and this often leads to a lack of understanding between the sensor providers and end users. Secondly is the industry's ability to interpret the results. For example, while regions of sudden excessive strain may give some indication of a problem the more usual subtler shifts over a period of time are more difficult to interpret. In the case of an embankment dam, settlement over time is expected and measuring the displacement over this period is likely to indicate significant change. So measuring strain across a system without knowing what is normal is not always helpful, especially given the inaccessibility of the regions under test. Thus with much more careful study of these effects using the OFS sensors now available, monitoring of these large structures can become much more effective.

3 Dams

Here as in the preceding section only a brief description of the highly diverse science of dam construction, operation and maintenance is given and readers requiring more detail are directed towards texts such as [3].

3.1 Dam Types

There are basically three fundamental types of dam based on their construction material[1]:

1. Masonary Dams. These are dams that are usually made form concrete sometimes along with stone or brick and are of one of two types:
   – Arch - where the arch geometry distributes the hydrostatic forces to prescribed locations (e.g. to the buttresses). These dams are particularly useful in narrow high regions of water containment such as steep river gorges.
   – Gravity - where the dam is made large enough that gravity holds the structure from being overturned or displaced. These dams are well understood and robust and used in a large variety of terrains.
     • Many masonry dams use a combination of arch and gravity construction.
2. Embankment Dams. These dams are constructed from naturally occurring materials in earth, usually locally sourced. The two main types are:
   – Earth Filled - rolled and compacted earth (often clay) material.
   – Rock Filled - Often earth with larger number and size of rock aggregate.
3. Composite Dams. A combination of the above two types.

3.2 Dam Failure

Dams fail due to one or more of three main actions:

1. Seepage - water permeating through the dam causing internal erosion.
2. Structural - the structural integrity is compromised due to cracking, internal erosion, settlement, slippage, design/material failure etc.
3. Overtopping - erosive action on the embankment due to water spill.

There are a number of causes for each of these actions that may include such things as design oversights, unusual weather conditions, failure of other dam's upstream and geological events such as earthquakes.

Monitoring for conditions leading to these failure events is still largely by visual inspection. For example seepage in embankment dams can be estimated from drainage system flows, wet areas and surface deformations such as cracks and sink holes. Unfortunately such monitoring is necessarily restricted in coverage and is dependent upon the quality and regularity of the observation. In many installations visual inspections are complemented by more qualitative measurements from specialty (mostly point) sensors. In general the parameters these sensors try to measure include:

[1] Dams are often categorized by other features including construction type and dam use.

- Strain (structural) – In core building components including concrete walls, embankment fill, abutments and foundations.
- Deformation, both horizontal and vertical (structural and seepage) – settlement of foundations and abutments.
- Water pressure (seepage) – both pore pressure (for compacted material such as soil) and joint pressure such as rock fill.
- Vibration (structural) – due to seismic activity and in some cases man made activity.
- Water level (overtopping and structural) – risk of overtopping and calculation of imposed strain.

Out of the above parameters, the first four have received some attention from optical fibre sensor developers in dam monitoring, mostly in strain and temperature.

4 Optical Fibre Sensors in Dams

While there are a number of commercial sensors available for measuring strain, temperature, pressure and displacement that may be suitable for use in monitoring dams, this section discusses only those sensors that have actually been used and widely reported. Qualitative information about the success of many of these installations is hard to find and this is partly due to the difficulty in collecting and analysing often long term results. More convincing evidence for the viability of OFS strain and temperature monitoring comes from other areas of engineering where more analysis has been done both in the laboratory and on site. In fact bridges have become the test ground for many OFS sensors and the technology in this area is reaching a level of maturity that is beginning to change the conceptions of the civil engineering industry.

One of the most widely researched applications of OFS to monitoring seepage in dams was carried out by measuring temperature changes within the downstream toe of an embankment dam, standpipe and drainage system. Small temperature changes due to water seepage can be monitored with either a Raman or Brillouin distributed fibre sensor to indicate variations in small flows (often around 10^{-6} m/s). Johansson [8] modelled the seepage by comparing seasonal changes in the surface water temperature to that inside the dam structure. In this process the lag and relative variation in temperature between the two give an indication to the amount of seepage. For example, a constant temperature within the dam wall over a seasonal cycle, where the surface water temperature changes considerably, indicates little seepage. The interpretation of non constant changes is a function of a number of factors including dam construction and the amount of surface water variation. HydroResearch have commercialised the modelling (DamTemp) of this interpretation and together with Sensornet, who offer a range of Raman (DTS – temperature) and Brillouin (DTSS – temperature and strain) OFS's, installed the system in a number of dams. Installations in new dams and retro-fitting in old dams (e.g. Bergeforsen power plant Sweden) were undertaken with both the Raman and Brillouin sensors for different configurations and compared. Comparison with standard thermocouples show good agreement but the results, in terms of seepage, are difficult to characterize by the nature of the environment.

The SOFO fibre interferometer has been commercially available from Smartec since the mid 1990's and employs an infrared LED as its light source. It has been used extensively to monitor strain on a number of civil engineering applications including bridges [2] (e.g. Colle Isarco bridge, Italy, Seggenthal bridge, Switzerland), tunnels and dams (e.g. Emosson dam Switzerland). The installation in the Emosson dam showed thermally induced creep was an important factor to resolve and a subsequent redesign of the SOFO configuration to mitigate against this produced measurements consistent with collocated extensometers. Smartec have also installed different OFS systems into number of other dams including the Nam Ngum dam in Laos (temperature – seepage), Kalivac Dam in Albainia (temperature – seepage), Koudiat dam in Algeria (Temperature – seepage) and Plavinu dam (Strain – structural). All these dams have a Brillouin distributed strain and temperature sensor installed (DiTeSt) along with a reference Raman distributed temperature sensor (DiTemp).

While results look promising for many of these implementations, the success of the overall procedure is difficult to quantify. Electricity of France (EDF) conducted extensive performance test both in the laboratory and at two field locations to monitor seepage through dykes by monitoring temperature changes [4]. They concluded that some of the commercially available Raman sensors could successfully be used to detect water flow (seepage) through Dyke walls over considerable distances provided that they were a) calibrated at the fibre extremities with conventional point temperature sensors, and b) the raw data was significantly post processed using modelled flow analysis. The work also provided an impressive in depth study of the practical requirements of using these distributive temperature sensors in real civil engineering structures. The same group also conducted tests on using Brillouin scattering distributed sensing to measure strain in concrete foundations and found that the uncoupling of strain and temperature was difficult to achieve in the field and that strain measurements were hampered by poor spatial resolution (i.e. location along the fibre using OTDR) and sensitivity to strain.

5 Modelling New FBG Configurations

There are many possible configurations for most of the OFS's discussed here. In particular FBG sensors offer a wide variety of possibilities. To consider the potential of such configurations initial assessment of its capabilities and design parameters can be cheaply explored by modeling its electromagnetic propagation and interaction characteristics. The method of Finite Difference Time Domain (FDTD) modeling initially proposed by Yee [21] is a well developed electromagnetic propagation modeling technique that can be adapted for this purpose [17][1]. FDTD has the advantage of being flexible enough to provide complex geometry and has been used to explore some of the more fundamental aspects of optical fibre propagation (e.g. [22][20][19]). To see how this modeling can be used to estimate the performance of envisaged sensors, two new Bragg configurations are simulated using FDTD.

5.1 Two New Configurations

For both of the examples described below the propagation can be well approximated by the meridional rays (i.e. those rays passing through the axis of the fibre) and so a 2-dimensional geometry can be used effectively to characterise the propagation within the fibre. This greatly reduces the processing time of the FDTD algorithms which is essentially an iterative process on small discrete "Yee" cells.

Platt and Woodhead [13] outlined a new approach to measuring strain using an FBG sensor that both decouples strain from temperature, reduces the requirements of the sensors housing and converts the measurement from an observation of a frequency shift to that of an amplitude change. Unlike other FBG sensors the core is free to move inside the cladding and the grating etched in both the core and cladding acts like a vernier that is sensitive to changes in length (see figure 4). Since temperature affects the refractive index in both core and cladding by the same amount there is no cross coupling between temperature and strain. To asses the potential of such an arrangement several key questions need to be resolved:

1. How sensitive is the Bragg Grating to evanescent modes in this region?
2. Directly related to the first point is; what is the resolution obtainable for the expected movement over strain over the active region.
3. What refractive index differences between the grating and cladding provide optimum performance?

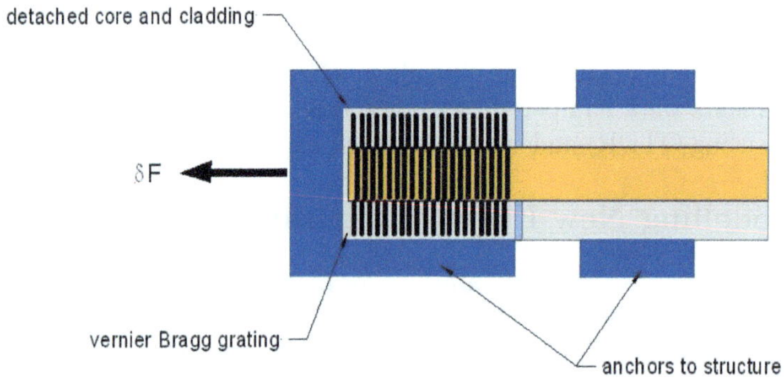

Fig. 4 The proposed vernier grating arrangement to measure strain. In the centre section the core and cladding are detached and free to move relative to each other.

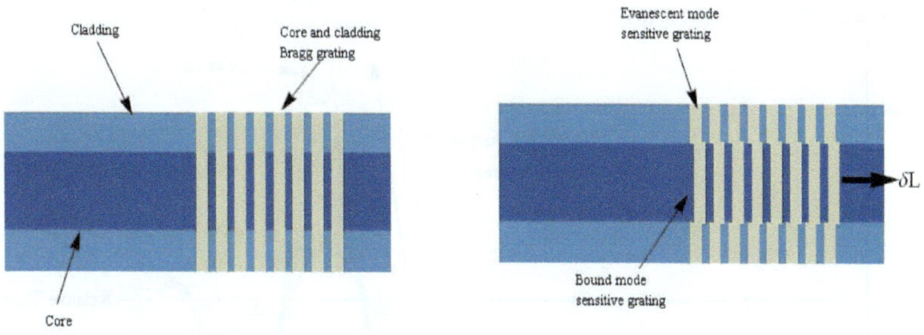

(a) Aligned gratings.

(b) Is an example of the displacement generated by strain, or relative length change δL.

Fig. 5 The Bragg grating methodology used in the FDTD simulation to measure the effects of displacement between the core and cladding gratings

A Gaussian pulse illuminates the aperture of a single mode fibre and propagates along the fibre towards the grating. After the transient region the pulse interacts with the Bragg grating of figure 4 to produce a backscattered signal whose amplitude is measured back at the initial aperture. Figure 7 is a clip from the FDTD solver showing the propagation as it moves toward the grating (not shown). Clearly visible in this figure are the modes associated with the core (bound) and cladding (evanescent) propagation. To test the vernier action the core grating is progressed longitudinally relative to that in the cladding. The situation is illustrated in figure 5.

The resulting amplitude changes (relative to the aligned case) due to this vernier action are shown in figure 6. Note that in the two cases discussed here δd refers to the number of "Yee" cells (or grid lengths) moved. The FDTD can be scaled in such a way that only its relationship to the incident wavelength need be considered when testing different fibre dimensions. The simulation of figure 6 clearly indicates that the amplitude changes are considerable as the two gratings move relative to each other so that, at least in theory, it is possible to measure strain via this configuration.

There are a number of variants possible to this vernier geometry and their relative effectiveness can be estimated via similar FDTD simulations.

As another example, water pressure measurement is of principal importance in monitoring seepage. For example, an increase in pore pressure in embankments of a dam indicates increased seepage and if the pressure goes from a negative to positive (relative to air pressure) serious water ingress is taking place with the potential to cause significant internal erosion. Little work has been reported in the monitoring of pressure with OFS's in this regard, though some has been undertaken in related fields.

OFS sensors used for this are of either Fabry-Perot or Bragg type, detecting the pressure change through variation in diaphragms, pistons [24][23] or other mechanically induced means (e.g. [15]). Both of these methods require some

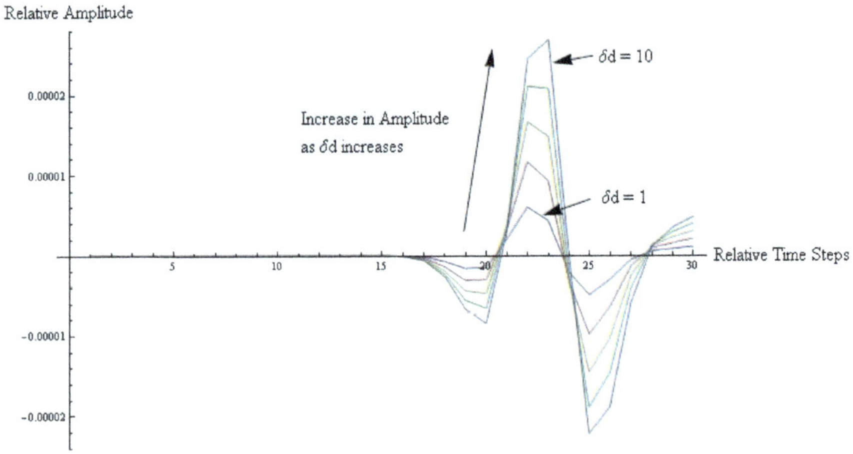

Fig. 6 Relative amplitude of backscattered signal from the vernier configured grating to measure strain. All measurements here are relative to the signal when the gratings are aligned. This difference amplitude increases as the gratings move away from alignment. When $\delta d = 0$ the gratings are aligned and at $\delta d = 10$ are at their maximum misalignment.

sort of moveable mechanical housing (or other structure) that in the case of Fabry-Perot alters the cavity size and in the Bragg grating imposes a strain that is transformed to interpret applied pressure. A different configuration to measuring pressure using an FBG is shown in figure 8.

In this construction the inline simplicity of the sensing region means that complicated mechanical housing is avoided thus keeping cross section low and the number sensing points per unit length high, compared to those already available. The main feature of this type of sensor is that the active part of the grating is in the cladding region, so only evanescent modes are involved in the backscatter. Asking the same questions as those for the previous modeling and using the same fibre parameters, a 2-dimensional FDTD solver is employed with the Bragg grating etched into the fibre cladding only. Figure 9 indicates the FDTD setup used to test this configuration and shows two examples, one where no force is applied and the second where a force is applied to the cladding to depress the grating closer to the core-cladding boundary. The main independent parameter here the change in distance between the grating and the core-cladding interface, δd.

Figure 10 shows the backscattered difference in amplitude between the case where no force is applied ($\delta d = 15$) and those where different amounts of force has been applied ($\delta d = 10, 5, 0$). Note here that there has been no application of a force to δd transformation since the compressible material in figure 8 has not been specified. It is thus tacitly assumed that the force will be directly proportional to a change in δd.

Results for this simulation show considerably less differentiation between the different displacement scenarios than did the previous example. Discrimination

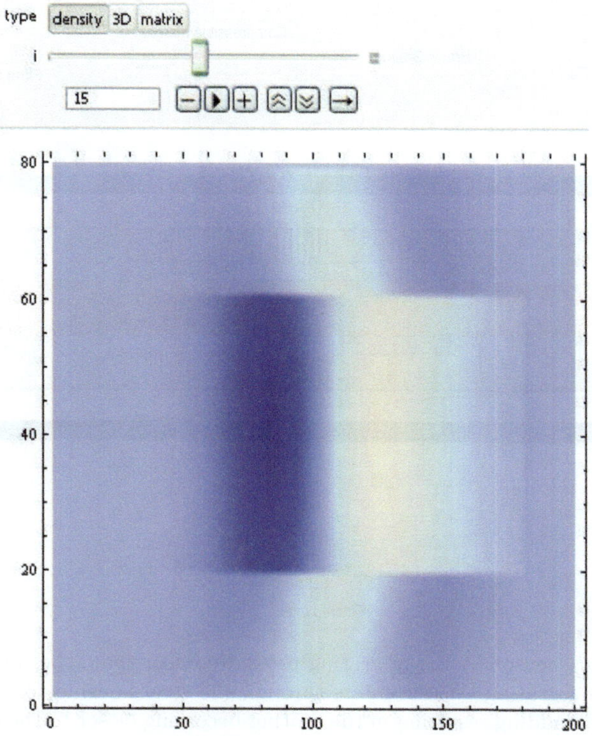

Fig. 7 Wave propagating in fibre core and cladding

becomes more difficult when the grating is further away from the core, corresponding to low pressures, and this is not entirely unexpected since fundamental theory tells us that the evanescent field falls of exponentially with distance away from the core. Thus the TDFD modeling here indicates that this configuration is likely to be problematic in monitoring pressure changes, especially low pressures. It may be that some clever re-arrangement of the gratings positioning can improve pressure resolution and these can be tested quickly using this modeling procedure.

So how much does this modeling really say about the viability of such sensors? The authors are reminded of the often quoted comment by George E. P. Box[2], "Essentially, all models are wrong, but some are useful". All that is known from the modeling done here is that there is no basic theoretical reason *within the scope of the model* why these configurations will not behave in a similar manner to that described. It is important to bear in mind however, that for the cases given above it is the relative differences between configurations that is most reliably modeled. For instance it is well known

[2] George Edward Pelham Box, born 18 October 1919. Statistician who made important contributions to many fields of statistics.

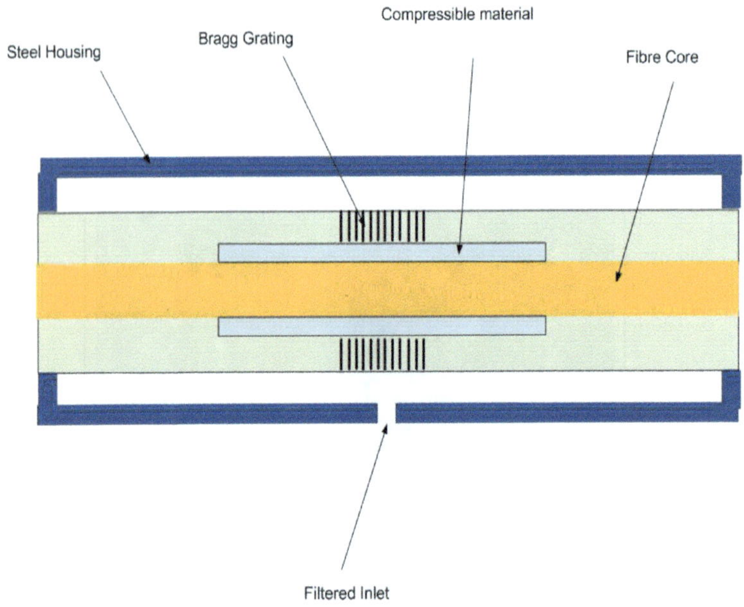

Fig. 8 Pressure sensor. A Bragg grating pressure sensor that relies on deformation of the cladding grating. Water enters through the steel housing to apply pressure to a region of cladding resulting in the grating becoming closer to the core-cladding boundary as the refractive index matching compressible material is depressed.

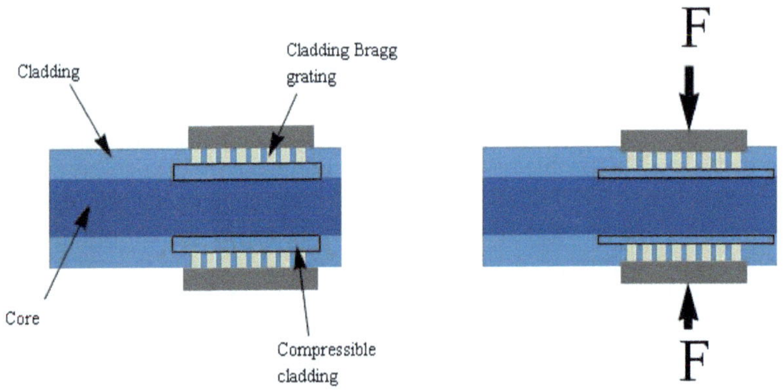

(a) No external force to the cladding is applied.

(b) External force of water pressure is applied to the cladding.

Fig. 9 The Bragg grating methodology used in the FDTD simulation to measure the effects of a grating in the cladding only where no external force to the cladding is applied

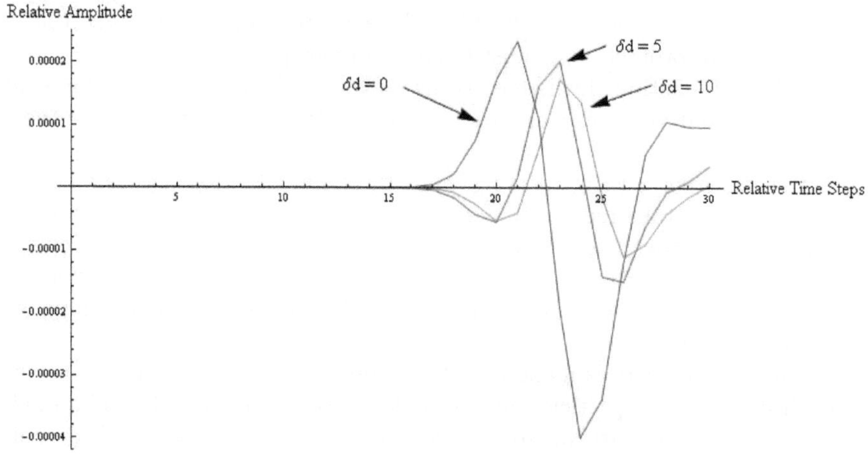

Fig. 10 Relative amplitude of backscattered signal from the pressure sensitive cladding grating

and documented in the literature referenced in this work that Bragg gratings in both the core and cladding can return a backscattered signal that is easily measurable. So varying the geometry somewhat to look for differences afforded by the two cases outlined here is not unreasonable. On the other hand attempting to obtain absolute values for backscattered signal will almost certainly fail to correctly predict those obtained from an operational system. In short, taken with due care modeling represents a small, but arguably, important part of the development process.

6 Future Work

Optical Fibre Sensor technology has advanced slowly over the past 20 years or so and much of its growth has been spurred on by the progress made in the much more heavily funded area of telecommunications. There have been many factors inhibiting the usefulness of the fibres full potential in the sensing industry including cross coupling between parameters to be measured, deployment problems and the high cost of associated equipment. This has added to the reluctance of the civil engineering community, who are rightly conservative in these issues, to be enthusiastic about their use. The OFS industry is now maturing along with the development of their sensors and these types of problems are diminishing. There are now in fact many OFS sensors on the market that are more than a match for the traditional varieties. Since the OFS sensors on offer now are capable of providing so much more data over longer and often embedded regions the issue becomes one of effectively using this data to monitor the important parts of the structure. In the case of dams there is much to learn about the physical processes leading to failure, especially the early warning signs. There is thus a great opportunity to use these sensors to better understand the early warning processes so that a greater level of protection against failure becomes possible.

As already mentioned, there is strong movement towards the development of fully distributive sensors and the reasons for this are clear. However these sensors, especially those used for strain, add another layer of operational complexity compared to Bragg gratings and the commonly used interferometers. It will therefore take more time for their impact to be felt in the civil engineering sector. Advances in areas such as microstructured fibres, equipment design will also add to the potential of OFS in distributive sensing for the civil engineering industry as well as a range of others such as manufacturing and hazard control.

Finally, while there is no substitute for prototyping a system such as the ones discussed in this article, there is a clear role for the use of careful modeling. As the capability in fibre optics has grown the mathematical tools available for simulating them has also grown. Used as a tool for evaluating potential and/or looking for unexpected issues, techniques like Finite Difference Time Domain can provide valuable insight into what the sensor is actually doing.

References

1. Davidson, D.B.: Computational Electromagnetics for RF and Microwave Engineering. Cambridge University Press, Cambridge (2005)
2. Glisic, B., Inaudi, D., Kronenberg, P., Vurpillot, S.: Dam monitoring using long sofo sensor. In: Proceedings of Hydropower Conference (1999)
3. Golze, A.R. (ed.): Handbook of dam engineering. Van Nostrand Reinhold (1977)
4. Henault, J.-M., Moreau, G., Blairon, S.: Truly distributed optical fiber sensors for structural health monitoring: From the telecommunication optical fiber drawling tower to water leakage detection in dikes and concrete structure strain monitoring. In: Advances in Civil Engineering 2010 (2010)
5. Idrissy, R.L., Kodindouma, M.B., Kersey, A.D., Davis, M.A.: Multiplexed bragg grating optical fiber sensors for damage evaluation in highway bridges. Smart Mater. Struct. 7, 209–216 (1998)
6. Inaudi, D.: Sofo sensors for static and dynamic measurements. In: Fibre Optic Workshop, pp. 1–10 (2004)
7. James, S.W., Dockney, M.L., Tatam, R.P.: Simulataneous independent temperature and strain measurement using in-fibre bragg grating sensors. Electon Letters 32, 1133–1134 (1996)
8. Johansson, S.: Seepage Monitoring in an Earth Embankment Dams. PhD thesis, Royal Institute of Technology, Stockholm (1997)
9. Li, E.: Characterization of a fiber lens. Opt. Lett. 31(2), 169–171 (2006)
10. Lopez-Higuera, J.M.: Handbook of optical fibre sensing technology. Wiley, Chichester (2002)
11. Nikles, M., Thevenaz, L., Robert, P.A.: Simple distributed fiber sensor based on brillouin gain spectrum analysis. Optics Letters 21, 758–760 (1996)

12. Pinet, E., Hamel, C., Glisic, B., Inaudi, D., Miron, N.: Health monitoring with optical fiber sensors: from human body to civil structures. In: SPIE Smart Structures and Materials & Nondestructive Evaluation and Health Monitoring 14 th International Symposium Health Monitoring of Structural and Biological Systems (SSN10 Conference), San Diego, California USA, March 18-22 (2007)
13. Platt, I.G., Woodhead, I.M.: The use of bragg gratings in the core and cladding of optical fibres for accurate strain sensing. Sensors and Transducers 90, 333–341 (2008)
14. Snyder, A.W., Love, J.: Optical Waveguide Theory. Chapman and Hall, Boca Raton (1983)
15. Song, D., Wei, Z., Zou, J., Yang, S., Du, E., Cui, H.-L.: Pressure sensor based on fiber bragg grating and carbon fiber ribbon-wound composite cylindrical shell. IEEE Sensors Journal 9(7), 828 (2009), doi:10.1109/JSEN.2009.2024035
16. Song, M., Lee, S.B., Choi, S.S.: Interferometric temperature insensitive strain measurements with different diameter fibre bragg gratings. Optic. Letters 11, 790–792 (1997)
17. Taflove, A., Hagness, S.: Computational electrodynamics: The Finite-Difference Time Domain method. wisc (2000)
18. Udd, E. (ed.): Smart Structures And Materials 2005: Smart Sensor Technology And Measurement System. Society of Photo Optical (2005)
19. Vu, N.H., Hwang, I.K., Lee, Y.-H.: Bending loss analyses of photonic crystal fibers based on the finite difference time domain method. Optic. Letters 33, 119 (2008)
20. Wu, F., Guo, S., Ikram, K., Albin, S., Tai, H., Rogowski, R.S.: Numerical analysis of bragg fibers using a compact 1d finite-difference frequency-domain method. Optics. Communications 249(1-3), 165–174 (2005)
21. Yee, K.: Numerical solution of inital boundary value problems involving maxwell's equations in isotropic media. IEEE Transactions on Antennas and Propagation 14(3), 302–307 (1966)
22. Yunming, W., Jingcao, D., Mingde, Z., Xiaohan, S.: Theoretical and experimental study on multimode optical fiber grating. Optics Communications 250(1-3), 54–62 (2005)
23. Zhang, W.T., Li, F., Liu, Y.L., Liu, L.H.: Ultrathin fbg pressure sensor with enhanced responsivity. IEEE Photonics Technology Letters 19(19), 1553–1555 (2007)
24. Zhang, Y., Feng, D., Liu, Z., Guo, Z., Dong, X., Chiang, K.S., Chu, B.C.B.: High-sensitivity pressure sensor using a shielded polymer-coated fiber bragg grating. IEEE Photonics Technology Letters 13(6), 618–619 (2001)

Optical Sensors Based on Fiber Bragg Gratings for Structural Health Monitoring

P. Antunes, H. Lima, N. Alberto, L. Bilro, P. Pinto, A. Costa, H. Rodrigues, J.L. Pinto, R. Nogueira, H. Varum, and P.S. André

Instituto de Telecomunicações
Departamento de Física
Departamento de Engenharia Civil
Institute of Nanostructures, Nanomodelling and Nanofabrication
University of Aveiro
Campus de Santiago, 3810-193 Aveiro
Portugal

Abstract. In this work we review the structural health monitoring techniques based on fiber Bragg gratings. The working principle of the fiber Bragg gratings sensors and the most common techniques to inscribe and interrogate these sensors are described. Several implemented examples are also presented, like the deformation monitoring of one historical building with reduced visual impact, the unidirectional acceleration measurements in a metallic bridge structure and the bidirectional acceleration monitoring in a 50 m mobile telecom tower. Finally, the implementation of an automated remote structural health monitoring system design to operate with optical sensors in a highway bridge is described.

The obtained results prove the applicability of optical fiber sensors, namely fiber Bragg gratings for structural health monitoring.

1 Introduction and Motivation

The main objective of the Structural Health Monitoring (SHM) is to observe the *in-situ* structural behavior under different loading conditions during a predetermined time period or during the structures lifetime and to detect structural or material properties deterioration. The health of the structure should be checked like the health of a human being, where the doctors evaluate the human body health using advanced medical equipment. Based on the results, health is evaluated and, if required, an intervention plan is established. In the same way, SHM uses advanced sensors in order to evaluate the "health" of the structure. Engineers, based on the collected data, can evaluate the structural integrity and durability. In any case, preventive evaluation can identify prematurely problems and point guidelines for the definition of the solution.

Several major natural disasters, such as earthquakes or hurricanes, have occurred in the last decades, causing a large number of victims and a considerable monetary lost, due to the collapse of civil engineering structures. Therefore, the need to identify structural damage and to monitor its evolution imposes the development of SHM techniques [1, 2]. These techniques are supported by data

S.C. Mukhopadhyay (Ed.): New Developments in Sensing Technology for SHM, LNEE 96, pp. 253–295.
springerlink.com

collected by a sensors network and related to the behavior and response of the structure, providing indicators about eventual structure damage or anomalies, which adversely affect the structure integrity. The data are collected in real time conditions, being considered a wide group of parameters related with the structure physical properties such as strain, stress or acceleration.

The present work intended to provide an overview of SHM techniques based on fiber Bragg grating (FBG) sensors. The intrinsic characteristics of FBGs make them one of the most promising technologies to be used in SHM. The FBG based sensors take advantage of the properties provided by optical fibers, namely low loss transmission, immunity to electromagnetic interference, electrical isolation and reduced weight. These characteristics make them attractive for use in hostile environments, where electrical currents might pose a hazard. Moreover, the intrinsic advantages of FBG itself should be also considered, like high signal to noise ratio, compactness, high linearity, high sensitivity, immunity to electromagnetic fields, resistance to hash environments, low noise (resulting from the information codification in the wavelength domain), and the possibility to multiplex a large number of FGB based sensors in the same optical fiber reducing the need of multiple and heavy cabling used in traditional sensing [3, 4].

Nowadays, the main advantage of traditional sensors when compared with the optical ones is the low complexity of the interrogation systems. In a near future, due to the maturity of FBG production and the cost reduction of the interrogation systems, these optical sensors technology will be widely commercialized for a large variety of applications, such as SHM. Moreover, in large infrastructures, where a high number of different types of sensors is required, the utilization of several multiplexed FBG sensors may provide an effective solution to simultaneously measure static and dynamic parameters.

In this work we describe the application of FBGs in the monitoring of three structures, namely: the church of Santa Casa da Misericórdia in Aveiro, built in the XVI and XVII centuries; a footbridge in the Aveiro University Campus and a mobile telecom tower. The application of a remote sensing platform used to monitor in real time a highway bridge will be described.

2 Structural Health Monitoring

The health of a structure should be checked regularly and the engineers, based on the collected data, can evaluate the structural integrity and durability. In any case, preventive evaluation during the life-time of the structure can detect prematurely any problem or defect and can help in pointing out guidelines for the solution definition and implementation.

A SHM system can be composed by a different number of subsets, like the data acquisition, communication, processing and data storage and diagnostic [5].

The data acquisition involves the definition of the monitoring plan and the installation of the sensors in order to acquire the information about the structural behavior.

The data communication depends on the SHM system and is associated with the information transfer between the acquisition system and the station where the data are storage. Additionally, the definition of the communication strategy is dependent on the complexity of the data acquisition system and on the location where the data are stored. The data can be communicated with wire systems or wirelessly.

The data processing system includes the direct verification of the measurements obtained by the sensors and its processing, in order to perform actions as, for example, thermal correction of the measurements or selection of the data to be stored or analyzed. For instance, in the monitoring of a tower response, only the values readings of wind speed at the sensors that are superior to a certain value are stored. Therefore, in many situations, the data processing should be performed prior to its storage.

The obtained data is then used for the diagnostic and current evaluation of the structure. For the analysis of the structural degradation and aging, the measured properties or structural response parameters should be recorded through time.

The diagnostic is the final phase of a SHM program that, combining individual measurements at each sensor, allows the analysis and interpretation of the structural behavior and could lead to an eventual recommendation for intervention on the structure.

2.1 Evolution of SHM

SHM is in development in the last two decades, especially for industrial applications in mechanical and aerospace engineering. Clearly, the importance of the integration of SHM in civil engineering structures is increasing. Important civil engineering structures were built in the last decades and, in many cases, the major difficulty in their design and construction was associated with the high level of uncertainties in geometry, materials and loads during the life-time of the structure. In most cases, structures have associated small safety margins and are public. Nowadays, the transportation infrastructures system is directly correlated to the economic development of a nation [6]. In particular, bridges are critical structures of the transportation system and the application of SHM systems is more often than in buildings.

Steven Lovejoy [7] presents eight key elements of success for a SHM system applied to highway bridges, but also extensible to all civil engineering structures:

i) the owner has to clearly understand the parameters that will be measured and how the measurements are related to the condition of the structure to be monitored;
ii) determine if there is a need of monitor system or a combination of a monitor with a early warning system (if the latter is chosen, a clear response plan has to be established);
iii) hardware redundancy especially in critical applications, such as in early warning systems;
iv) use of high quality components and installation practices including environmental demands protection;

v) optimize the number of sensor sites (excessive data can often hamper a clear understanding of the basic response parameters of the structure or system);
vi) the data must be easily collected, stored, manipulated and presented to the end-user;
vii) inspect routinely the data to monitor for faulty or degrading sensor components, preventing lost or bad data; and
viii) provide periodic inspection and maintenance on the hardware and installation materials.

The evolution of the civil engineering constructions introduces the need for larger and geometrically more complex structural systems, but also lighter and safer. This is only possible with the use of new construction materials and techniques. This issue introduces several new difficulties and needs in the SHM systems for applications in civil engineering structures.

One of the main target applications of SHM systems for civil constructions is the historical buildings. The identification of defects and damages in existing ancient buildings can be very difficult, as well as their causes, which makes the rehabilitation intervention very difficult. For such type of structures, the data collected from structural monitoring is often the unique way to understand their behavior, and to allow an adequate intervention in the structures.

As an example, it is cited the main nave of Santa Maria of Belém Church of the Monastery of Jerónimos, in Lisbon, where two monitoring systems where implemented to characterize the static and dynamic behavior of the structure, aiming the damage detection and the improvement of the seismic capacity of the monument. The adopted health monitoring system was based on the observation of the changes in the static and dynamic response parameters, combined with environmental actions measurements [8].

2.2 Field Testing

The main objective of health monitoring is to track any aspect of performance or condition of structures in a proactive manner, using the measured data and simulations to identify possible problems or deficient behavior due to severe loading events (caused by natural disasters like earthquakes, strong wind, or man-made as explosions) and deterioration due to environmental effects. The damage identification is performed based on changes in the properties of the structure or materials and provides useful information to help owners to take appropriate decisions at an early stage [2].

The deterioration of civil infrastructures in North America, Europe and Japan has been well documented and publicized. In the United States, 50% of all bridges were built before the 1940's and approximately 42% of these structures are structurally deficient [9, 10]. These statistics underline the importance of the development of reliable and cost-effective methods for the massive rehabilitation and renewal investments in the years ahead [11].

The definition of the main objectives and the expected results from the SHM has implications in the design of the system. Experimental technologies can be divided as: geometry monitoring, controlled testing (which may be static or dynamic, non-destructive or destructive), and continuous monitoring [12].

Geometry monitoring is not continuous, can be performed with longer intervals, and have the objective of verify the changes in the geometry as an indication of phenomena, such as foundation settlements.

Controlled testing (static and dynamic) aims the application of controlled loads and/or the measurement of ambient inputs to structures while its corresponding response is monitored. This type of test has specific time duration. It can be a static test, like a proof-load test to verify the load capacity of the global structure or of a particular element, or a dynamic test to identify dynamic properties of the structure, namely, the natural frequencies, mode shapes and damping.

The long-term monitoring is now possible due to the recent advances in sensors, computing and communications technologies, allowing the monitoring of structures during years and, eventually, for their entire life cycle. In this type of monitoring is important to divide the required measurements into two categories[12]:

i) the low-speed monitoring, to measure and record, for example, the displacements and deformations of the structure during its life;
ii) the monitoring of high-speed events that occurs over a short time-window, like earthquakes, fires or explosions. Each category requires different sensors, data acquisition systems, post-processing, interpretation and information management strategies.

Static and dynamic tests are frequently used before setting new bridges into service, in order to verify the real structure behavior and to compare it with the numerical results obtained in the design phase. They allow a real representation of the structures response under static or dynamic loading and a data record of the original undamaged basic structural parameters, which can be useful for a future condition assessment. The sensing network implemented in the circular pedestrian steel bridge recently constructed in Aveiro, Portugal, combines strain and temperature sensors. The monitoring plan was established according to the previously obtained numerical analysis results of the structure response [13]. It was expected that the optical fiber strain sensing network provided the stress distribution in the most important structural elements of the bridge, namely the suspension cables. The measurements obtained with the installed sensing network allowed the improvement and calibration of the predicted numerical models, as well as the real-time monitoring of the bridge structural health during loading tests and structure service. One of the key-objectives of two series of static loading tests performed on the bridge was to evaluate the eventual variation of the axial force in the cables.

2.3 Monitored Parameters

Health monitoring can be divided into two major groups: material and structural health monitoring. For a specific structure in service, it could be of interest to assess the properties of the materials used. This is classified as Material Health

Monitoring (MHM) and covers the measurement of the elasticity modulus, material stiffness or density and the analysis of their influence in the structures durability [14]. If a very large number of these sensors are installed at different points, it is possible to extrapolate information about the behavior of the whole structure from these local measurements [15]. The SHM includes the monitoring of loadings applied to a structure and the assessment of their influence in terms of strains, deformations or vibrations. The structural monitoring approach may detect material degradation, like cracking or deformation under constant loading, if they have an impact on the shape of the structure. This approach usually requires a reduced number of sensors when compared to the material monitoring approach [15]. In the monitoring of the church of Santa Casa da Misericórdia, in Aveiro, Portugal, described in section 5.1, only SHM was adopted (with displacement and temperature sensors). After the visual inspection, it was observed that the critical zones were located in the main arch and in the structural walls above it. The sensors were strategically located, after the structural damage analysis, in points where the most important deformations were found or expected [4].

In the case of bridges, the deterioration due to aging or due to the increase of traffic loads raise concerns about their reliability. One of the ways to check the reliability of the existing bridges is based on proof loading tests. A successful proof loading test may demonstrate immediately if the capacity of a bridge is adequate for the structure loading and service [16]. In some cases, a damage-state assessment of the structure has to be done considering both SHM and MHM actions. For example, in the interventions of the Tele Castle and Prague New Town Hall, in Czech Republic, the evolution of the cracks opening in masonry walls was monitored jointly with temperature and humidity variations [17].

Typically, in civil engineering SHM applications, the most common monitored parameters include the characterization or measurement of strain, displacement, load, impact, pH-level, moisture, crack-width, vibrations, accelerations and presence of cracks [18].

The geometric monitoring is a key point. The change in the shape of a structure, and its cause, can be associated with a variety of direct or indirect agents. Examples include known forces applied to a structure during loading tests or unknown forces like traffic, wind, earthquakes or snow [19].

Deformations, like cracking, flow, relaxation or a change of temperature, can also result from changes in the constituent materials of the structure. A deformation is usually associated by a change of the strain distribution in the structure [20]. Deformation measurements may allow the material properties characterization at a local level, as well as the global structural response characterization based on a deformation/displacement in a representative point/section. Deformations can be measured with embedded sensors installed during the construction phase (e.g. in concrete elements/structures before casting), or placed on the exterior surface of the structure after its construction. However, to obtain global structural displacements, embedded sensors may be no effective, since there is a need of displacement measurements relatively to external reference points. For these cases, sensors to capture global displacements, such as global positioning systems (GPS), inclinometers, linear variable differential transformer (LVDTs), among others, may be used [20].

Monitoring global forces may be important for structures where a load superior to the design values is expected and affects the structural safety or performance. So, in many cases the load distribution and stress level in load-carrying members of a structure should be measured. As examples, the bridges where the loads associated to heavy trucks may be expected or for a seismic event are referred.

The dynamic response of a structure for ambient induced vibrations can be assessed by different methods, based on the measurement of motion, deformations, or forces in representative points. Concerning motion monitoring, the most common methods are based on the acquisition of displacements, velocities or accelerations time-histories. Even if these parameters are related by single integration or differentiation rules, in current practice, the acceleration are the more often parameter measured through accelerometers, because a good accuracy is achieved with a single monitoring scheme. Acceleration sensors are commonly used to determine the axial forces in cable elements, by the calculation of the eigen-frequencies from the accelerations measurements. This procedure can be used for the long-term monitoring of cable bridges, or for the imposition of the desired initial tension in the cables [13].

For the majority of the structural instrumentation programs, the measurement of temperature variations is included. For certain sensors, these measurements are also required for data correction and essential for the determination of temperature gradients or heat of hydration effect on material properties.

Besides the mechanical characterization, in civil engineering applications there are other physical and chemical properties and processes which measurement can be required in order to fully understand the structural response of certain constructions. For example, in some structures, it might be necessary to measure temperature, humidity and electrochemical phenomena to ensure a holistic surveillance concept in the structural assessment. In recent civil engineering structures, concrete and steel are the most common materials used. Monitoring of concrete carbonation and steel reinforcement corrosion are essential to assess the structural integrity and durability [19]. Carbonation and corrosion are normally gradual processes and the detection of these deteriorations in their early stages is crucial to repair the structural systems. Carbonation can reduce the alkalinity of concrete permitting corrosion to occur in the reinforcing steel bars. Carbonation occurs when carbon dioxide from the air reacts with the concrete reducing the pH. Carbonation of the concrete may also induce additional shrinkage, which causes crack formation. The corrosion of reinforcing bars induces an early deterioration of concrete structures and reduces their service life [21]. In particular, the increased use of de-icing salts in severe climates and the attack from sea salt in coastal areas enhance the steel reinforcement corrosion. Several methods have been developed for detecting and evaluating the effects of steel corrosion and concrete carbonation. The classic techniques include visual inspection, or collection of samples to be tested in the laboratory in order to determine the pH level. However, these techniques are destructive, requiring repair of the concrete and reinforcement steel after samples extraction. Also, the results are limited to the analyzed samples, which may not represent the overall structure [19]. Remote inspection techniques with embedded sensors for measurement of the pH in concrete and evaluation of the reinforcing bars corrosion can facilitate the early detection of their pathologies.

2.4 SHM and Non-destructive Testing

There is a large number of non-destructive evaluation (NDE), non-destructive testing (NDT), and non-destructive inspection (NDI) techniques to identify local damage and detect incipient failure in critical structures or simply to characterize materials properties [22].

NDT can be seen as the offline implantation of non-destructive evaluation for assessing the damage-state of a structural material or component without introducing new damage. Both SHM systems and NDT, allow the characterization of the materials' properties, the determination of the structural response parameters, and the identification of damage. However, SHM may perform it on-line and continuously, allowing a estimation of the structural performance and, eventually, early warnings for structural intervention needs [23].

NDT techniques are normally used to complement results of a previous visual inspection, helping in prioritizing rehabilitation, maintenance and emergency repairs interventions. NDT includes vibration analysis, infrared thermography, acoustic emission analysis, ultrasonic imaging, X-ray computer tomography, ground penetrating radar, digital radiography, optical testing methods, eddy current imaging, magneto-inductive cable testing, among others [24].

NDTs should be view as complementary to SHM systems because it can be used for a more detailed analysis in a material or structural component, where the SHM systems have detected damage. In cases where is not expected a significant variation of the materials' properties, the SHM system can be designed to measure the global structural response parameters, while the materials' properties can be evaluated through NDT techniques.

2.5 Numerical Models and SHM Systems

SHM systems associated to the numerical modeling of the structures may allow a better representation of the civil engineering structural response. With the recent advances, the available numerical models for simulation of civil engineering structural response can reproduce accurately the behavior of the constructions. The instrumentation distribution and accuracy implemented in the monitoring plan, and the complexity of the numerical finite element model can vary based on the purpose of the analyzed problem. Thus, the selection of the monitoring scheme and of the modeling approach should be made based on the type of structure, its importance, intervention urgency, economical impact of service interruption, etc. [12].

The interaction between SHM and the numerical models may work in both senses. For example, results from a numerical model of a structure may help in the design of the monitoring instrumentation scheme. In the other sense, results from dynamic tests with identification of the structure natural frequencies and mode shapes allow the calibration of the structural numeric model. Currently, for example, in cable-stayed bridges the association of SHM and numerical models are commonly adopted, allowing to detect eventual damages in the bridges based on dynamic identification models [25]. Using an interactive relation between a SHM system and the numerical model of the structure, a strategy may be outlined allowing: to capture, in more detail, damages or performance limitations; to evaluate structural vulnerability as a function of changes in demand or increases in performance requirements; to estimate the influence of different values of live loads, seismic demands or other unanticipated hazard; and to assist in the design of a structural modification/retrofitting due to an observed damage or to changes in its use [12].

2.6 Decision Support Systems

A SHM system may allow the evaluation of the ability of the structure to behave as designed or the assessment of the remaining service-life of the structure. A prognostic in terms of the estimated remaining life of the structure is essential for the construction owner, who has to decide on the maintenance process to be adopted, or on the eventual substitution of the structure.

A SHM system can comprehend a large number of sensors collecting data continuously. However, only part of this data is normally used in the decision-making process. Decision Support Systems (DSS) can filter the data and convert it into information. Therefore, the operator receives the converted and filtered data and can make options and take decisions on the strategy to be followed. In the last decades, there were efforts to develop systems to support experts of various fields in taking their decisions. DSS represent an approach that tries to integrate many different disciplines into the field of computer science. A reason for the emerging of DSS was the wish to have a system helping to manage very complex situations. The adoption of a DSS will allow to make decisions based on a better understanding and preparation of several tasks, which leads the user towards a more rigorous evaluation and choosing of alternatives [26]. Due to the different problems that can be found associated to civil engineering structures, there is no ideal solution for DSS and therefore the DSS should be designed according to each problem [27].

3 Optical Fiber Based Sensors

Buildings, bridges, dams, aircraft, ships, among others, are complex engineered structures essential for the society. Unfortunately, these structures are many times subjected to severe environmental aggressions and harsh loads, which result in long term structural degradation. To ensure the safety and durability of these structures, engineers exploit the advantages of the sensing technologies to rapidly identify structural damages and adjust maintenance. SHM offers a new paradigm for tracking the health status of a structure, combining sensors and monitoring systems with damage detection algorithms, to ensure safety and durability.

One of the most promising sensing technologies for this purpose is based on optical fiber sensors, specifically, FBG sensors. The use of these devices in SHM has increased significantly due to its innumerous advantages over the conventional sensing solutions.

The first application of FBGs in sensing was on strain and temperature measurements, however with the continuous development of the FBG technology, novel sensors and applications are being reported by the scientific community. Nowadays, FBG sensors are used to measure acceleration, humidity, chemical parameters, among others. A short review of the state of the art for the most important SHM parameters are here presented.

3.1 Acceleration

Accelerometers are essential devices in the detection of changes on the dynamic properties of infrastructures, including buildings, dams, bridges and tunnels. In the last years, the number of reports on fiber based accelerometers has increased. The configuration of the FBG based accelerometers is diverse, however in a simplistic way, it is based on a mass-spring system, as described in [28].

In this case, it was used a single degree-of-freedom structure consisting of a mass resting on a layer of compliant material, which contains the grating, and is supported by a rigid base plate. When subjected to an external acceleration the compression or expansion of the compliant resulting in the FBG central wavelength shift. With this approach, the minimum detectable signal was $\approx$1 mg/$\sqrt{}$Hz.

Todd *et al.* proposed an accelerometer similar to [28]; however they used a hexagonal mass welded between two thin parallel plates [29]. As the FBG is only fixed to the bottom surface of the lower plate and is not embedded in a material, as happens in [28], the probability of transverse strain-induced and birefringent splitting of the FBG reflection peak is lower. This device has several accelerometer desirable features, including good acceleration sensitivity (2-12.5 $\mu\varepsilon$/g), high resonance frequencies (on the order of 1 kHz) and low noise ($\approx$1 mg/$\sqrt{}$Hz, near 1 Hz).

The sensor proposed by Antunes *et al.* comprises, beyond a FBG, an inertial mass, supported by a L-shaped aluminum cantilever beam, connected to the structure base through a steel leaf spring [30]. The operating mechanism also relies on the contraction/expansion of the fiber, as a result of the inertial mass movement. The proposed interrogation system is based on a bandpass optical filter, which represents a low cost solution when compared to the demodulation schemes normally employed for this purpose (spectrum analyzers, interferometric techniques or scanning Fabry-Pérot filters). The Bragg wavelength shift induces variations in the optical power transmitted and measured at the filter output. This is related with the convolution of the filter transfer function and the FBG reflection spectrum. The implemented accelerometer was used to estimate the structure eigenfrequencies of a metallic footbridge located at University of Aveiro Campus, in Portugal (see section 5.2).

In the case of the previously reported accelerometers, the cross thermal sensitivity is a problem, since the FBG responds to both temperature and strain variations. The addition of a temperature compensation scheme will increase the system cost. However, the monitoring of this parameter is also essential for some applications. For example, the natural frequencies of a bridge vary with structural temperature and cracking is also temperature dependent.

Zhu *et al.* developed a temperature-insensitive FBG accelerometer without any additional component [31]. They attached a FBG in a rectangular stainless steel cantilever, which had a mass on the end. When acceleration was applied, the strain varied linearly and, since initial FBG had a uniform period, a linear chirped grating was obtained. The acceleration was measured detecting the reflected power. As the photodetector collect the total reflected power, a Bragg wavelength shift caused by thermal variation will not influence the results, turning the sensor insensitive to this parameter. With the proposed approach, a linear output range of 8 g could be detected.

Recently, Antunes *et al.* also proposed a temperature insensitive acceleration measurement system based on a brass piece and two FBGs placed in opposite positions [32]. The system consisted in an inertial mass, supported by an L-shaped cantilever beam and connected through a thin element. The variation of the acceleration moves the inertial mass, contracting one FBG and expanding the other. In the presence of temperature variations, both gratings are affected in the same way, making this system immune to thermal effects.

The accelerometer described in [33] used a grating glued in a slanted direction onto the lateral side of a right-angled triangle cantilever beam. The application of an acceleration leads to a variation of the bending curvature along the beam length. Consequently, the FBG becomes chirp and the vibration values are given by the reflection bandwidth and optical power of the grating.

The devices described above can only determine the acceleration in one dimension. Nevertheless, some applications require monitoring two or three dimensions. The most common solution for this purpose consists in using individual accelerometers to measure the vibration in each direction. The system complexity, and also the cost, increase with this procedure.

In the literature, few papers report accelerometers for multidimensional monitoring. However, in 2002, Morikawa *et al.* demonstrated a triaxial temperature insensitive FBG accelerometer based on one mass and six FBGs, acting as spring elements [34]. Each direction was monitored by one fiber containing two FBGs, for compensation of the temperature effects. Although the authors proposed a triaxial sensor, only a one direction solution was implemented. In 2008, Fender *et al.* proposed a two-axis temperature-insensitive accelerometer relying on a fiber cantilever [35]. This was based on an optical fiber with four cores, each one containing a FBG. Acceleration induces curvature of the fiber cantilever and could be measured through the difference between the Bragg wavelength shifts of two gratings in the plane of the bend.

3.2 Strain and Temperature

The analysis of the strain performed in civil engineering structures is essential to avoid their failure. Usual structures maintenance of relies on scheduled visual inspections, supported by few conventional sensors for damage monitoring. However, these maintenance routines are expensive, the precision of visual inspections is poor and traditional sensors are not always well suited for the harsh conditions that they are subjected to. SHM systems have become a valid tool to study the stability of structures and to identify the design limits of similar structures. In this context, FBG sensors demonstrated to be a suitable cost effective tool to perform SHM in structures, from newly built oil platforms, where sensors can be embedded in the structure during the construction, to ancient restored buildings, where the sensors can easily be attached to the surface of the structure.

3.2.1 FBG Strain Sensors in SHM Applications

FBG strain sensors can be applied to recent structures, such as the Tsing Ma Bridge [36], or during restoration interventions in historical buildings, such as in the Church of Misericórdia in Aveiro, Portugal [4]. In some situations, sensors can also be embedded in the concrete in order to measure strains and loads during the construction and to monitor the structure during its lifetime, as Kister *et al.* reported for a 13 floors building in Bankside, London [37]. This building had FBG sensors in the foundations, measuring the cure of the concrete and the load while the floors were constructed.

Nowadays, the Tsing Ma Bridge is the longest suspended bridge in the world, with 1377 m in a double deck configuration. The bridge is monitored using a traditional wind and SHM system (WASHM). In 2006, Chan *et al.* published the results of their work comparing the performance of a assembly of FBG strain sensors to the existing WASHM system [36]. The tests were carried out in three specific locations: hanger cables, rocker bearings and a supporting structure of a lower deck. Twenty one FBG strain sensors were used to monitor the traffic load. Other FBG sensors measured temperature and allowed a compensation of the strain-temperature cross sensitivity. The conclusions attained from this work proved that the results from the optical fiber system agreed with the resistive strain gauges from the WASHM system.

Bragg sensors were also used to monitor the West Mill Bridge, the first Europe all-fiber reinforced composite bridge [38]. In this work, 40 FBGs were used to monitor, remotely and real time the strain on the bridge. This work aimed to be a tool to remotely assess the structural integrity of the bridge, validating the design codes and providing additional information for maintenance scheduling.

Another application in bridges was realized by Maaskant *et al.* where the long term stability of the pre-stressing tendons used in the Beddington Trail Bridge, Canada, was evaluated [39]. A strain precision of 40 $\mu\varepsilon$ was achieved and the results revealed that, over a 19 month period, the carbon fiber reinforced plastics (CFRP) tendons lost less 25% of pre-stress than the equivalent steel tendons, justifying the advantages of using CFRP material in bridges.

Fiber sensors are essentially used in buildings, but also in boats [40], railways [41], oil platforms [42], tunnels [43] and in geodynamic studies [44]. Due to their small size, weight and integration capabilities, FBG sensors also have the competitive advantages over traditional sensors for integration in smart composite structures. Therefore, it is natural that the number of structures being monitored by FBG strain sensors is increasing and diversifying.

3.2.2 Strain and Temperature Discrimination

When a FBG sensor is subjected simultaneously to strain and temperature variations, the Bragg wavelength shifts as a response to these variations. Therefore, a method to perform parameter discrimination is required.

The most common scheme to perform parameter discrimination consists in using two FBGs: one subjected to strain and temperature variations, while the other is isolated from strain, measuring only temperature. The wavelength shift of the second grating allows the determination of the temperature variation, which can be then subtracted from the wavelength shift of the first FBG, allowing to obtain the strain value.

Other methods for temperature and strain discrimination have been proposed over the years, and are still an interesting research area, with new solutions reported every year. The first sensing head for strain and temperature discrimination, proposed by Xu *et al.* in 1994, was based on two superimposed FBGs with very distant wavelengths, 850 and 1300 nm [45]. This experimental setup, as can be seen in figure 1, explored the different thermo-optic and photoelastic coefficients of the two FBGs to obtain a matrix with four different strain and temperature coefficients.

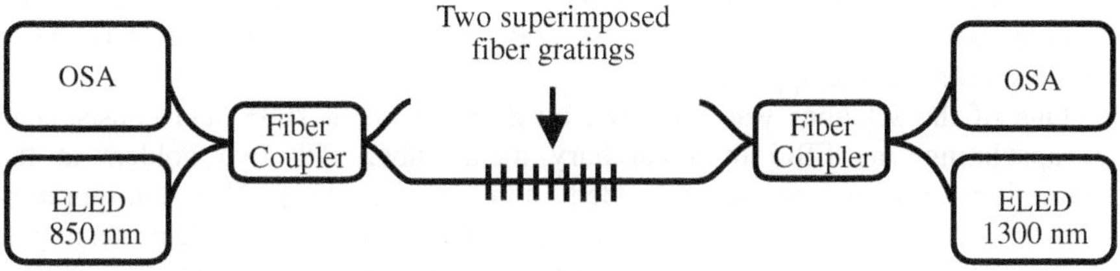

Fig. 1 Experimental set-up for strain-temperature discrimination using a dual-wavelength

This idea of exploring the different temperature and strain coefficients was followed by other authors. In 1996, James *et al.* created a sensing head by splicing two FBGs inscribed on optical fibers with different diameters, achieving distinct strain coefficients [46]. A similar approach, but for different temperature sensitivities, was later presented using FBG sensors written in the spliced region of fibers with different dopants [47]. This formula was repeated for a sensing head based on fibers doped with different concentrations [48] and for a sensing head obtained by splicing different FBG types [49].

More recently, a sensor based on two FBGs with distinct polymeric coatings was proposed [50]. The coating imposes different optical responses of the gratings and the sensitivity of the sensor to an individual parameter can be exactly determined. Mondal *et al.* employed an embedded dual FBG mounted on opposite sides of an arc-shaped steel strip [51]. The compressive and tensile strain effects were explored for thermal and strain discrimination.

In 2010, Lima *et al.* gave a step further in the strain and temperature discrimination by encoding strain information in the bandwidth of the Bragg signal [52]. They used a single FBG written in an optical fiber taper with a linear diameter variation, as represented in figure 2. When subjected to tension and due to the different cross sections of the fiber along its length, different values of strain occur, causing the broadening of the FBG signal and allowing the use of the information contained in both peak wavelength and spectral width.

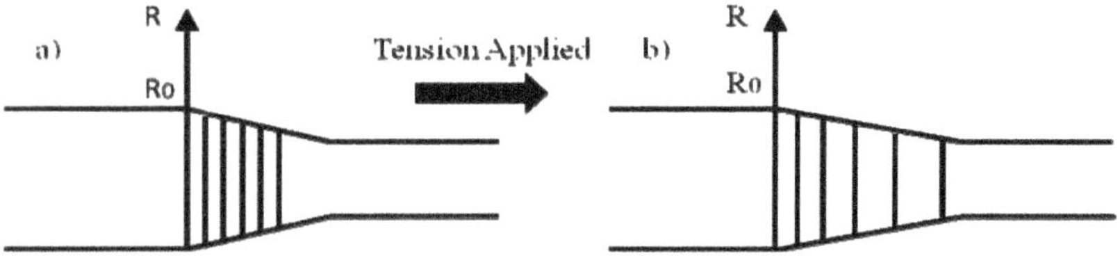

Fig. 2 Illustration of a tapered FBG (a) and tapered FBG after positive strain (b)

3.2.3 FBG Encapsulation

The low mechanical resistance of a FBG sensor arises by the direct inscription in the optical fiber. Thus, a suitable protection is required, for practical and long-term installation in infrastructures. Several encapsulation techniques have been proposed for specific applications.

One of the schemes was proposed by Zhou *et al.* in 2003, and consisted in encapsulating one FBG in a capillary metal tube, with two holders at the extremities designed to be embedded in a structure [53]. This configuration transfers the deformation from the structure to the FBG sensor, while protecting it. A year later, Slowik *et al.* also presented a similar design that added a concrete proof plastic house for extra protection against the cement alkaline environment [54]. For surface mounting on metal or concrete structures, a common FBG protection technique consists in gluing an optical fiber with the FBG sensor between two metal slices, as described in [53]. In this technique, since the fiber is encapsulated between the metal layers, the sensitivity is different from the original FBG, and so a calibration of the sensors is required before installation. Various designs for FBG sensor protections were also proposed by Leng *et al.*, in 2006 [55]. These included FBG sensors protected by CFRP, steel tubes and steel rebars. This work evaluated the strain transfer efficiency between the sensor protection and the sensing region using non-linear finite analysis. Experimental validation of the proposed protection techniques allowed the comparison between the performance of FBG based sensors and electrical resistance strain gauges, revealing a good agreement between the two sensing technologies.

Some encapsulation techniques provide protection of the bare FBG sensors, but also handle with the strain-temperature cross sensitivity. Athermal packaging designs for FBGs capable of compensating the thermal induced wavelength shift have been proposed [56, 57]. This is accomplished using a quartz substrate with the extremities of the FBG inscribed fiber attached and where part of the optical fiber has a copper coating. Because the quartz has a lower thermal expansion coefficient then copper, when the temperature increases, the high expansion of the copper compresses the FBG and creates a negative strain on it, compensating the temperature effect on the Bragg wavelength shift.

3.2.4 Concrete Cure Monitoring

Concrete cure is a complex process, dependent on the water to cement ratio, curing temperature, humidity and type of cement used, among others. The cement hydration is responsible for the gain in strength, but is also accompanied by water evaporation and re-arrangement of particles within the mix, resulting in a decrease of the concrete volume and in the development of internal strains. The strain in early age concretes is known as shrinkage strain and is responsible for the small cracks that appear after the curing process. The small cracks can grow in size and penetrate the structure at later ages, with the consequent implications to the structure health.

Traditional strain gauges can only be attached once the concrete is ready to be demoulded when it a minimum strength has been reached. However, there are some methods capable of determining the volume changes in concretes during the plastic phase. The most common technique consists in measuring the settlement of fresh mortar in a cone-shaped form [58], but this only allows discrete readings. For a continuous monitoring of the volume changes during the plastic phase, Slowik *et al.* proposed a method using FBG strain sensors to measure shrinkage strains of cement paste at early age, between 0 and 12 h after mixing [54]. Portland cement was placed into a prismatic form (9 cm x 3 cm x 3 cm) and the acrylate coated FBG sensors were embedded in the center of the specimen. Temperature discrimination was achieved using the data from the embedded thermocouples. The results from this work revealed a significant shrinkage between 3 and 6 h after mixing. After that, a temperature increase was detected induced by the exothermic nature of the hydration reaction. After 12 days, the total measured strain was 2700 $\mu\varepsilon$. The traditional measurement tests, started 24 h after the mixing, revealed 2000 $\mu\varepsilon$. The authors also concluded that the early age shrinkage depends on the concrete composition, environmental factors and the geometry of the specimen in study.

3.3 Pressure

The integrity of infrastructures depends on the exposure to several external conditions, including excessive use, overloading and insufficient maintenance. In the field of pressure sensing, the first FBG sensor was developed by Xu *et al.*, in

1993 [59]. In their experiments, a Bragg wavelength shift of 0.22 nm was obtained for a pressure of 70 MPa. A pressure sensitivity of -2.02 x 10^{-6} MPa^{-1} was achieved. In [60] the Bragg grating was embedded in a polymer-filled metal cylinder. The polymer was silicon rubber and the metal an aluminum cylinder, with one side open to enhance the pressure sensitivity. When pressure was applied the grating was strained by the polymer. With this configuration, the FBG only responds to axial pressure. The sensitivity obtained was -3.41 x 10^{-3} MPa^{-1}, which is about 1720 times higher than the reported in [59].

More recently, Liu *et al.* used a similar scheme, however the FBG was only partially embedded in the polymer (organic silica gel) filled copper tube [61]. As in [60], the sensor only responds to axial pressure. When pressure was applied the reflection wavelength was splitted into two peaks, with one steady peak and the other shifting to lower wavelengths. The pressure value is obtained from the wavelength difference of these two peaks. The obtained sensitivity was -2.44 x 10^{-3} MPa^{-1}, which corresponds to 1200 times enhance compared with the value acquired with a bare FBG. In addition to the significant improvement in the sensitivity, this sensor also provides immunity to thermal variation, within a temperature range of 18-24 ºC. Beyond the action as a transducer, the polymer used in these sensors also protects the physical integrity of the grating. This is an important feature, since the building monitoring occurs in some cases, under extreme conditions.

3.4 Moisture/Humidity Measurement

The water molecules can act as a transport medium for aggressive ions, including chloride, sulfate, carbonate and ammonium. The existence of such species in the building structures and in concretes represents a risk for their deterioration and corrosion. Thus, relative humidity (RH) sensors can be a useful diagnostic tool for the civil engineers in SHM.

RH is defined as the ratio of the quantity of water vapor present in atmosphere to the maximum quantity that atmosphere can hold. The number of traditional methods used to detect this parameter is high and includes resistive, capacitive and hygrometic humidity sensors. Regarding to optical fiber technology, since a bare optical fiber is immune to RH, it is required to coat the fiber with a humidity sensitive material. This material will act as a transducer to convert the RH into a measurable perturbation.

The influence of humidity on a polymer–coated FBG was first described by [62]. The sensing principle relies on the strain effect induced on the Bragg grating resultant of the swelling of the sensitive material. With the present sensor and using a polyimide coating, the authors obtained a linear response over a wide humidity ranging, from 10% to 90% RH. Due to temperature cross sensitivity, it is required an additional scheme to compensate the temperature effects in the humidity measurements. This can be easily obtained using a bare FBG, which is not RH sensitive.

The investigation in this field developed towards the study of the influence of coating thickness in several sensing characteristics, including the RH and temperature sensitivity, the time response and the hysteresis effect. Yeo and his collaborators concluded that the RH sensitivity of the sensor can be enhanced with the use of a thicker sensing polymer layer, inducing a higher strain effect on the Bragg grating [63]. However, in this case, the sensor response is slower and the susceptibility to temperature disturbances increases. A small degree of hysteresis was observed in all tested cases.

In 2009, Venugopalan *et al.* designed a RH FBG sensor for SHM [64]. The sensing principle is similar to the presented in [63], however, the sensor was embedded in a stainless steel tube containing multiple holes allowing the entrance of moisture. To compensate the thermal effect on the humidity sensor, an uncoated FBG was also included in the tube. This configuration provides resistance to the sensor that is essential to survive to the hash working conditions of structural monitoring. Additionally, the thermal cross sensitivity is also solved.

In 2008, the same research group had already proposed a humidity sensor for the same purpose, based on a Long Period Grating (LPG) [65]. The grating was coated with polymer polyvinyl alcohol (PVA) due to its affinity to water and ease of deposition onto the optical fiber. The sensing principle relies on the variation of the PVA refractive index and, consequently, wavelength shift as a result of the physical effect of swelling. A simple comparison of relative humidity FBG and LPG based sensors showed a superiority of the LPG device in the sensitivity and response time when compared with the FBG system.

Recently, other schemes based on optical fiber technology have been proposed to sensing the RH, as for instance references [66] and [67]. In the first case it was used a tilted FBG (TFBG) also coated with PVA. The sensing principle is similar to [65], however in this situation it is the TFBG transmission power that codifies the humidity levels, instead of the wavelength shift. This appears as a low-cost sensor since it was used a photodetector that is a cost-effective demodulation process. In [67], an etched superstructure FBG coated with a thin film of sol-gel was used. Its operation principle relies in the refractive index change of the sensing material with the presence of water molecules that is detectable through a Bragg wavelength shift.

3.5 Inclinometers

Tilt sensors, also known as inclinometers, are frequently used in many fields, including civil engineering. Important applications rely on the monitoring of the inclination of towers and bridge holders and detection of earthquakes. Traditionally, tilt measurement is accomplished converting the inclination into electrical signals through a magnetic or capacitive effect. However, in the last years, several FBG sensors for one or two dimensional tilt measurement have been reported in the literature.

One of these was proposed by Guan *et al.* and is based on a vertical pendulum and two pairs of FBGs, each monitoring the inclination in one dimension [68]. When the system was tilted, the pendulum moved and changed the strain induced in the fibers. The tilt angle was given by the wavelength separation between two FBGs, overcoming the problem of temperature cross-sensitivity. With the proposed sensor, an accuracy and resolution of $\pm 0.1^{\circ}$ and 0.007° were achieved, respectively, for the measurement range [-9°, 9°].

In [69], the same scheme was applied, however only three FBGs were used. The inclination was obtained from the reflected optical powers of the gratings, whose bandwidths increased as a result of the nonuniform strain effects from the inclination. Tilt angle measurement accuracy of ± 0.13° and resolution of 0.02° were obtained with this temperature-insensitive sensor, for the measurement range [-3°, 3°].

Recently, a novel two-dimensional temperature-insensitive FBG tilt sensor with a large measurement range was demonstrated [70]. The device was comprised by a vertical cylindrical cantilever-based pendulum, a mass and four FBGs, glued parallel on its surface. With the tilt of the system the cantilever was bended due to the weight of the mass. Consequently, the gratings experienced different strains values, depending on the bending direction and curvature of the cantilever. The tilt angle of the 2D inclination was calculated from the wavelength separation of two orthogonal groups of FBGs. The proposed sensor provided an accuracy and resolution of ± 0.2° and 0.0013°, respectively, in a measurement range [-40°, 40°]. Comparing with the two previous sensors, a similar resolution and accuracy values were obtained, but the analysis range increased considerably.

3.6 Ultrasonic Structural Health Monitoring

One non-destructive method used to monitor the health of structures, particularly composite structures, is based on ultrasonic inspection. This technique relies on shear waves generated by a probe at a given point of the structure and sensed by another at a different point. These waves are generated by a piezoelectric transducer and have frequencies up to the MHz range. As ultrasonic waves propagate in a structure, the damaged areas affect their propagation, resulting in a large number of mixed modes. The damages can be detected through the analysis of the detected waves.

Piezoelectric transducers have been the most common detection devices, however recent works used successfully FBG sensors as ultrasound detectors to monitor the health of metallic structures [71-73] and even in composite (CFRP) structures [74-76]. They were able to distinguish between ultrasonic waves passing though an undamaged or a damaged area, in situations where the conventional piezoelectric sensors had failed.

There are, however, some limitations to the use of FBG as ultrasonic sensors, namely because the radial resonances in the fiber will constrain the temporal bandwidth, limiting the sensitivity. The principle of operation of this method is illustrated in figure 3. A piezoelectric device produces the shear waves that propagate in the structure and reach the FBG detector. Light from a broadband light source passes through an optical circulator and illuminates FBG 1. The reflected light, after passing the optical circulator, is filtered by an FBG 2 that has a slightly higher Bragg wavelength. When the shear wave propagates, strain is induced to FBG 1 and the changes in the power output after FBG 1 and FBG 2 are detected by a photodetector. The power output of this configuration increases during tension and decreases during compression.

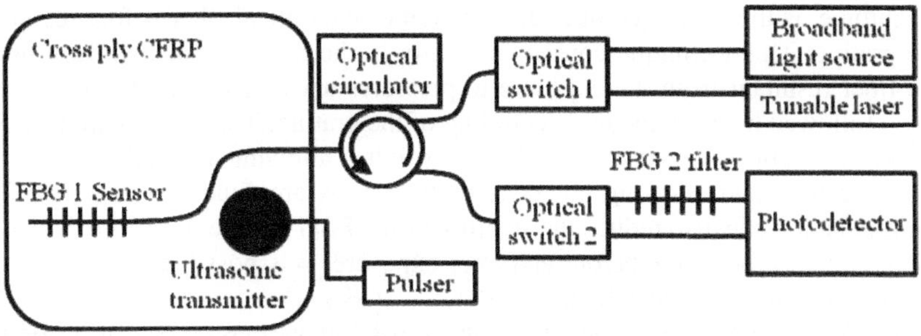

Fig. 3 Experimental setup in the ultrasonic non-destructive testing of structural health in cross ply CFRP and schematic illustrating the variation in reflectivity of the FBG sensor with applied strain [76]

4 Fiber Bragg Gratings Description

Fiber Bragg gratings are passive optical devices with application in the field of sensing and optical communications. Mainly due to the possibility of optimizing their spectral characteristics, the low insertion loss and the low implementation cost. Although they are rather complex devices, their characteristics depend on a large number of controllable parameters such as the grating length, the index modulation amplitude, the periodicity of the refractive index and the shape of apodization. A proper optimization of these parameters allows the shaping of the grating spectral characteristics, particularly in the reflection wavelength, reflectivity and spectral width, adapting the grating to the desired application.

The recording of permanent gratings was first demonstrated by Hill *et al.* at the Canadian Communications Research Centre (CRC), in 1978 [77, 78]. This team of researchers used an optical fiber, doped with germanium, which was illuminated by the radiation emitted from an argon ion laser (480 nm). After a few minutes, they observed that the intensity of the reflected light increased with the exposure time until the situation of total reflection. Later experiments proved that this increase in reflectivity resulted from the formation of a photoinduced periodic modulation of the refractive index in the optical fiber core [79]. During the following decade, it was found that the magnitude of the photoinduced disturbance in the refractive index was dependent on the square of the laser power. This suggested that photosensitivity would be a process resultant from two photons absorption phenomena, more specifically caused by the presence of germanium in the silica matrix oxygen centers. The maximum absorption occurs for a wavelength around 240 nm. The presence of these centers is due to the manufacturing process of optical fibers, during which the fiber core is doped with GeO_2 to slightly increase the core refractive index.

The standards optical fibers have low photosensitivity. However, there are techniques to increase it, such as co-doping of the core or increasing the concentration of Germanium. But one of the most widely used technique, for its simplicity, allowing an increase of the photosensitivity in about two orders of magnitude, is the technique of hydrogenation of the optical fiber before recording the grating. This technique consists basically in the diffusion of hydrogen inside the fiber resultant from the exposure to pressures above 100 atm during several days, followed by an immediate recording of the grating. The fiber hydrogenation, before irradiation, increases the photosensitivity, allowing the reduction of the exposure time and allowing higher refractive index amplitude modulations. The hydrogenation can also reduce the stability of the FBG with temperature, however, using certain procedures before and after exposure, it is possible to improve this stability, like thermal annealing.

In telecommunications, the FBG can be used at various points of an optical transmission system. They are used at the emitter elements as reflectors in semiconductor lasers, in order to obtain single-mode emission with high stability. In optical amplifiers, acting as the recirculation pump, the spectral gain of the diode pumping is equalized and stabilized, in dispersion compensation and filtering schemes. At the receiver, FBGs can act as filters and demultiplexers for multi wavelength networks.

4.1 Working Principle

The FBGs are structures created in the core of an optical fiber by exposure to an optical interference pattern of ultraviolet radiation. Through exposure, a longitudinal periodic perturbation of the refractive index is formed along the fiber core. The conversion of ultraviolet radiation on this spatial modulation is caused by a nonlinear mechanism called photosensitivity. The contrast of the refraction fringe modulation depends on the exposure time to radiation. Fibers with higher coefficient of photosensitivity require lower exposure times for the grating recording.

The principle of operation of a Bragg grating is illustrated in figure 4. When the wavelength of the incident signal satisfies the Bragg condition, the back scattered components on each plan of the structure are added constructively, resulting in a reflected signal. When the Bragg condition is not verified, the components scattered by the plans become progressively out of phase, and eventually vanish [80].

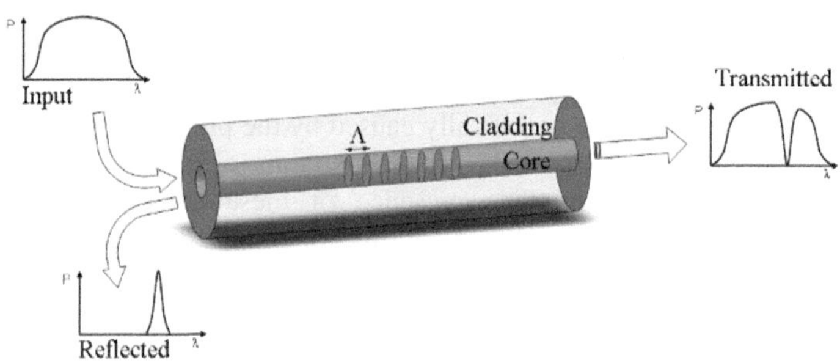

Fig. 4 Basic principle of operation of a fiber Bragg grating

The wavelength of the reflected mode, or the Bragg wavelength λ_B, is given by the first order Bragg condition:

$$\lambda_B = 2\Lambda n_{eff} \tag{1}$$

where Λ is the period of the refractive index modulation and n_{eff} is the effective refractive index of the guided mode.

The length of a FBG can vary from a few millimeters to several centimeters. The modulation amplitude of the refractive index, Δn, does not usually exceed values in the order of 10^{-2}, with typical values of $\Delta n \approx 10^{-4}$. For a FBG operating in the 1500 nm spectral region, a frequency modulation of $\Lambda \approx 0.5$ µm is typical. Any variation in the physical properties of the optical fiber, where the grating is recorded, such as stress or temperature variation, leads to changes in the grating structure and therefore changes in the Bragg wavelength.

As previously mentioned, the exposure of an optical fiber to ultraviolet radiation, with a suitable wavelength and intensity, induces a permanent change in the refractive index of the fiber core. The disturbance induced in the n_{eff} along the axis of propagation z is given by:

$$\delta n_{eff}(z) = \overline{\delta n_{eff}}\, f(z)\left\{ n_{th} + \upsilon \cos\left[\frac{2\pi}{\Lambda} z + \phi(z)\right]\right\} \tag{2}$$

where $\overline{\delta n_{eff}}$ represents the amplitude of the index modulation, $f(z)$ is the apodization shape (normalized to 1), ν the contrast between the recorded fringes that can have values between 0 and 1, Λ the period of the grating, $\phi(z)$ describes the grating chirp (variation of the period) and n_{th} is the deviation of the average refractive index perturbation [81].

4.2 Sensitivity to External Perturbations

The change of the reflected signal wavelength by the grating when subjected to external disturbances, allows the use of such devices as sensors. According to equation(1), the Bragg wavelength depends on the effective refractive index of fiber core and on the period of the interference pattern. Therefore, any external perturbation acting on these parameters can be quantified by the consequent shift in the Bragg wavelength. The application of a mechanical stress or temperature variations results in a change in the refractive index and on its period. These changes are quantified by the thermo-optic, thermal expansion and photoelastic coefficient.

The change in Bragg wavelength due to temperature variations, ΔT, and mechanical deformations, Δl is given by [80]:

$$\Delta\lambda_B = 2\left(\Lambda\frac{\partial n_{eff}}{\partial T} + n_{eff}\frac{\partial \Lambda}{\partial T}\right)\Delta T + 2\left(\Lambda\frac{\partial n_{eff}}{\partial l} + n_{eff}\frac{\partial \Lambda}{\partial l}\right)\Delta l \tag{3}$$

The first term of equation (3) represents the effect of temperature variation in the reflected wavelength, while the second term represents the effect of mechanical disturbance.

For a grating, free of mechanical disturbances ($\Delta l = 0$), the effect of temperature on Bragg wavelength is described by [80]:

$$\Delta\lambda_B = S_T \Delta T \tag{4}$$

where S_T is the thermal sensitivity, given by:

$$S_T = \lambda_B(\alpha_\Lambda + \alpha_n) \tag{5}$$

$$\alpha_\Lambda = \frac{1}{\Lambda}\left(\frac{\partial \Lambda}{\partial T}\right) \tag{6}$$

$$\alpha_n = \frac{1}{n_{eff}}\left(\frac{\partial n_{eff}}{\partial T}\right) \tag{7}$$

where α_Λ is the thermal expansion coefficient (in the case of silica, $\alpha_\Lambda \approx 0.55\times10^{-6}$ $^{\circ}C^{-1}$) and α_n the thermo-optic coefficient (in the case of Ge doped silica, $\alpha_n \approx$ 8.6×10^{-6} $^{\circ}C^{-1}$). For FBGs whose λ_B is centered at 1550 nm, we expect a thermal sensitivity of approximately 13 pm/°C.

For a grating not subjected to thermal perturbations ($\Delta T = 0$), the effect of mechanical disturbances in the Bragg wavelength can be described by [80]:

$$\Delta\lambda_B = S_{\Delta l}\varepsilon_z \tag{8}$$

where $S_{\Delta l}$ is the sensitivity to deformation along the longitudinal axis (z), and ε_z is the relative elongation according to the same longitudinal axis. The sensitivity to mechanical deformations can be represented by:

$$S_{\Delta l} = \lambda_B(1 - p_e) \tag{9}$$

being the effective photoelastic constant, p_e, defined as:

$$p_e = \frac{n_{eff}^2}{2}[p_{12} - \upsilon(p_{11} + p_{12})] \tag{10}$$

In equation (10), υ represents the silica Poisson coefficient and p_{11} and p_{12} are components of the photoelastic tensor. For a typical germanosilicate fiber the typical values are 0.16, 0.113 and 0.252, for υ, p_{11} and p_{12}, respectively. The use of these values in the previous expressions results in a strain sensitivity of 1.2 pm/1 με [80].

The characterization of a Bragg grating can be accomplished by the analysis of its reflection and/or transmission spectrum. Usually, a reflection scheme is used, as showed by figure 5, requiring the connectorization of only one fiber end. In order to minimize reflections at the free end of the fiber and to minimize background noise, a refraction index adapter gel is used, thereby decreasing the optical power reflected. The reflection spectrum can be obtained with the setup presented in figure 5, using an optical spectrum analyzer (OSA) and a broadband optical source.

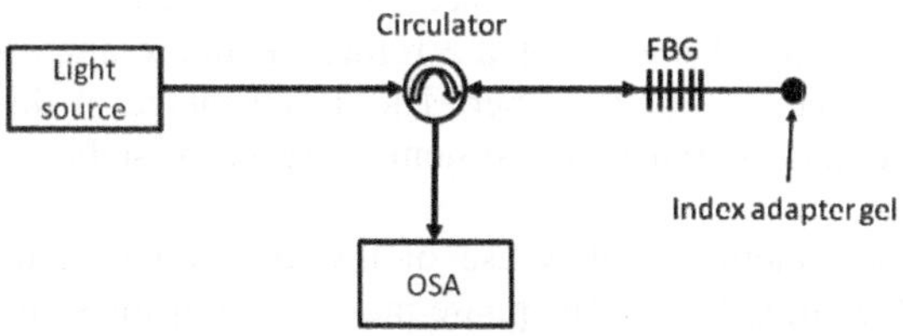

Fig. 5 Experimental setup to acquire the reflection spectrum of a FBG

A typical spectrum of an FBG is showed in figure 6, for a grating recorded by the interferometric method with phase mask.

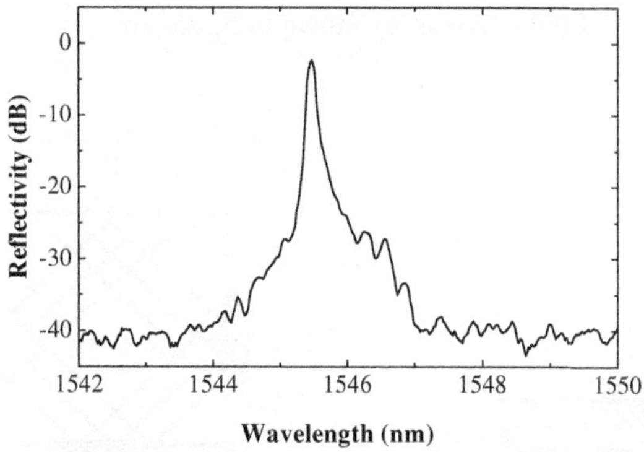

Fig, 6 Reflectivity spectrum, for a grating with a Bragg wavelength of 1545.46 nm

4.3 Writing Processes of FBGs

Hill used an internal method for FBG recording which consisted on the injection of radiation from an argon ion laser into the optical fiber core. In this case, the interference of the propagating wave with the counter-propagating wave resultant from the Fresnel reflection at the cleaved optical fiber end forms a standing wave occurs in the fiber core. The points where the maximum intensity of the standing wave lead to a regular and permanent change of the refractive index of fiber core, with a spatial periodicity equal to the wavelength. The major disadvantage of this approach lies in the weak amplitude modulation of the refractive index [82].

The commonly used external methods are based on the following techniques: interferometric processes, recording point to point and phase mask. Interferometric methods are based on dividing the laser beam into two beams with identical amplitudes, followed by recombination to form an interference pattern. When photosensitive fiber is exposed to this pattern, disturbances in the refractive index of the fiber core are induced with the periodicity of the interference pattern.

In the point to point method a pulsed UV laser is used and focused into the fiber. After recording a point, the fiber is translated a distance corresponding to the periodicity of the grating. This method allows each plan to be recorded independently, allowing a choice of the refractive index amplitude modulation along the longitudinal axis of the fiber. The disadvantage of this method is the difficulty to obtaining a translation system sufficiently stable and accurate for small translations.

The phase mask method makes use of this diffractive element to spatially modulate the UV writing beam. The phase mask is a transmission optical element, with a sequence of disturbances on the surface of a silica substrate and is usually produced by holographic processes or by lithographic processes with scanning electron beam [82]. The operating principle of this technique, showed in figure 7a, consists of the incidence of two overlapping orders on the fiber core, forming an interference pattern. Typically, the phase masks used are designed to maximize the diffraction orders -1 and 1 and to minimize the zero order.

It is also possible to use an interferometric method with a phase mask. The latter acts as an amplitude divisor, as shown in figure 7b.

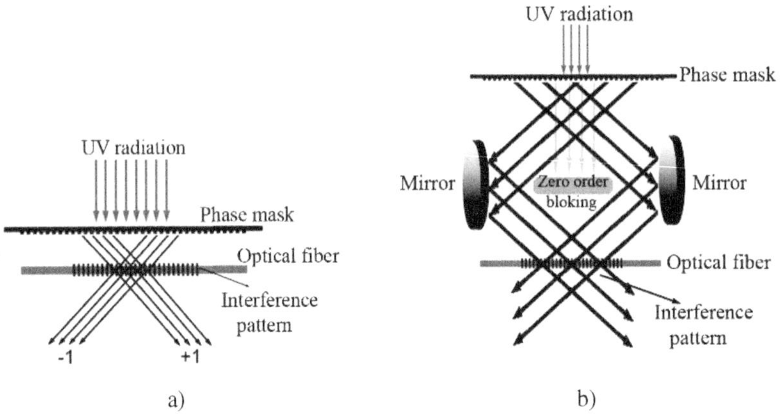

Fig. 7 Schematic representation of two methods used for recording Bragg gratings: a) phase mask and b) interferometric method with phase mask

4.4 Sensoring with FBGs

Over the last two decades, following the first successful manufacture of an FBG, an intense effort in research has been observed to improve FBG based sensors. FBG based sensors are now one of most promising sensing technologies due to the advantages over traditional electronic sensing. Namely, they form an intrinsic part of the fiber optic cable that can transmit the measurement signal over several tens of kilometres, the reduced weight and volume, the immunity to electromagnetic interference, the electrical isolation (no interference with electromagnetic radiation, so they can function in many hostile environments where conventional sensors would fail), do not make use of electrical signals, being explosion safe, have the ability to multiplex many sensors using only one optical fiber (driving down the cost of complex sensing systems) and due to its small size they are suitable to be embedded into many kinds of structures [83]. Although we are focusing our attention on SHM sensors, FBGs can have much more applications, such as in: aerospace, marine, medical, nuclear power, power transmition lines, among others [82, 84].

In structural sensing FBGs can be used for: strain monitoring in reinforced concrete beams, strain monitorization in civil infrastructures, strain monitoring in smart beams, pile load monitoring, early age cement shrinkage, moisture and humidity measurements in civil applications, geodynamic applications and ultrasonic non-destructive testing of structural health, see [83] and references therein. Although these types of sensors are usually applied in static measurements, they could simultaneously measure static and dynamic parameters in order to derive the structures eigenfrequencies, such as acceleration. The information provided by dynamic measurements is essential to calibrate numerical models and to infer about the structures integrity, since the global structure stiffness is directly related with its eigenfrequency [30, 79]. The FBGs present also a high response speed, only limited by the acquisition interrogation system.

A typical Bragg grating, recorded by interferometric method with a phase mask in a photosensitive fiber, was subjected to external disturbances, including variations in temperature and in strain. From the reflectivity spectrum, the Bragg wavelength can be estimated for different temperatures and applied strains. Figure 8 shows the wavelength shift for a typical Bragg grating, demonstrating a good linearity over practical wavelength ranges.

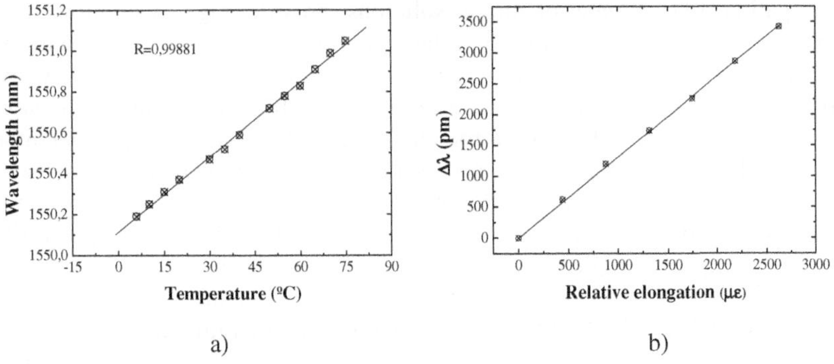

Fig. 8 Wavelength shift for a typical Bragg grating exposed to a) temperature variations and b) different strains. The points are experimental data and the lines represent the linear fit (r>0.99).

A linear fit to the data in figure 8 could be used to derive the FBG sensitivity to temperature and strain. For silica fibers, values of 12.21±0.12 pm/ºC and 1.307±0.008 pm/με (derived from figure 8) are typical for temperature and strain sensitivities, respectively.

One of the advantages of FBG sensing is the inherent capability to place several and different kinds of sensors in the same optical fiber. This multiplexing capability can be accomplished by different methods, commonly time division multiplexing (TDM) and wavelength division multiplexing (WDM). The TDM system employs a pulsed broadband light source and identifies different gratings by the time taken for their return signals to reach a detector. The pulses from closer gratings are received before those from more far away FBG. If the grating is subjected to some type of perturbation the time taken for its returning signal is changed. Because there are no spectral limitation, and thus gratings with the same wavelength can be used, the number of sensors in the same optical fiber can be as high as 100 sensors [85]. Because the sensors can be written in the same wavelength, they need to have low reflectivity to allow the signal to pass through the gratings and illuminate the gratings downstream. This is as setback of this demodulation system, because it will imply the use of amplifiers and the sensitivity could be reduced [86]. The other method, and the most usual, is the WDM method, in which each FBG has a different Bragg wavelength. In this system, several sensors can be implemented in the same optical fiber with different nominal centre wavelengths, each wavelength separated from the next by a few nanometers. The sensors are addressed individually by its Bragg wavelength which changes due to the environmental changes.

To use an FBG as a sensor, it must be illuminated by a broad band spectrum light source and the reflected wavelength must be measured and related to the local parameters of interest. The shifts in the Bragg wavelength can be monitored by several methods, including techniques based on simple interferometry [87], Fabry–Perot filters [88], matched gratings [89], acoustic–optic tunable filters [90], long period gratings [91, 92], Sagnac loops based on the chirped fiber Bragg gratings [93] or multi-port fiber Mach-Zehnder interferometer for multi sensors interrogation [94]. Some of these solutions provide high resolution in the measured wavelength domain, but they are rather complex or present high implementation costs. The interferometer technique may be used to convert wavelength shifts into phase shifts, measuring variations in the light intensity as the path difference in the interferometer is varied. This technique potentially allows high sensitivities, but the necessary equipment is expensive and can be sensitive to environmental interference. One of the most used and simple techniques can be implemented using a linear wavelength dependent optical filter. Due to its simplicity, high speed and lower implementation cost, this technique is appropriate for dynamic measurements, *e. g.* to demodulate an optical FBG accelerometer data. This method was firstly proposed by [95] and includes a band pass optical characterized by a linear spectral transfer function in the tuning range of the FBG. When the Bragg grating wavelength changes, a variation in the optical power transmitted thought the optical filter will be induced.

5 Experimental Implementation and Results

A SHM based on optical fiber sensors was implemented in several civil engineering structures. In this section we describe in detail the obtained results.

5.1 SHM in a Historical Building

The church of Santa Casa da Misericórdia of Aveiro is an important part of the architectural and historical heritage of the city of Aveiro in Portugal. Built in the XVI and XVII centuries, this building presents several construction techniques and, despite the presence of several construction materials, it is made mainly of masonry stone.

The detection of some reasonably sized cracks during an inspection drove the necessity to evaluate the structural stability of the structure and to monitor the structural movement control parameters (deformation and temperature).

A SHM system, designed to have a minimal visual impact, was implemented to monitor the structural health of this historical building. This SHM system aimed to monitor the main structural damages in the structure, and to obtain a continuous record of the structural health of the church and keeping the system as invisible and least intrusive as possible.

The blueprint of this building presents two rectangles that are the central nave and the long chapel. Between these, an arch is formed by two rows of stones, which is fixed on tuscane pilasters, see figure 9.

The technical inspections performed to this structure allowed the identification of the main structural problems. The critical zones were located in the centre of the arch and above it. The location of the gaps in the arch was homogenously

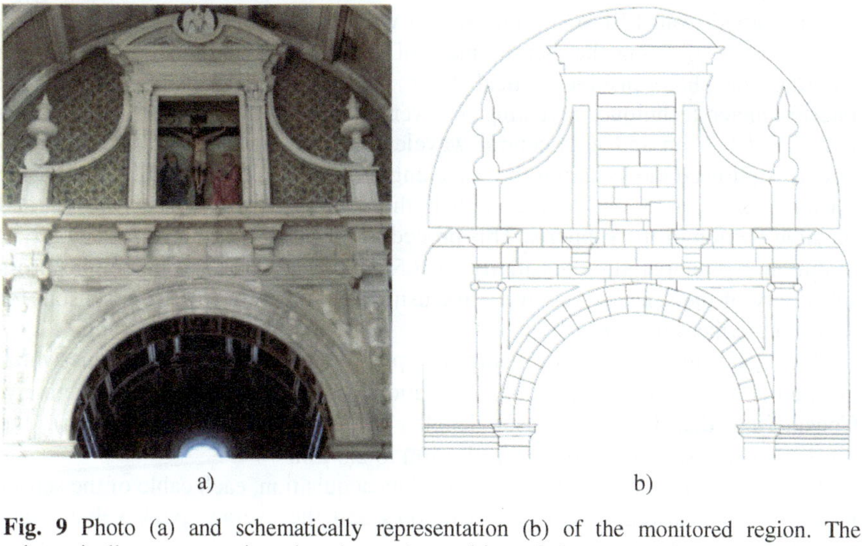

a) b)

Fig. 9 Photo (a) and schematically representation (b) of the monitored region. The schematically representation also shows the position of the stones hidden by decorative elements.

distributed, but their dimensions were variable from point to point, presenting, although, some symmetry. Furthermore, in some of the analyzed regions, the stones had suffered both horizontal and vertical movement. Additionally, the technical inspection revealed that the arch presented some abatement by decompression and, as result of this, some zones of the structure presented irregular alignments.

This project required the sensors installation with minimum visual impact and damage to the structure. In order to achieve that, the sensors were bonded to the blocks using epoxy resin and after the sensors installation only the small size supports could be seen (figure 10).

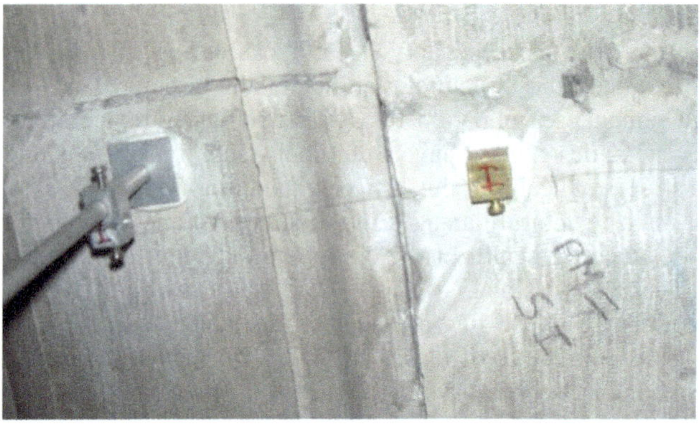

Fig. 10 FBG sensor after installation

The length of the FBG sensors was about 2 mm and the sensors total gage lengths varied from 140 to 300 mm with a working displacement range of ±0.2% of the length, allowing the measurement of gap opening and closing. They were recorded in photosensitive optical fiber (Fibercore PS1250/1500) using the interferometer technique, revealing an average peak reflectivity of 80% with a FWHM of 0.3 nm and with central wavelengths ranging from 1535 nm to 1555 nm. This allowed the system to be wavelength multiplexed. The calibration of the sensors was carried out to accomplish the effects of thermal expansion and possible flexion of the supports. This procedure revealed a strain response of 1.32 pm/$\mu\varepsilon$ and a temperature sensitivity of 8.5 pm/ºC. The strain-temperature cross sensitivity of the sensors was overcome using several strain free FBG sensors for temperature measurement.

Data acquisition was made using an optical sensing interrogator unit which allowed a strain and temperature resolution of 8 $\mu\varepsilon$ and 0.1 ºC, respectively. Considering the different sensor lengths (from 140 mm to 300 mm), the displacement resolution varied from 1.1 μm to 2.3 μm.

To decrease the uncertainty during the data acquisition, each cable of the sensor network was measured for a period of 60 s and the average peak values were recorded.

Displacements with two different origins were expected to be measured: thermo-mechanical displacements, which occur due to the expansion/retraction of the materials when subjected to temperature variations, and structural displacements, which are characterized by an effective movement between the stones where the sensors are mounted. Both can be caused by a great number of factors, such as traffic vibrations, earthquakes, and stresses accumulated during temperature variation cycles.

The measured displacements for the sensors are related to both described displacements. Sensors located at the extremities of the arch present a good correlation with the temperature evolution, as presented in figure 11a). In these locations, the monitored displacements were mainly due to temperature variations, and the structural displacements were negligible.

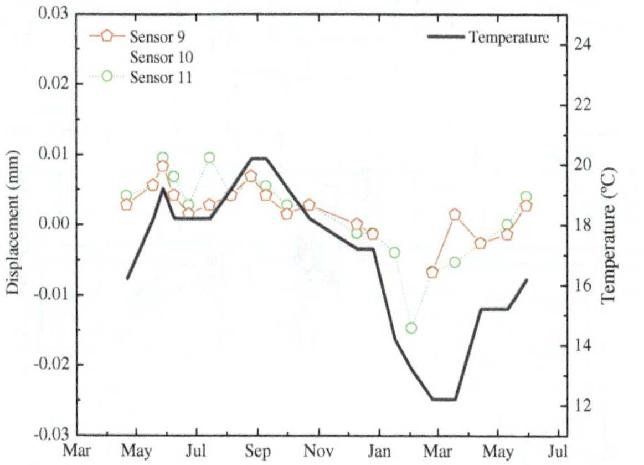

a)

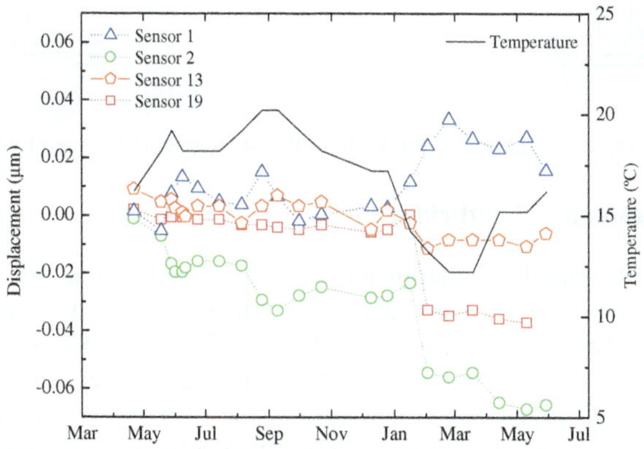

b)

Fig. 11 Measured displacements and temperatures for some of the sensors located at the extremities of the arch (a) and above the center of the arch (b)

The sensors located above the center of the arch revealed a distinct behavior, as pictured in figure11b). These sensors measured some sudden structural displacements, especially the ones caused by a 5.9 magnitude earthquake that occurred on the12th February 2007, with the epicenter located 500 km from the building.

The remaining sensors revealed a mixed behavior, showing the presence of thermo-mechanical displacements and effective structural displacements.

The information provided by the sensors allowed to identify the most sensitive regions of the structure and conclude that most of the displacements occur as a result of the load over the arch, and that is observed by the abatement of the centre of the arch, as represented in figure 12.

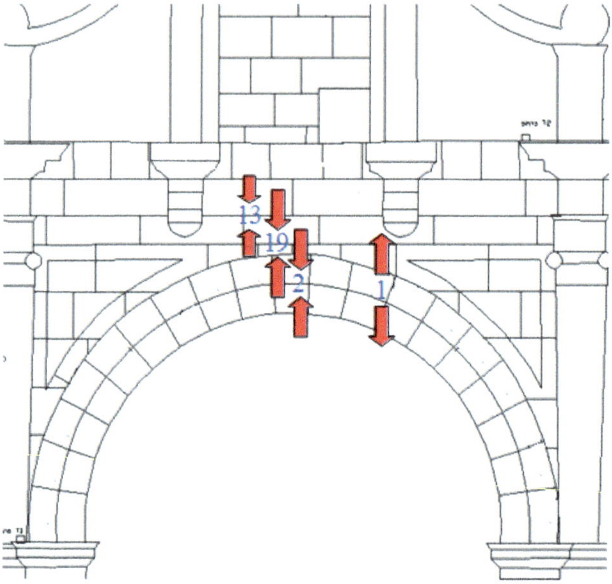

Fig. 12 Location and direction of the structural displacements induced by the earthquake

5.2 Acceleration in a Footbridge

A uniaxial FBG based accelerometer was developed and tested in an existing footbridge to evaluate its performance in full-scale structures at real loading conditions. The footbridge is deployed over the "Esteiro de São Pedro", located at the University of Aveiro (figure 13). The footbridge was constructed in 2001 to connect the two Campus of the University site, over the Aveiro estuary branch "Esteiro de São Pedro". The main structure is a straight continuous tubular steel truss, simply supported at the abutments at its ends and in 8 intermediate steel piers. The 9 spans of the bridge have an average length of 36 m, and the total length of the footbridge is 324 m. The bridge deck is a reinforced concrete slab connected to the steel tubular structure [30].

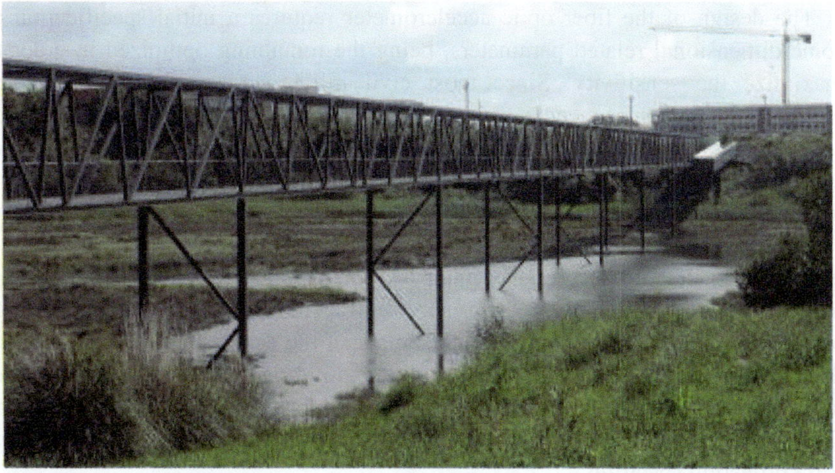

Fig. 13 Photo of the University of Aveiro steel footbridge over the Esteiro de S. Pedro

The sensor element of the developed accelerometer is a Bragg grating, written in a photosensitive single mode optical fiber, which was anchored in two points (A and B in figure 14). The structure of the accelerometer consists in an inertial mass, supported by a L-shaped aluminum cantilever beam, connected to the structure base by a steel leaf spring and a fiber Bragg grating element. When exposed to an external acceleration the inertial mass moves in the vertical direction, imposing a contraction/expansion of the optical fiber. This deformation induces variations on the λ_B. Since the vibration amplitude is small when compared to the cantilever dimensions, it can be considered that the movement of the inertial mass occurs only in the vertical direction.

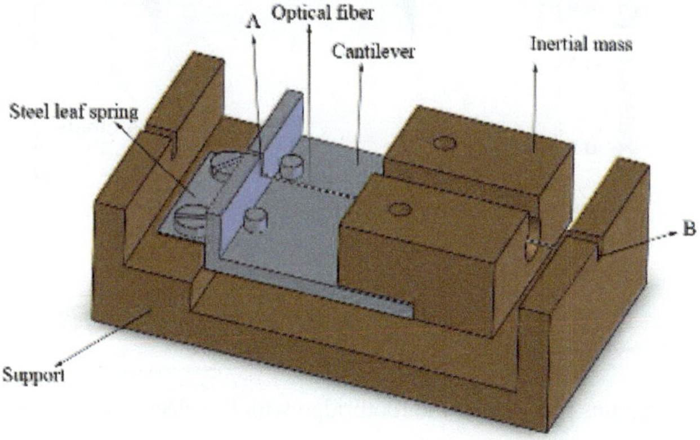

Fig. 14 Diagram for the FBG based accelerometer

The design of the fiber optic accelerometer requires a initial specification of some dimensional related parameters, being the remaining optimized in order to maximize the sensitivity. Since most civil infrastructures present the mains fundamental eigenfrequencies in the 0-20 Hz range, the implemented accelerometer should present a natural frequency higher than this value, but lower enough to maximize its sensitivity and keep the noise minimized. To measure the response of this optical accelerometer, with a sample rate compatible with the unit spectral response, it was also required the development of a low cost and fast interrogation unity. The proposed interrogation system is based on a band pass optical filter, which presents a linear spectral transfer function in the tuning range of the Bragg grating. Due to the displacement of the accelerometer inertial mass, the grating Bragg wavelength changes, inducing variations in the optical power transmitted through the optical filter. This optical power variation, measured at the filter output, is related with the convolution of the filter transfer function and the FBG reflection spectrum.

In the full-scale bridge structure, the implemented acceleration fiber optic sensor was tested and compared to a reference sensor, namely an electronic accelerometer. The tested sensors were attached to a heavy (5 kg) steel plate placed at the bridge over the measuring point. Therefore, it was assumed that the steel plate and the footbridge, at the measuring point, have the same displacement and acceleration components.

Figure 15 shows the acceleration data collected by the optical accelerometer and the electronic accelerometer, in which two mechanical impulses were applied by the simultaneous impulsion of five persons over the footbridge at a point close to the measuring position.

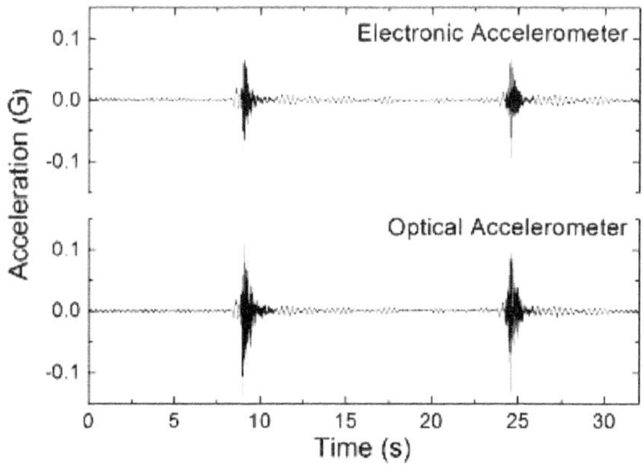

Fig. 15 Accelerograms recorded at the footbridge with the electronic accelerometer and the optical accelerometer

The root mean square error of the measured optical accelerometer data, when compared with the data from the electronic accelerometer, is 2.53×10^{-5} g and can be related to the system noise.

In figure 16, the frequencies spectra obtained from the data recorded during 40 seconds are shown, allowing the identification of the principal footbridge eigenfrequencies. These are summarily presented in table 1.

The optical accelerometer spectrum is very similar to those obtained from the electronic devices, in the 0-20 Hz range. For frequencies higher than 30 Hz an enhancement on the amplitude is obtained from the data recorded with the optical accelerometer, due to the proximity to the device natural frequency.

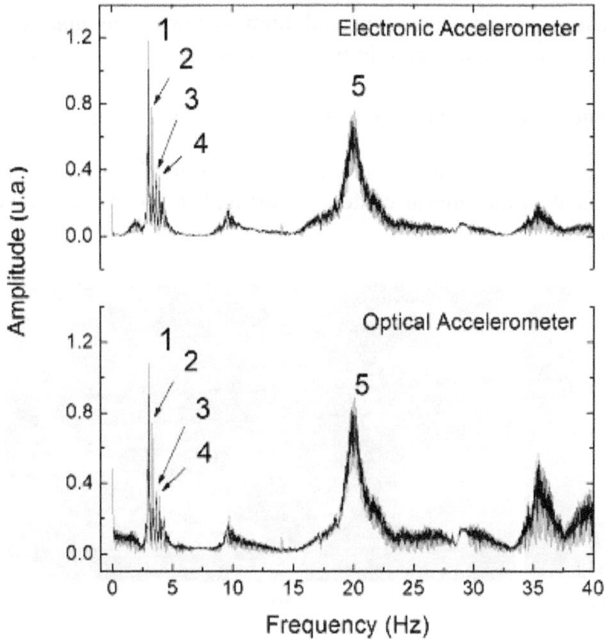

Fig. 16 Footbridge frequencies spectra

From the data presented in table 1, it is possible to compare the eigenfrequencies obtained with the optical accelerometer and with the electronic device. The optical accelerometer allows the identification of the footbridge main eigenfrequencies with a maximum relative error smaller than 0.01 % for the first resonant frequency, when compared with the values obtained with the electronic accelerometer data.

Table 1 Eigenfrequencies estimated

n	*Optical Accelerometer* *Frequency (Hz)*	*Electronic Accelerometer* *Frequency (Hz)*
1	3.02154	3.02154
2	3.34888	3.34888
3	3.70139	3.70139
4	3.92801	3.92801
5	20.04290	20.04290

These results confirm the expected high performance that results from the introduction of the optical technology in the structures dynamic characterization.

5.3 Dynamic Measurements in a Mobile Network Tower

The dynamic monitoring was extended to a mobile network tower. The studied tower is located in the littoral center of Portugal in the Aveiro region, as can be seen in figure 17.

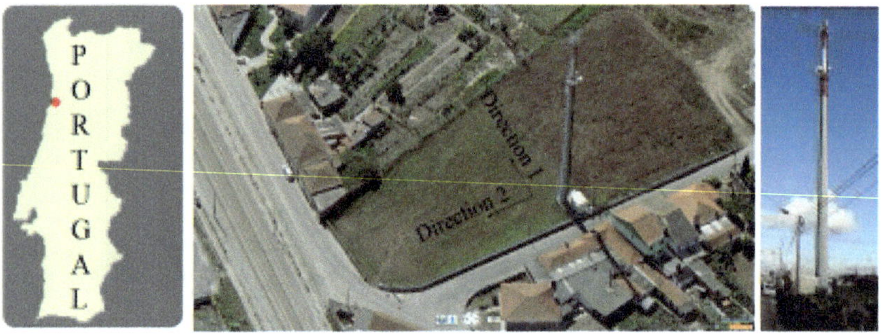

a) b) c)

Fig. 17 a) Location of the studied tower in the Portugal map; b) Studied tower and indication of the directions for which the acceleration sensor is sensitive (the picture was obtained through Bing Maps on 29th November 2010) and c) Photography of the tower.

For this test a FBG based biaxial accelerometer was used to characterize the resonant frequencies in the horizontal plane. The accelerometer was fixed in the top of the tower, with the axis align accordingly with figure 17b). The tower is a self-supported metal tower with 50 meters high and consists of seven distinct sections made of metal hexadecagonal cross-section profiles, joined by forced fit and fixed into the ground through a semi-deep foundation of reinforced concrete, with dimensions in plan 3.30x3.30 m and 3.60 m deep.

The acceleration data over time was acquired during the application of dynamic impulses on the tower at a height of 25 m. The data was acquired during 105 s using an experimental setup similar to the one showed in figure 5. The used spectrometer was an I-MON E-USB Interrogation Monitor Unit from Ibsen, acquiring at a rate of 950 Hz. The collected data is presented in figure 18.

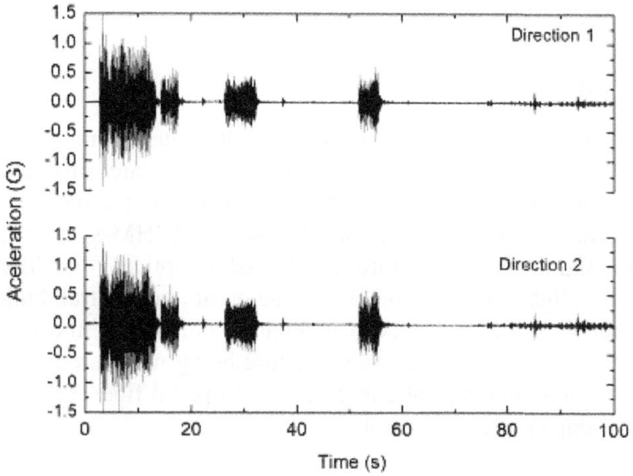

Fig. 18 Acceleration data over time in the two measurable directions

The natural frequencies of the tower are obtained by Fast Fourier Transform of the acceleration data over time. Figure 19 shows the frequency spectrum obtained for each direction, allowing the identification of several eigenfrequencies.

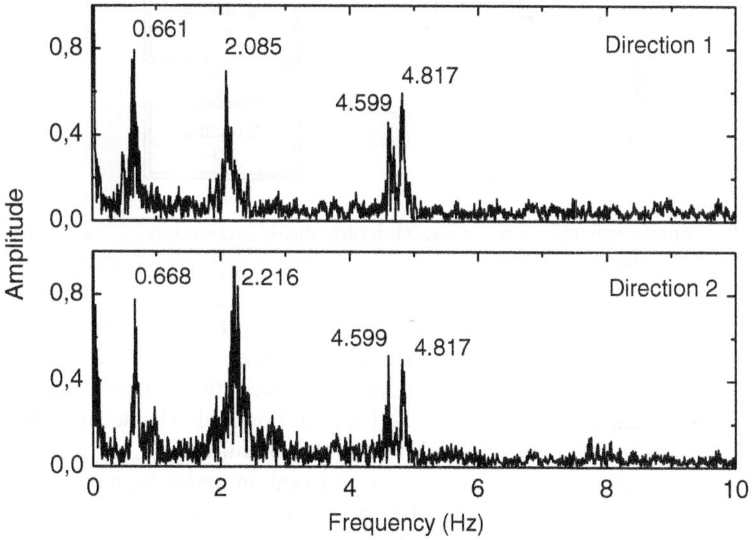

Fig. 19 Telecom tower frequencies spectra

The results shown that the first natural eigenfrequencies measured in both directions have similar values. The first natural frequency measured is within the limits of current values for this type of structures. These measured frequencies will be used to calibrate a numerical finite element model to represent the structural behavior of the tower. With the calibrated model, eventual structural damages or deficiencies in these towers can be identified [96].

5.4 Remote Structural Health Monitoring

In SHM, it is usually necessary to have an automated remote structural health monitoring (RSHM) and data access. The main reasons are: difficult access to the structure, cost reduction, automatic alarm triggering and possibility of monitoring different structures in a central station. A possible RSHM system may include a central station and different structures connected by optical fiber. The fiber is used to transport the light between the interrogator at the central building and the remote structures. Each fiber link is a separate channel of the interrogator, but each channel can have more than one structure being monitored. Figure 20 shows an example of a possible RSHM connected with optical fiber, based on 2 channels and three different structures to monitor.

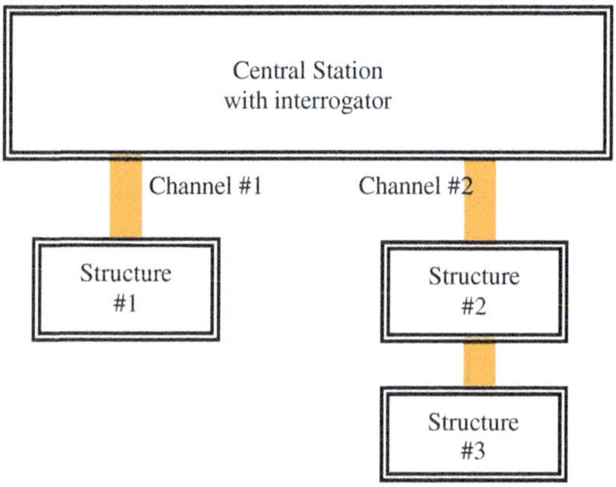

Fig. 20 Example scheme of a remote structural health monitoring system based on 2 channels and 3 structures to monitor

In some circumstances, it is not viable to connect the central station to the structures to monitor, thus a wireless data transmission between the sensors and the central station might be a solution. This was the solution used for the monitoring of one bridge in the A17 highway in Portugal. The access was limited and there was neither any optical fiber infrastructure nor any power supply available. Therefore the solution was developed in order to have a complete autonomous monitoring system. The full system is based on the following subsystems: autonomous power supply, optical fiber sensors, optical interrogation unit, communication unit and remote server, as illustrated in figure 21.

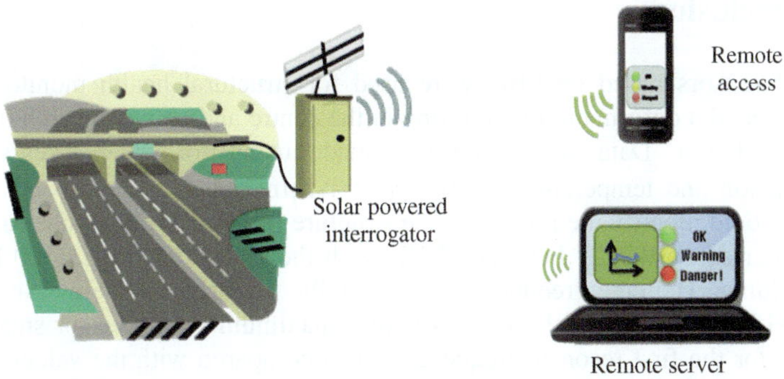

Fig. 21 Scheme of the installed remote structural health monitoring system, based on a solar powered interrogator and a remote server

The autonomous power supply is based on solar panels and a rechargeable battery. The system was dimensioned in order to be able to operate during more than five days without recharging. This is more than enough for the typical Portuguese weather. The optical fiber sensors are based on FBGs for displacement, deformation and temperature measurement. The displacement sensors can measure up to 8 cm displacements and have an additional FBG for temperature compensation and measurement. These sensors measure the relative movement of the bridge. The deformation and independent temperature sensors are standard FBGs with an external packaging for protection. The optical interrogator unit is based on an optical grating and a CCD with 512 pixels, operating in the C band. The measurement resolution is increased by software processing. The optical source is a broadband superluminescent LED. The interrogation sub-system is temperature controlled in order to minimize fluctuations and increase accuracy. The control system of the interrogator was designed in order to switch on and off the system in an automated way. In this way, the interrogator is generally on a hibernated state. After a pre-determined amount of time, in this case is 60 minutes, the temperature control system is switched on and, after a delay, the interrogator is also switched on, retrieving the info from the sensors. The data is then stored in the memory and the interrogator goes again to hibernated state. This procedure is repeated continuously. At a fixed time of the day, the interrogator sends the stored data to the remote server through a GPRS connection. The data sent is pre-processed to reduce data transmission. With these procedures, the power consumption is minimized. The remote server collects the data and processes the information taking into account the position of each sensor in the structure. It can also change the measurement parameters. It is also possible to have different alarms that can be triggered after a certain displacement or deformation is above the threshold. The data can also be used to give important information about the aging of the bridge, by analyzing the dynamics of the bridge over the years. The system will certainly give important information about the health of the bridge and can pave the way for next generation intelligent buildings.

6 Conclusion

Optical sensors based on FBG were used for structural health monitoring. We implemented a deformation monitoring in the centre and above the arch of a XVII century church. Data acquisition was made using for several years with a deformation and temperature resolution of 1.1 μm and 0.1 ºC, respectively. The system could identify the impact on the structure from a 5.9 magnitude earthquake that occurred on the12th February 2007, with the epicenter located 500 km from the building. The eigenfrequencies of a metallic footbridge were measured using an FBG base optical accelerometers with a maximum relative error smaller than 0.01 % for the first resonant frequency, when compared with the values obtained with the electronic accelerometer data. A bidirectional optical accelerometer was used to measure the resonant eigenfrequencises in a mobile telecom tower, allowing the identification of structural damage in the structure symmetry. Finally, the application of a remote sensing platform used to monitor in real time a highway bridge was described.

These results illustrate the applicability, maturity, flexibility and performance of FBG based sensors for structural health monitoring.

Acknowledgments

P. F. C. Antunes, H. F. T. Lima, N. J. Alberto and L. Bilro acknowledge the financial support from Fundação para a Ciência e Tecnologia (FCT) through the Ph.D fellowships SFRH/BD/41077/2007, SFRH/BD/30295/2006, SFRH/BD/30551/2006 and SFRH/BD/28607/2006. The authors gratefully acknowledge the collaborations of Santa Casa da Misericórdia de Aveiro, Vodafone Portugal, JustBit and Aveiro University for the access to the studied facilities.

References

[1] Sohn, A.H., et al.: A Review of Structural Health Monitoring Literature form 1996-2001, Los Alamos National Laboratory (2004)

[2] Culshaw, B., et al.: Smart structures and applications in civil engineering. Proceedings of the IEEE 84, 78–86 (1996)

[3] Rao, Y.-J.: In-fibre Bragg grating sensors. Measurement Science and Technology 8, 355 (1997)

[4] Lima, H.F., et al.: Structural health monitoring of the church of Santa Casa da Misericordia of Aveiro using FBG sensors. IEEE Sensors Journal 8, 1236–1242 (2008)

[5] ISISCanada, Guidelines for Structural Health Monitoring, Design Manual No. 2 (2001)

[6] Helmut Wenzel, P. F.: SHM at the Civil Infrastructure: Applications, recent Progress and future Demands (2010), http://www.brimos.com/Brimos/HTML/FRAMESET/Frameset_Downloads.htm

[7] Lovejoy, S.: Applications of structural health monitoring to highway bridges (2010), http://www.oregon.gov/ODOT/HWY/BRIDGE/index.shtml
[8] Oliveira, D.V., et al.: Structural monitoring of the Monastery of Jerónimos. Presented at the International Conference on the 250th Anniversary of the 1755 Lisbon Earthquake, Lisbon (2005)
[9] Aktan, E., et al.: Monitoring and Managing the Health of Infrastructure Systems. In: SPIE Conference on Health Monitoring of Highway Transportation Infrastructure. SPIE, CA (2001)
[10] Stallings, J.M., et al.: Field Performance of FRP Bridge Repairs. Journal of Bridge Engineering 5, 107–113 (2000)
[11] Fraser, M., et al.: Elements of an integrated health monitoring framework - Smart Nondestructive Evaluation and Health Monitoring of Structural and Biological Systems II. Presented at the Proceedings of the SPIE (2003)
[12] Aktan, A.E., et al.: Development of a Model Health Monitoring Guide for Major Bridges, Report Submitted to: Federal Highway Administration Research and Development (2002)
[13] Barbosa, C., et al.: Weldable fibre Bragg grating sensors for steel bridge monitoring. Journal of Measurement Science and Technology 12, 125305–125315 (2008)
[14] Jayant, D.M.: Health Monitoring of Civil Engineering Materials, Master Thesis, Purdue University, West Lafayette, Indiana (2008)
[15] Inaudi, D., et al.: Structural monitoring by curvature analysis using interferometric fiber optic sensors. Smart Mater. Struct. 7, 199–208 (1998)
[16] Faber, M.H., et al.: Proof load testing for bridge assessment and upgrading. Engineering Structures 22, 1677–1689 (2000)
[17] Drdácký, M.: Structural and Material Health Monitoring of Historical Objects. In: Ansari, F. (ed.) Sensing Issues in Civil Structural Health Monitoring. Springer, Heidelberg (2005)
[18] Kuang, S.C., et al.: Plastic Optical Fibre Sensors for Structural Health Monitoring: A Review of Recent Progress. Journal of Sensors (2009)
[19] FIBTaskGroup5.1, Monitoring and Safety Evaluation of Existing Concrete Structures - State-of-the-Art Report (2002)
[20] Inaudi, D., et al.: In-line coherence multiplexing of displacement sensors: a fiber optic extensometer. Presented at the SPIE, Smart Structures and Materials, San Diego, USA (1996)
[21] Rodríguez, J., et al.: Assessing Structural Conditions of Concrete Structures with Corroded Reinforcement. Presented at the nternational Congress: Concrete in the Service of Mankind, Conference No. 5 Concrete Repair Rehabilitation and Protection, Dundee, UK (1996)
[22] Giurgiutiu, V., Cuc, A.: Embedded Non-destructive Evaluation for Structural Health Monitoring, Damage Detection, and Failure Prevention. The Shock and Vibration Digest 37, 83–105 (2005)
[23] Adams, D.: Health Monitoring of Structural Materials and Components: Methods with Applications. John Wiley & Sons Inc., Chichester (2007)
[24] Pines, D., Aktan, A.E.: Status of structural health monitoring of long-span bridges in the United States. Progress in Structural Engineering and Materials 4, 372–380 (2002)
[25] Caicedo, J.M., Dyke, S.J.: Implementation of a SHM method on a numerical model of a cable-stayed bridge. Presented at the Proceeding of the 2004 American Control Conference, Boston, Massachusetts (2004)

[26] Freudenthaler, B., et al.: Case-based Decision Support for Bridge Monitoring. Presented at the The Third International Multi-Conference on Computing in the Global Information Technology. IEEE, Los Alamitos (2008)
[27] Wenzel, H.: Health Monitoring of Bridges. John Wiley & Sons, Ltd., Chichester (2009)
[28] Berkoff, T.A., Kersey, A.D.: Experimental demonstration of a fiber Bragg grating accelerometer. IEEE Photonics Technology Letters 8, 1677–1679 (1996)
[29] Todd, M.D., et al.: Flexural beam-based fiber Bragg grating accelerometers. IEEE Photonics Technology Letters 10, 1605–1607 (1998)
[30] Antunes, P.F.C., et al.: Optical Fiber Accelerometer System for Structural Dynamic Monitoring. IEEE Sensors Journal 9, 1347–1354 (2009)
[31] Zhu, Y., et al.: Temperature-insensitive fiber Bragg grating accelerometer. IEEE Photonics Technology Letters 15, 1437–1439 (2003)
[32] Antunes, P., et al.: Uniaxial fiber Bragg grating accelerometer system with temperature and cross axis insensitivity. Measurement 44, 55–59 (2011)
[33] Zhou, W., et al.: Temperature-independent vibration sensor with a fiber Bragg grating. Microwave and Optical Technology Letters 52, 2282–2285 (2010)
[34] Morikawa, S.R.K., et al.: Triaxial Bragg grating accelerometer. In: 15th Optical Fiber Sensors Conference Technical Digest, OFS 2002, vol. 1, pp. 95–98 (2002)
[35] Fender, A., et al.: Two-Axis Temperature-Insensitive Accelerometer Based on Multicore Fiber Bragg Gratings. IEEE Sensors Journal 8, 1292–1298 (2008)
[36] Chan, T.H.T., et al.: Fiber Bragg grating sensors for structural health monitoring of Tsing Ma bridge: Background and experimental observation. Engineering Structures 28, 648–659 (2006)
[37] Kister, G., et al.: Methodology and integrity monitoring of foundation concrete piles using Bragg grating optical fibre sensors. Engineering Structures 29, 2048–2055 (2007)
[38] Gebremichael, Y.M., et al.: Integration and assessment of fibre Bragg grating sensors in an all-fibre reinforced polymer composite road bridge. Sensors and Actuators a-Physical 118, 78–85 (2005)
[39] Maaskant, R., et al.: Fiber-optic Bragg grating sensors for bridge monitoring. Cement & Concrete Composites 19, 21–33 (1997)
[40] Todd, M.D., et al.: Bragg grating-based fibre optic sensors in structural health monitoring. Philosophical Transactions of the Royal Society a-Mathematical Physical and Engineering Sciences 365, 317–343 (2007)
[41] Tam, H.Y., et al.: Utilization of fiber optic Bragg Grating sensing systems for health monitoring in railway applications. Structural Health Monitoring 2007: Quantification, Validation, and Implementation 1& 2, 1824–1831 (2007)
[42] Ren, L., et al.: Health monitoring system for offshore platform with fiber Bragg grating sensors. Optical Engineering 45, 084401 (2006)
[43] Okundi, E., et al.: Structural health monitoring of underground railways. Structural Health Monitoring and Intelligent Infrastructure 1& 2, 1039–1046 (2003)
[44] Ferraro, P., De Natale, G.: On the possible use of optical fiber Bragg gratings as strain sensors for geodynamical monitoring. Optics and Lasers in Engineering 37, 115–130 (2002)
[45] Xu, M.G., et al.: Discrimination between Strain and Temperature Effects Using Dual-Wavelength Fiber Grating Sensors. Electronics Letters 30, 1085–1087 (1994)
[46] James, S.W., et al.: Simultaneous independent temperature and strain measurement using in-fibre Bragg grating sensors. Electronics Letters 32, 1133–1134 (1996)

[47] Cavaleiro, P.M., et al.: Simultaneous measurement of strain and temperature using Bragg gratings written in germanosilicate and boron-codoped germanosilicate fibers. IEEE Photonics Technology Letters 11, 1635–1637 (1999)
[48] Frazao, O., Santos, J.L.: Simultaneous measurement of strain and temperature using a Bragg grating structure written in germanosilicate fibres. Journal of Optics a-Pure and Applied Optics 6, 553–556 (2004)
[49] Shu, X.W., et al.: Dependence of temperature and strain coefficients on fiber grating type and its application to simultaneous temperature and strain measurement. Optics Letters 27, 701–703 (2002)
[50] Lu, P., et al.: Resolving cross sensitivity of fiber Bragg gratings with different polymeric coatings. Applied Physics Letters 92, 171112–171112-3 (2008)
[51] Mondal, S.K., et al.: Embedded Dual Fiber Bragg Grating Sensor for Simultaneous Measurement of Temperature and Load (Strain) with Enhanced Sensitivity. Microwave and Optical Technology Letters 51, 1621–1624 (2009)
[52] Lima, H.F., et al.: Simultaneous Measurement of Strain and Temperature With a Single Fiber Bragg Grating Written in a Tapered Optical Fiber. IEEE Sensors Journal 10, 269–273 (2010)
[53] Zhou, D.P., et al.: Techniques of advanced FBG sensors: fabrication, demodulation, encapsulation and their applications in the structural health monitoring of bridges. Pacific Science Review 5, 6 (2003)
[54] Slowik, V., et al.: Experimental investigation into early age shrinkage of cement paste by using fibre Bragg gratings. Cement & Concrete Composites 26, 473–479 (2004)
[55] Leng, J.S., et al.: Structural NDE of concrete structures using protected EFPI and FBG sensors. Sensors and Actuators a-Physical 126, 340–347 (2006)
[56] Johnson, A.E., et al.: Athermal package for fibre Bragg gratings with two or more bonding regions, US Patent Patent 6,856,730 (2005)
[57] Lo, Y.L., Kuo, C.P.: Packaging a fiber Bragg grating with metal coating for an athermal design. Journal of Lightwave Technology 21, 1377–1383 (2003)
[58] Greim, M., Teubert, O.: Vorrichtung zur Erfassung des frühen Dehn-und Schwindverhaltens von Baustoffen, German Patent Patent DE 10046284 A1 (2002)
[59] Xu, M.G., et al.: Optical in-fibre grating high pressure sensor. Electronics Letters 29, 398–399 (1993)
[60] Zhang, Y., et al.: High-sensitivity pressure sensor using a shielded polymer-coated fiber Bragg grating. IEEE Photonics Technology Letters 13, 618–619 (2001)
[61] Liu, L., et al.: Temperature-independent FBG pressure sensor with high sensitivity. Optical Fiber Technology 13, 78–80 (2007)
[62] Giaccari, P., et al., Influence of humidity and temperature on polyimide-coated fiber Bragg gratings, p. BFB2 (2001)
[63] Yeo, T.L., et al.: Characterisation of a polymer-coated fibre Bragg grating sensor for relative humidity sensing. Sensors and Actuators B: Chemical 110, 148–156 (2005)
[64] Venugopalan, T., et al.: Evaluation and calibration of FBG-based relative humidity sensor designed for structural health monitoring, p. 750310 (2009)
[65] Venugopalan, T., et al.: Long period grating-based humidity sensor for potential structural health monitoring. Sensors and Actuators A: Physical 148, 57–62 (2008)
[66] Miao, Y., et al.: Relative Humidity Sensor Based on Tilted Fiber Bragg Grating With Polyvinyl Alcohol Coating. IEEE Photonics Technology Letters 21, 441–443 (2009)
[67] Ai, L., et al.: Humidity fiber sensors based on superstructure fiber Bragg gratings coated with porous sol gel. Microwave and Optical Technology Letters 51, 40–42 (2009)

[68] Guan, B.-O., et al.: Temperature-independent fiber Bragg grating tilt sensor. IEEE Photonics Technology Letters 16, 224–226 (2004)

[69] Dong, X., et al.: Temperature-insensitive tilt sensor with strain-chirped fiber Bragg gratings. IEEE Photonics Technology Letters 17, 2394–2396 (2005)

[70] Bao, H., et al.: Temperature-insensitive FBG tilt sensor with a large measurement range. Optics Communications 283, 968–970 (2010)

[71] Sorazu, B., et al.: Optical generation and detection of ultrasound. Strain 39, 111–114 (2003)

[72] Tsuda, H., et al.: Fatigue crack propagation monitoring of stainless steel using fiber Bragg grating ultrasound sensors. Smart Materials & Structures 15, 1429–1437 (2006)

[73] Tsuda, H., et al.: Investigation of fatigue crack in stainless steel using a mobile fiber Bragg, grating ultrasonic sensor. Optical Fiber Technology 13, 209–214 (2007)

[74] Lee, J.R., et al.: Single-mode fibre optic Bragg grating sensing on the base of birefringence in surface-mounting and embedding applications. Optics and Laser Technology 39, 157–164 (2007)

[75] Takeda, N., et al.: Development of smart composite structures with small-diameter fiber Bragg grating sensors for damage detection: Quantitative evaluation of delamination length in CFRP laminates using Lamb wave sensing. Composites Science and Technology 65, 2575–2587 (2005)

[76] Tsuda, H.: Ultrasound and damage detection in CFRP using fiber Bragg grating sensors. Composites Science and Technology 66, 676–683 (2006)

[77] Kawasaki, B.S., et al.: Narrow-Band Bragg Reflectors in Optical Fibers. Optics Letters 3, 66–68 (1978)

[78] Hill, K.O., et al.: Photosensitivity in Optical Fiber Waveguides - Application to Reflection Filter Fabrication. Applied Physics Letters 32, 647–649 (1978)

[79] Antunes, P.: Análise dimânica de estruturas com sensores de Bragg, MSc Dissertation, Departamento de Fisica, Universidade de Aveiro, Aveiro (2007)

[80] Othonos, A.: Fiber Bragg gratings. Review of Scientific Instruments 68, 4309–4341 (1997)

[81] Lima, M.J.N., et al.: Simultaneous filtering and dispersion compensation in WDM systems using apodised fibre gratings. Electronics Letters 36, 1412–1414 (2000)

[82] Othonos, A., Kalli, K.: Fiber Bragg Gratings: Fundamentals and Applications in Telecommunications and Sensing. Artech House, Boston (1999)

[83] Majumder, M., et al.: Fibre Bragg gratings in structural health monitoring–Present status and applications. Sensors and Actuators A: Physical 147, 150–164 (2008)

[84] Jose, M.: Manuel Menendez and G. Alfredo Guemes. SHM Using Fiber Sensors in Aerospace Applications, p. MF1 (2006)

[85] Chung, W.H., et al.: Time- and wavelength-division multiplexing of FBG sensors using a semiconductor optical amplifier in ring cavity configuration. IEEE Photonics Technology Letters 17, 2709–2711 (2005)

[86] Zhou, Z., et al.: Techniques of Advanced FBG sensors: fabrication, demodulation, encapsulation and their application in the structural health monitoring of bridges. Pacific Science Review 5, 116–121 (2003)

[87] Kersey, A.D., et al.: Fiber-optic Bragg grating strain sensor with drift-compensated high-resolution interferometric wavelength-shift detection. Optics Letters 18, 72–74 (1993)

[88] Kersey, A.D., et al.: Multiplexed fiber Bragg grating strain-sensor system with a fiber Fabry - Perot wavelength filter. Optics Letters 18, 1370 (1993)

[89] Jackson, D.A., et al.: Simple multiplexing scheme for a fiber-optic grating sensor network. Optics Letters 18, 1192–1194 (1993)

[90] Volanthen, M., et al.: Simultaneous monitoring of multiple fibre gratings with a single acousto-optic tunable filter. Electronics Letters 32, 1228–1229 (1996)

[91] Jung, J., et al.: Novel interrogation system for dynamic strain measurement based on fiber Bragg grating sensor using long period grating pair and EDF. Presented at the Lasers and Electro-Optics Society 2000 Annual Meeting, Puerto Rico (2000)

[92] Zhang, L., et al.: Large-Dynamic-Range and High Resolution From a Strain Sensing System Using Long-Period Grating Interrogating FBG Strain Sensor. Presented at the ECOC 1998, Spain (1998)

[93] Zhao, D., et al.: Sensor interrogation technique using chirped fibre grating based Sagnac loop. Electronics Letters 38, 312–313 (2002)

[94] Jiang, Y.: Four-element FBG acceleration sensor array. Optics & Lasers in Engineering 46, 695–703 (2008)

[95] Melle, S.M., et al.: A passive wavelength demodulation system for guided-wave Bragg grating sensors. IEEE Photonics Technol. Lett. 4, 516–518 (1992)

[96] Travanca, R.: Torres de radiocomunicações: Patologias e dimensionamento Msc, University of Aveiro (2010)

Polymer Optical Fiber Sensors in Structural Health Monitoring

Sascha Liehr

BAM Federal Institute for Materials Research and Testing,
Unter den Eichen 87, 12205
Berlin, Germany

1 Introduction

This chapter summarizes the recent development in the relatively new and emerging field of structural health monitoring using polymer optical fiber (POF) sensors, also referred to as plastic optical fiber sensors. The extraordinary mechanical properties of POF in terms of strainability and ruggedness allows for measurement applications that could not or only insufficiently be solved with existing techniques. A great number of measurement parameters relevant for structural health monitoring applications, such as strain, displacement, crack width, vibrations or moisture can be measured with POF sensors. Numerous sensing principles have been proposed during the last 20 years and the most promising techniques and developments for SHM will be introduced. The focus is on the measurement of physical quantities for early damage detection and propagation, structural surveillance and analysis of dynamic processes.

The general advantages of optical fiber sensors over traditional measurement techniques are well-known. Being immune to electromagnetic interference, chemically inert, lightweight, small in size, easy to integrate and providing galvanic isolation often make them the only option for certain sensing applications. Silica fiber-based and already matured technologies such as fiber Bragg gratings (FBGs) for point-wise or quasi-distributed strain and temperature sensing are already a downmarket product. But especially fiber optic sensors for distributed measurement of strain or temperature have advantages over existing sensor techniques and are already common practice in various fields of structural health monitoring. Their ability to measure for example strain continuously distributed along the whole length of the fiber substitutes for thousands of standard electrical transducers. The benefit of these sensors in addition to an increase of safety is also a commercial one since damages can be detected and repaired at an early stage, thus decreasing maintenance costs. Sensor systems based on stimulated Brillouin scattering in silica optical fibers provide precise strain resolution and good spatial resolution and have been commercially used for many years already [1,2].Coherent backscatter measurement techniques have been proposed for precise and high spatial resolution measurement of short fiber sections [3].

S.C. Mukhopadhyay (Ed.): New Developments in Sensing Technology for SHM, LNEE 96, pp. 297–333.
springerlink.com

All these silica fiber-based sensor systems however, suffer from the relatively low break-down strain of the fibers of about 1%. Here, polymer optical fibers with their extraordinary mechanical properties come into focus. It has been shown that standard POFs can measure strain up to 45 % [4] or even more than 100 % [5,6]. This ability provides a solution for many monitoring problems that cannot be solved with traditional measurement techniques and opens new fields of applications where high-strain measurement is necessary. Moreover, POFs are very rugged, easy to handle and interconnect due to their relatively large core diameters and numerical apertures. Standard fibers and cables for data transmission can be used for many sensor applications and are available at a low price.

Also the mechanical parameters of POFs are favorable for sensing applications. The very low Young's modulus of POFs (3.2 GPa of PMMA compared to 72 GPa of silica) is beneficial, especially when deformations in materials or structures of low Young's modulus have to be measured. The implementation of a ductile and mechanically continuous fiber does not induce mechanical discontinuities in the structure and prevents possible measurement inaccuracies caused by mechanical interaction of the sensor with the structure itself.

The development of POF-based fiber sensors is still at a relatively early stage but recent years saw a series of very promising developments that already proved its applicability in SHM in successful field tests. The topic has seen increasing interest and thorough review of POF sensing techniques have been presented [7,8]. The focus of this chapter is on distributed sensor systems and measurement techniques that are already an option for structural health monitoring schemes or have proved applicability in field tests. Promising techniques and developments that might become an option for special applications are also introduced.

2 Sensing Techniques

This section gives an overview over the various POF-based measurement techniques applicable for structural health monitoring and summarizes its current state of development. The potential for SHM and possible fields of application of the single techniques are discussed in each section. The development of POFs, fiber materials and structures is ongoing and considerable improvements are expected [7,8] promising further improvement of the sensor performance. Various fiber types with partly very different characteristics such as attenuation, spectral transmission windows, core diameters or dispersion properties are currently being used for sensing. The different fiber types require different measurement techniques and also provide different interrogation possibilities.

Most of the more advanced sensor systems are based on commercially available multimode (MM) POFs. These fibers have larger core diameters ranging from 50 μm to 1 mm, are easy to handle and interconnect and are generally used for incoherent detection schemes. Single-mode (SM) POFs however, are still rather a subject of research and are used for coherent detection techniques.

The various measurement and interrogation techniques presented in this chapter are introduced along with the POF types in the corresponding section.

2.1 Distributed Backscatter Measurement Techniques

Optical backscatter measurement techniques provide the advantage of distance-resolved detection of extrinsic influences that interact with the propagating light waves in the optical fiber. The measurement principle is similar to the well-known radar technique. Here, the light's runtime in reflection provides the spatial information of the light's interaction with the measurand. Therefore, only one end of the fiber is needed for interrogation which facilitates multiplexing and remote sensing. This fully distributed measurement technique has great potential for spatially resolved strain detection and evaluation for the monitoring of extended structures. Until now, mostly optical time domain reflectometry (OTDR) devices have been used for this purpose.

The development of different fiber types with different properties and geometries resulted in various sensing principles and interrogation techniques used for strain measurement.

Basically two different multimode fiber types are being used for distributed backscatter measurement. Standard polymethylmethacrylat (PMMA) POFs with a relatively high attenuation of about 150 dB/km and large core diameters up to 1 mm are being used for distributed strain detection up to about 100 m fiber lengths [5]. Advantages of this fiber type are their very strong strain sensitivity, their ruggedness, high strainability and the ease of connection due to the large core diameters and numerical apertures.

The recent development of low-loss perfluorinated (PF) gradient index (GI) POF types based on poly(perfluorobutenyl-vinylether), also known as CYTOP, allows for higher spatial resolution measurement and extended measurement lengths up to 500 m [9,10].

Both fiber types are mass products for optical in-house data transmission systems and are commercially available at a low price. Due to the different interrogation and evaluation techniques associated with these two fiber types, distributed PMMA POF sensors and PF POF sensors are presented separately in section 2.1.1 and 2.1.2 respectively.

2.1.1 Standard PMMA POF Backscatter Sensors

Husdi et al. showed for the first time, that the local backscatter level of strained standard PMMA fiber sections increases as a function of strain applied [11]. This effect only occurs in polymer fibers and has later been applied for distributed strain measurement using the optical time domain reflectometry (OTDR) technique [12,13,14]. OTDR devices are standard tools in the telecommunication industry for fault detection and characterization of fiber optic networks. Short laser pulses are launched into the optical fiber and all backscattered light, mainly caused by Rayleigh scattering, is recorded as a function of time. Knowing the group velocity of the light travelling in the optical fiber, the average of a great number of backscattered pulses calculates into the backscatter signal as a function of distance. For the subsequently presented measurements in PMMA POF, a high-resolution photon-counting OTDR device with a 650 nm light source has been used [14]. Depending on the interrogation device, fiber length and demanded accuracy, the typical measurement time is between seconds to several minutes. Fig. 1 shows a series of OTDR measurements of the same PMMA POF with a 1.4 m long section at 43 m being strained up to 16 %. The local increase of backscattered light with increasing strain can clearly be detected. The strong peak at 53 m is caused by a Fresnel reflection at the end of the fiber.

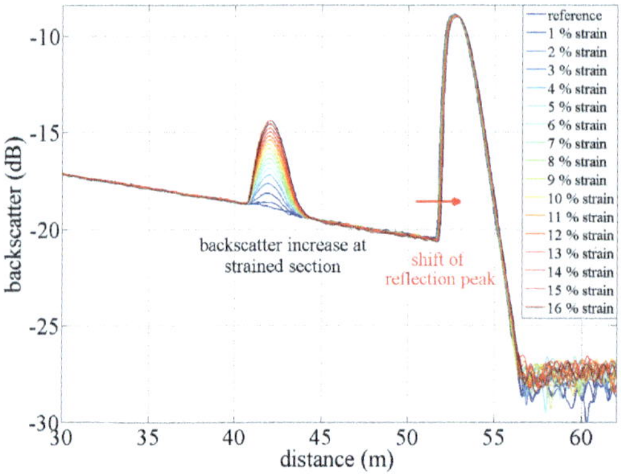

Fig. 1 OTDR plots of a 1.4 m long fiber section strained at 42 m from 0 % to 16 % showing increase of backscatter. The Fresnel reflection at the fiber end at 53 m causes a strong reflection which can be evaluated as a function of length change

By comparing the backscatter signal of a strained fiber section with the reference measurement of the same fiber, the backscatter change relative to the reference can be evaluated as a function of strain. The location of a strain event can be detected and the occurring strain value can be estimated.

Another evaluation technique is to measure the overall length change of a fiber section. The shift of characteristic reflection peaks in the fiber, for example originating from Fresnel reflections at fiber connectors or open fiber ends can be evaluated to give an absolute length change of a fiber section, see Fig. 1. Using this evaluation technique provides precise length change measurement better than 1 mm resolution for standard PMMA POF giving important additional information of the overall length change of the structure to be monitored. In order to use standard PMMA POFs as a reliable strain sensor medium in SHM, numerous investigations on strain response and external disturbances have been conducted. The backscatter increase relative to a reference measurement of an unstrained fiber is evaluated as a function of strain. This backscatter increase with strain is expressed as a factor calculated by integrating the increased backscattering of the strained fiber section relative to the reference measurement and normalizing it to the length of the strained fiber section. Fig. 2 shows the sensor characteristic, backscatter increase versus applied strain, for two different strain ranges. Depending on the rate of strain increase, the measurable strain rate can be 40 % or more for standard PMMA POFs [5].

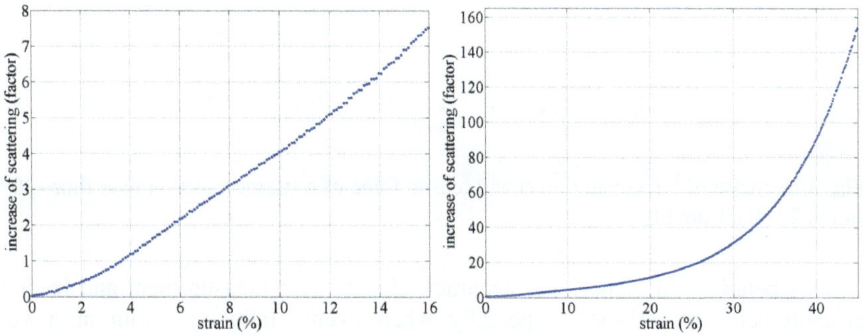

Fig. 2 Increase of backscatter with strain (factor) up to 16 % (left) and backscatter increase up to 45 % (right), from [5]

The observed strain characteristic was measured to be reproducible for independent measurements of different fibers showing maximum variances equivalent to 0.5 % strain. Mitsubishi's GH4001 fiber was found to be most suitable for strain measurement. The 980 μm step index PMMA and a thin fluorinated cladding is protected by a 2.2 mm diameter PE jacket. This fiber type also exhibits negligible loss up to 15 % strain and only 0.4 dB loss per meter strained fiber at 40 % strain [4] and has therefore been used for most of the investigations and field tests presented in this section.

Further advantages of this fiber type are its large core diameter and numerical aperture of 0.3 to 0.5 which allow for easy interconnection and handling on construction site without the need of expensive or sensitive equipment. It has to be noted that the step index profile of the fiber and the high numerical apertures causes considerable mode dispersion which results in a reduced spatial and strain resolution with increasing fiber lengths. Strain events at short distances can be measured with spatial resolutions of 20 cm whereas the spatial resolution is about 1 m at 100 m fiber lengths. A signal processing algorithm to increase the spatial resolutions at longer fiber lengths by compensating for the pulse dispersion along the fiber has successfully been developed and is being used [15].

As relaxation plays a role in polymer mechanics, a decrease of the backscatter level of a strained fiber section over time has been observed. Fig. 3 shows the decrease of backscatter and tensile strain in the fiber over time after applying 20 % strain to a fiber section.

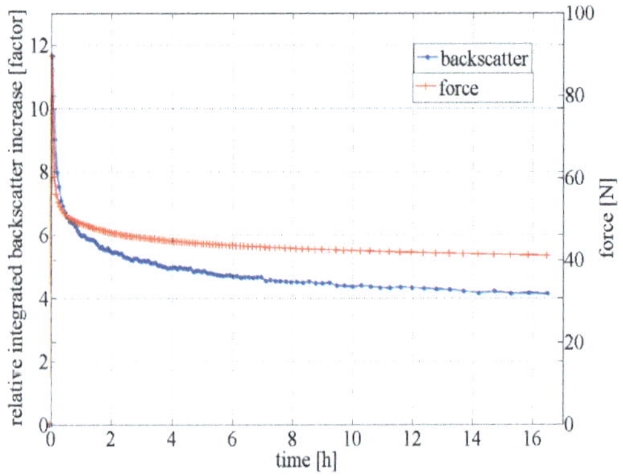

Fig. 3 Decrease of backscatter level and tensile force of a strained section over time (20 % strain, 23 °C), from [4]

This behavior influences the accuracy of the strain measurement and leads to measurement inaccuracies, especially when events inducing strain at a very low rate are to be measured. For strain measurements of unknown time-strain exposure, the actual strain can only be estimated. Under laboratory conditions, instantaneous strain events can be measured with a high strain resolution up to 0.1 % [4].

As for any sensor type, cross-sensitivities like temperature have an impact on the sensor response. The observed temperature influences on the OTDR signal were measured to be relatively small and appeared as change of the backscatter level and change of the light's runtime in the fiber. Both dependencies are approximately linear with temperature. The observed change of the light's runtime in the fiber with temperature was measured to be in the order of $15 \cdot 10^{-6}$ K^{-1} for the GH4001 fiber and a temperature change of 10 K would translate into a backscatter change corresponding to about 0.2 % strain [4].

The operation range of the investigated standard PMMA POFs is between -55 °C and + 85 °C. The use for high-temperature applications is therefore restricted but the recent development of high-temperature POFs promises to extend the temperature range. Fibers from polyarylate (PAR) with elevated glass transition temperatures of 170°C to 195°C and relatively low attenuation of 1 dB/m and 0.6 dB/m at 650 µm and 760 µm respectively have been presented [18].

The biggest market for distributed POF sensors is expected to be in the monitoring of civil engineering structures. Especially interesting are applications where very high strain is expected as it is the case in the geotechnical field for deformation measurement in earthwork structures or crack detection in concrete and masonry structures.

These applications have been targeted by the European project POLYTECT (Polyfunctional Technical Textiles against Natural Hazards), where POF sensors integrated into geotextiles or architectural fabrics have been used for health monitoring and strain detection in various fields. The integration of fiber optic sensors into these textiles is a logical step. Technical textiles are widely being used in various fields fulfilling different tasks from reinforcement to drainage. Thanks to their ruggedness, POFs can be directly integrated into the textiles on industrial scale during the fabrication process. The sensor-equipped textiles do not only fulfil their designated tasks for example as reinforcement element, but also facilitate easy sensor installation into the area of interest and guarantee direct transfer of deformations from the structure to the sensor fiber. Additional costs are negligible since the fibers are low-cost and no additional working steps during fabrication or installation have to be conducted. Several examples of POF-integrated technical textiles can be seen in Fig. 4.

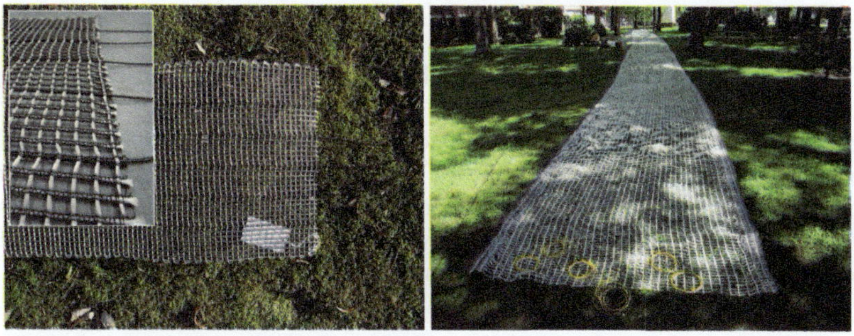

Fig. 4 Technical textiles with integrated POF sensors (left) and POFs/silica fibers (right), from [5] (© [2009] IEEE)

Several laboratory tests and field tests with POF sensor textiles have been conducted. Grid-like textiles for geotechnical applications, or geo-grids, have been used to measure the displacement of soil and textiles with strengthening capabilities have been applied on masonry buildings for reinforcement purposes as well as damage (crack) detection and localization.

In order to test different sensor textiles intended for use in geotechnical applications and investigate the interaction during forced displacement of soil, a series of model tests has been conducted. A lifting cushion was placed at the bottom centre position of a 9 m long wooden box and different sensor textiles were installed between layers of model sand. Stepwise inflation of the lifting cushion caused a lateral displacement simulating a local subsidence resulting in measurable local strain in the overlying sensor textiles. Fig. 5 (left) shows the model box, the lifting cushion and the forced displacement of soil at the surface. The resulting backscatter increase in the POF sensors at the position around the lifting cushion has been calculated into a strain distribution along the fiber. This strain distribution is shown in Fig. 5 (right) for 12 different measurements for different values of vertical displacement.

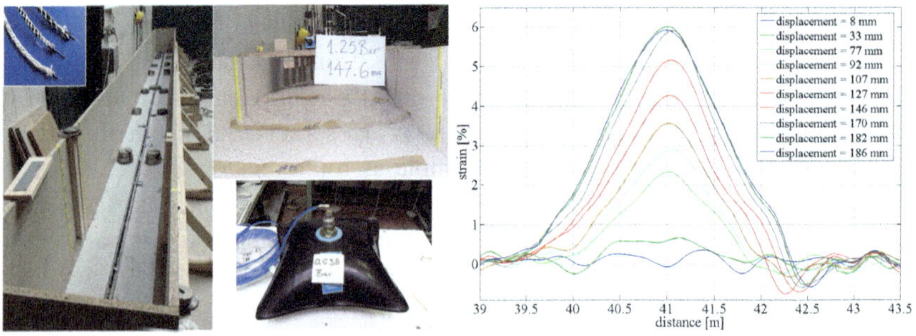

Fig. 5 Model box with textile-integrated POF sensors, lifting cushion (left) and calculated strain distribution for different displacements caused by the lifting cushion (right), from [5] (© [2009] IEEE)

Due to the good strain transfer from the soil to the sensor fiber, ensured by the geotextile, a well-resolved strain profile with a maximum strain of about 6 % has been detected, see Fig. 5 (right). The backscatter increase can also be used to estimate the overall length change of the fiber section by integrating the strain distribution over the strained section. The so calculated length change is plotted with the measured length changes obtained by the peak shift evaluation (compare Fig. 1) of the four POF sensors that have been installed in the textile, see Fig. 6.

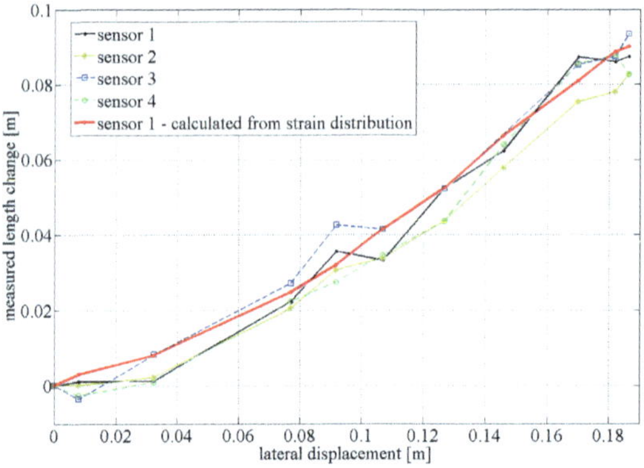

Fig. 6 Length change obtained by the peak shift evaluation (sensor 1 – 4) and calculated length change from the backscatter increase plotted versus the measured lateral displacement of the lifting cushion, from [5]

Before conducting the first field test with this technique, a long-term installation test of various sensor textiles into a railway embankment has been conducted [5]. This test proved that the sensors can survive the installation on a construction site involving heavy machinery without any damage or additional attenuation. Measurable strain was not expected but regular measurements over a period of more than three years show that long term installation and monitoring is possible with these fibers. Apart from a slight increase of attenuation of the fibers over time, presumably due to water absorption owing to humidity in the soil, no negative long term effects have been measured.

A first field test using the distributed POF OTDR sensor has been conducted in an open brown coal mine near Belchatow, Poland. A 10 m long and 2 m wide geogrid with an integrated standard PMMA POF was installed at the top of a creeping slope bridging the tear-off edge of the slope perpendicular to the sensor fiber. The sensor textile was installed in a slightly corrugated way simulating realistic installation conditions and covered with a 10 cm thick layer of sand, see Fig. 7.

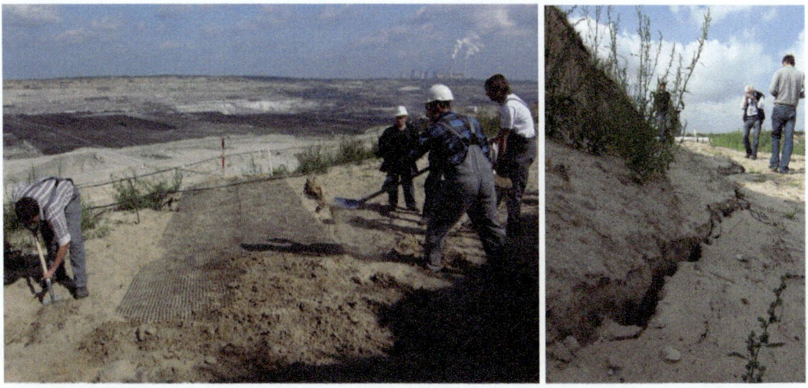

Fig. 7 Installation of the geogrid at the coal pit and cleft at the top of the creeping slope, from [19]

After installation, measurements were conducted in irregular intervals. The first three measurements show a steady increase of the strain signal extending over a length of about 7 m, see Fig. 8. The shape of the backscatter signal of the last two measurements shows that the strain distribution along the textile is not symmetric. The peak at 35 m indicates a very high local strain in the textile, possibly caused by rupture of the textile. The strain magnitude corresponds to strain value of more than 10%.

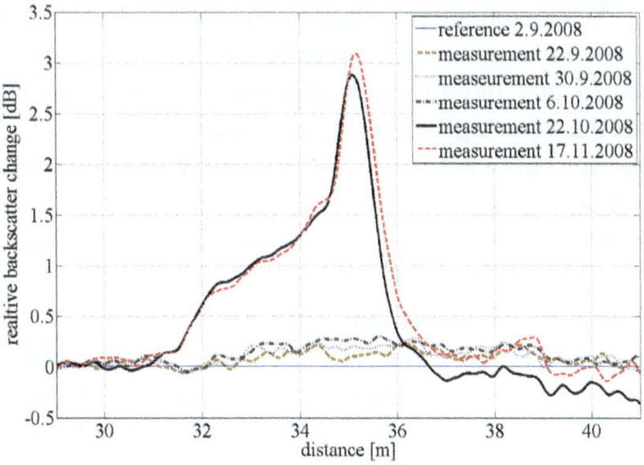

Fig. 8 Change of the backscatter signal relative to the reference measurement, from [19]

An additional evaluation of the total length change of the sensor textile has been conducted between reflection peaks at the beginning and the end of the sensor fiber. The relative shift of the reflection peaks is an indication of the creep rate of the slope. Fig. 9 shows the relatively linear increase of the sensor length with time.

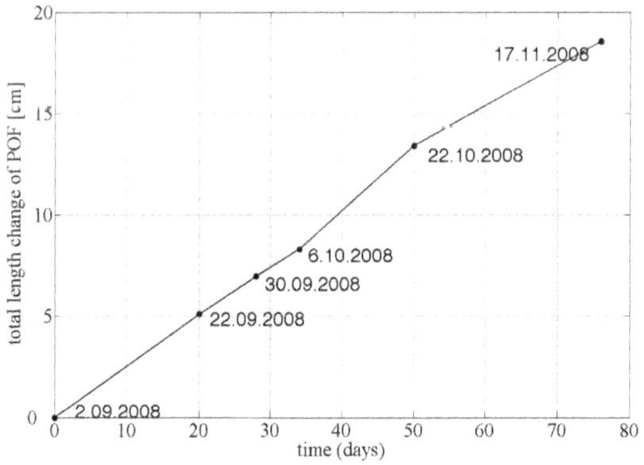

Fig. 9 Total elongation of the POF sensor fiber obtained by peak shift evaluation, from [19]

From these data, the average creep velocity of the slope has been calculated to be about 2 mm per day. This field test showed that even extreme geotechnical deformation and movement of soil can be detected and localized using this technique. This measurement stripe approach can provide valuable information on the location of deformation, absolute deformation and creep rate. A multiplexed online monitoring system could considerably contribute to the risk assessment as part of geotechnical monitoring schemes.

Another subtask covered by POLYTECT was the development of sensor-integrated textiles for retrofitting of masonry structures. The motivation for this application arose from the need for earthquake protection and monitoring of historical buildings. Sensor-integrated textiles are applied to structures for reinforcement purposes and to increase the ductility of the structure. Typical faults that have to be detected and monitored in masonry structures are cracks in vertical direction. Due to the very high local strain caused by the cracks, distributed POF sensors with their very high breakdown strain and their ability to locate such faults are the only suitable solution.

To prove this ability, a series of model tests has been conducted [5]. Various grid-like textiles with integrated POF sensors were applied to one side of two-stone samples, see Fig. 10. These specimen were placed in the set-up in Fig. 10 and the opening of a crack in a masonry structure was simulated by forcing a displacement to the upper side of the specimen so that a crack opened perpendicular to the sensor fiber on the bottom side of the sample where the textile was applied, see Fig. 10.

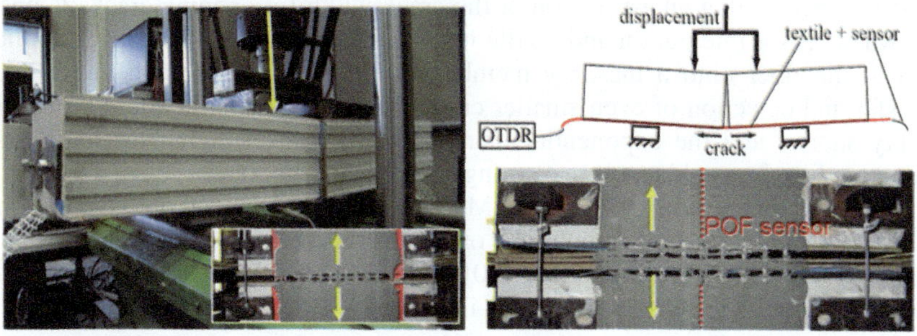

Fig. 10 Test set-up and schematic: two-stone sample with sensor textile on the bottom side in the set-up, from [4]

Displacement transducers continuously recorded the width of the opening crack whereas the backscatter signal of the sensor fiber was recorded for different crack width. Due to the good integration of the sensor into the textile and the matrix, the gauge length of the sensor is very short resulting in a very high local strain in the fiber. Only polymeric fiber sensors can endure the occurring strain levels and can therefore be used for continuous and distributed crack detection with very good spatial resolution.

Crack openings from 1 mm width could clearly be detected and also the width of the crack could be estimated from the sensor signal under laboratory conditions. Fig. 11 (left) shows the relative backscatter change of OTDR measurements for different crack widths. Various sensor textile samples with different mechanical properties and sensor integration techniques have been tested. The relative backscatter changes for one measurement series of increasing crack width is shown in Fig. 11 (left). Fig. 11 (right) shows the integrated backscatter increase versus crack width for two measurement series with different textile types.

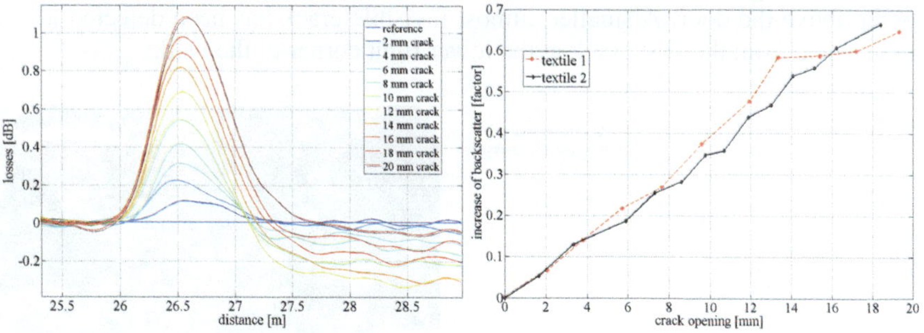

Fig. 11 Relative change of the OTDR signal to the reference measurement for a stepwise opening crack (left) and sensor signal (integrated backscatter increase vs. crack opening) for two different textile types (right), from [4]

It is expected that an estimation of the crack width for opening cracks is possible when sensor integration and textile installation is standardized. Direct application of the fiber onto a masonry member would allow for a more direct strain transfer and detection of even smaller cracks. The gauge length would be considerably shorter and the exponential increase of the sensor signal for high strain (compare Fig. 2) would result in a stronger backscatter increase.

A large scale test with standard PMMA POFs directly bonded onto the masonry walls of a one storey brick building on a seismic shaking table for distributed crack detection has been conducted [20]. Fig. 12 shows the structure with indications where the POF sensors have been installed.

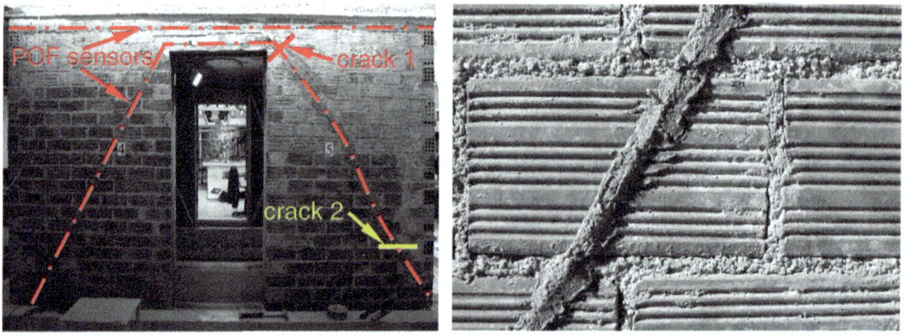

Fig. 12 Brick building on the shaking table with POF sensors installed horizontally and diagonally, from [20]

The testing procedure included several strong shocks, which resulted in structural damage at several locations of the building. All cracks that occurred in the structure could be detected and localized by the POF OTDR sensors.

Fig. 13 shows a measurement result of one of the sensor fibers installed diagonally on the wall. Two cracks were detected by this sensor at the locations indicated in Fig. 12. The stronger signal at 27 m is caused by a 2 mm crack at the corner above the door. A smaller, almost invisible crack has been detected at 150 cm distance from the first crack at the lower right corner of the wall.

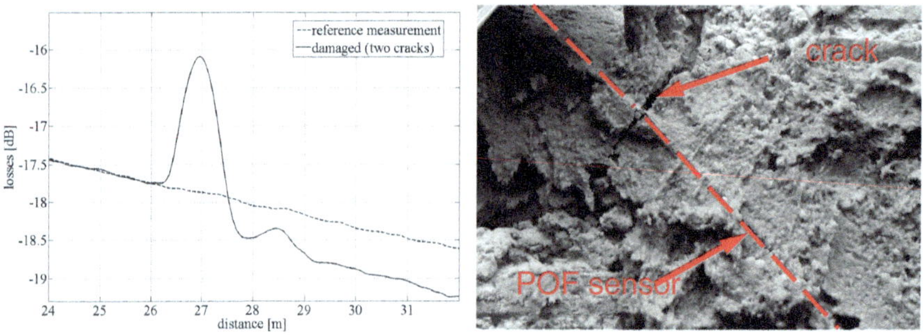

Fig. 13 OTDR result showing two cracks at 27.0 m and 28.5 m (left) and the corresponding crack 1 at 27.0 m (right), from [20]

This test shows that the distributed POF OTDR technique can be used for instant crack detection and localization. Sensor application is intended for heritage structures and buildings in earthquake-prone regions using sensor-integrated textiles as measurement stripes or full-cover solutions.

Another backscatter change measurement application has been presented by Fukumoto et al. Local backscatter increase has been evaluated at predetermined locations to detect deformation of a wooden structure, Fig. 14 [21]. Short gauge lengths at four joints at the corners of a rectangular structure were chosen for strain evaluation.

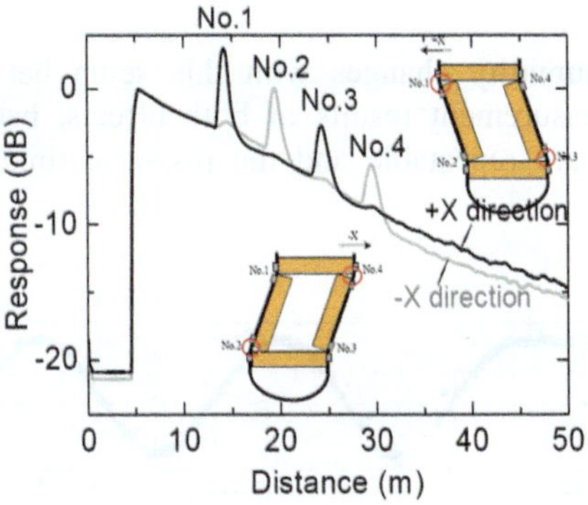

Fig. 14 OTDR responses for deformations of the rectangular frame, from [21]

By evaluating the backscatter increase of the single sensor sections, the direction and magnitude of the frame deformation could be determined.

Not only mechanical properties can be measured and spatially resolved using POF backscatter techniques. Standard PMMA POFs exhibit a relatively high water absorptivity which leads to small but measurable changes of the backscatter level (decreasing) and attenuation (increasing) with increasing water content [22]. Distributed relative humidity measurements have been conducted using standard PMMA POF and OTDR.

Fig. 15 (left) shows the measurement setup with an unjacketed PMMA POF of which a 10 m long section from 30 m to 40 m is subjected to changing relative humidity values. To measure the relative humidity change, the rest of the fiber was immerged into water and held at a constant, saturated humidity of 100 %. The relative backscatter change, obtained from OTDR measurements, clearly shows a local increase of the section of lower relative humidity which could be used for spatially resolved relative humidity measurement [23], see Fig. 15 (right).

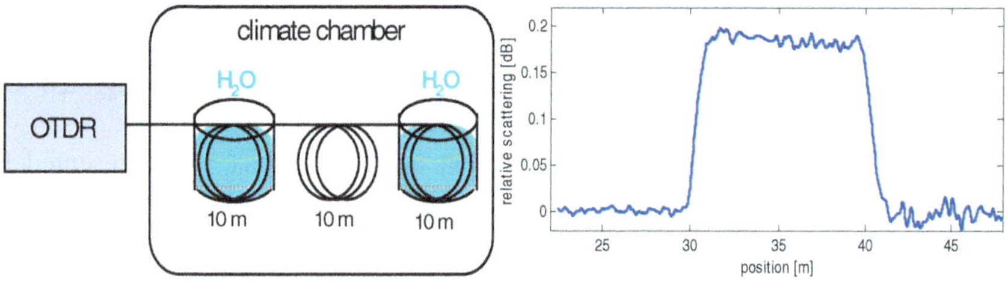

Fig. 15. Measurement setup (left) and relative backscatter plot of a low humidity fiber section between 30 m and 40 m (right), from [23]

Cyclic relative humidity changes with this setup between 20% and 80% showed that the measurement results of both effects, backscatter change and attenuation change, are repeatable and the response time is about 1 day, see Fig. 16.

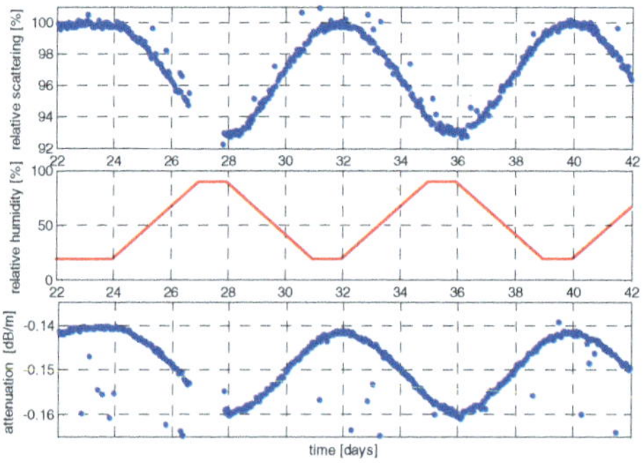

Fig. 16 Changes of attenuation and scatter intensity with relative humidity for Eska GK 40 PMMA POF, from [23]

The measurements indicate that the level of relative humidity could roughly be resolved. A distributed humidity sensor would be useful for various applications in the geotechnical and underground construction field to measure for example seepage lines or ground-water levels. Further applications are humidity measurement in foundations, concrete or wood structures.

2.1.2 Low-Loss GI POFs

The commercialization of low-loss perfluorinated (PF) POFs during the last few years and the recent availability of more rugged fibers and cables enabled practical use of this fiber type as a sensor for health monitoring applications. These fibers exhibit favorable properties for distributed strain sensing. Commercially available fibers have with about 30 dB/km considerably lower attenuation than standard PMMA POFs. This allows extending the maximum measurement range from about 100 m to about 500 m [12]. The theoretical lower limit of the attenuation of this fiber material is with 0.3 dB/km at 1.3 μm and 0.15 dB/km at 1.5 μm considerably lower and comparable to values of silica fiber [24]. Optimized production processes might further improve transmission values of commercially available PF POFs. Fibers with attenuation levels of about 10 dB/km are available [25], extending the theoretical maximum measurement range to more than 1 km. Another advantage of these fibers is their gradient refractive index structure and very low material dispersion which results in very low signal dispersion. Therefore, these fibers provide for maximum spatial resolution over the whole length of the fiber. Typical fiber core diameters are between 50 μm and 120 μm and the temperature range is specified between -30°C and +70°C [26]. Also, PF GI POFs operate at the commercially attractive transmission windows between 850 nm and 1310 nm.

The core material of PF GI POFs (CYTOP) is thermally very stable and chemically resistant. Investigations on cross sensitivity effects of this fiber type showed little influences. It has been shown that temperature has very little effect on attenuation and backscatter change [4,12]. Only the measured change of the light's runtime in the fiber with temperature is significant but has a linear dependency of $22{\cdot}10^{-6}\,K^{-1}$ [12], see Fig. 17.

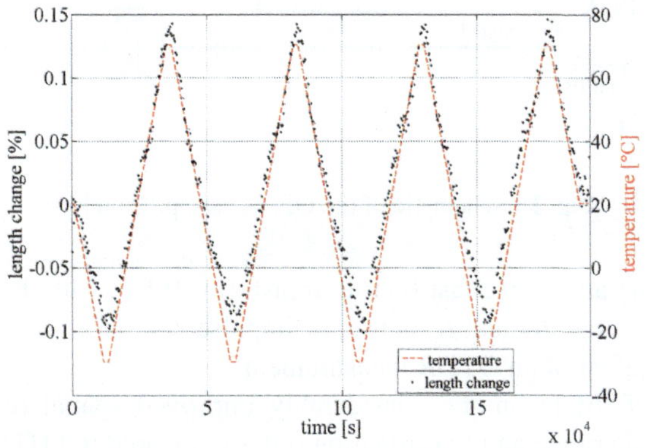

Fig. 17 Measured length change with temperature, 4 cycles between – 30 ° C and + 70 °C (Chromis GigaPOF 50SR), from [12]

As the water absorptivity of CYTOP is very low (<0.01 % compared to 0.3 % for PMMA [26]), no measurable change of backscatter or attenuation has been detected.

The fiber is relatively insensitive to bends; only fiber bends smaller than 10 mm result in scattering and loss and are to be avoided during sensor operation [4]. Recent development of double cladding fibers showed that even lower bend radii and even knots in the fibers can be tolerated [9], which is advantageous for loss-free sensor integration and installation.

Owing to the differences in core diameter and transmission spectrum of PF POFs and PMMA POFs, different OTDR systems at 1310 nm wavelength are used for interrogation. Due to the great potential for distributed strain measurement using this fiber type, a technology based on incoherent optical frequency domain reflectometry (OFDR) has been advanced and adapted to interrogate PF POFs [27].

The OFDR technique is based on measurement in the frequency domain by using a vector network analyzer (VNA) to measure the complex transfer function of the fiber under test (FUT), see Fig. 18. A continuous wave laser source is sinusoidally amplitude-modulated using an electro-optic modulator (EOM). This amplitude-modulated signal is then fed to the FUT using an optical circulator. All backscattered light from the fiber under test (FUT) is detected by a photo diode and the resulting electrical signal is coupled to the VNA to measure the frequency response over a wider frequency range up to 3 GHz [27].

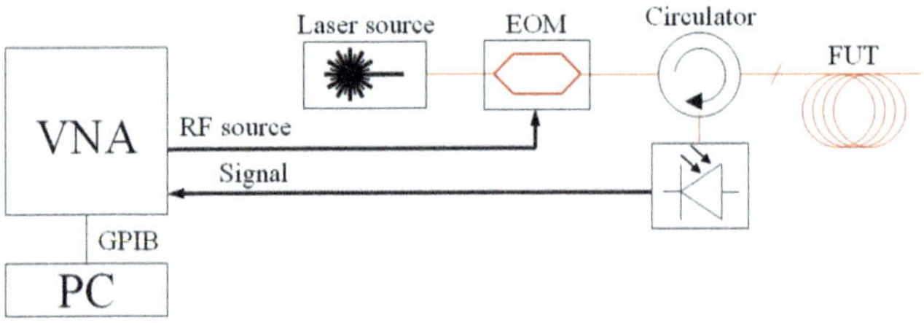

Fig. 18 Schematic of the OFDR set-up, from [28]

By conducting an inverse fast Fourier transform (IFFT) with the complex transfer function, the time domain response, or impulse response, is obtained. This result is the equivalent of an OTDR measurement.

Using the OFDR technique considerably improved spatial resolution, signal stability, dynamic range and interrogation times compared to OTDR measurement [27]. The spatial resolution could be improved to about 3.7 cm in PF POF. Fig. 19 shows a direct comparison of a PF POF between a high-resolution OTDR and an OFDR measurement. PF POFs typically exhibit a great number of randomly distributed scatter centers and impurities causing reflections or scatter centers along the fiber. These disturbances in the backscatter signal can better be resolved using the high-resolution OFDR technique.

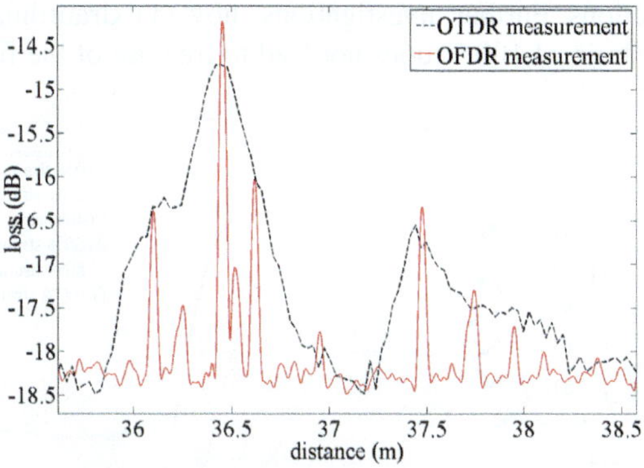

Fig. 19 Comparison of OTDR measurement and OFDR measurement in PF GI POF exhibiting random impurities, from [28]

Also the interrogation time could be reduced so that low dynamic measurement up to 1 Hz can be conducted [28]. The sensing mechanism for PF POFs is similar to PMMA fibers. As it has been shown for PMMA POFs in Fig. 1, strained fiber sections of PF GI POFs exhibit an increase of the backscatter level which can be detected using OTDR or OFDR. This effect however, is not linear with strain and is only evident between about 1.5 % and 3 %. Fig. 20 (left) shows the relative change of the backscatter level of a strained PF GI POF section measured with OTDR. Independent measurements of different fiber sections showed that this observed backscatter increase with strain is reproducible, see Fig. 20 (right).

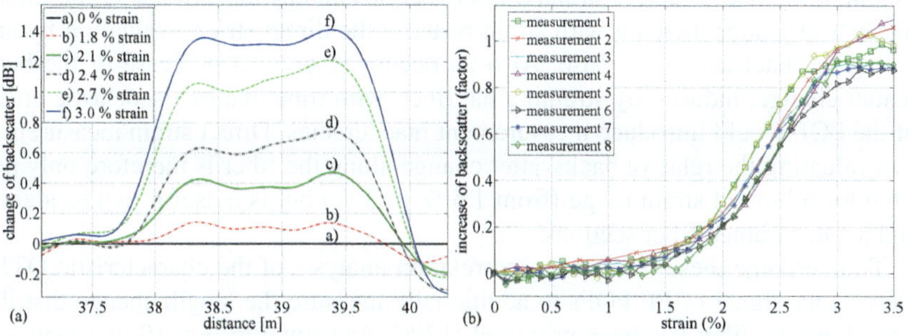

Fig. 20 Change of backscattering relative to a reference measurement along a 1.8 m long stretched fiber section (left) and increase of backscatter (factor) with strain for eight independent measurements of different fiber sections (right) (Chromis GigaPOF 50SR), from [28]

Due to the not linear sensor characteristic, direct strain measurement is only possible for a limited strain range from about 1.5 % to 3 % strain. For strain values higher than about 1.5 %, this technique is a very useful tool to detect and localize strained fiber sections. Further investigations showed extraordinary ductility of PF POF [28]. Even strain of 100 % does not lead to fracture of the fiber, Fig. 21.

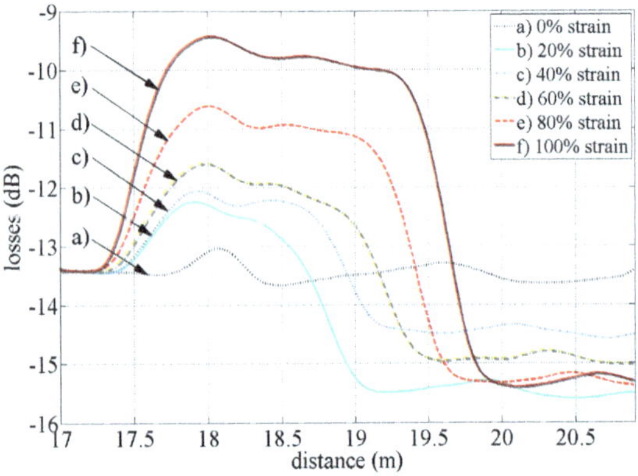

Fig. 21 OTDR signal of a 1 m long fibre section strained in steps up to 100 % (perfluorinated POF by Asahi Glass), from [28]

The occurring intrinsic loss is, even at 100 % strain very low, see Fig. 21. Recently, a more rugged PF POF sensor cable, capable of measuring very high strain up to 125 %, has been investigated for possible field application [6]. The availability of such a suitable sensor cable is the basic requirement for practical applicability in high-strain monitoring.

Although the evaluation of the local backscatter increase caused by strain is an excellent method to detect strained fiber sections and estimate local strain, the not linear backscatter increase with strain restricts the direct strain evaluation by analyzing the backscatter increase. Also an occurring gradual decrease of the backscatter change, induced by straining the fiber, with time due to viscoelastic effects of the POF would introduce measurement inaccuracies. Direct strain measurement by evaluating the relative backscatter change along the fiber is therefore only possible for a limited strain range (from 1.5 % to 3 %) but is a useful tool to identify and locate strained fiber sections.

To overcome these limitations, correlation analysis of the characteristic OTDR backscatter signal of PF POFs to additionally measure the length change distribution along the fiber has been proposed [12,5]. As shown in Fig. 19, the randomly distributed scatter centers along the fibre can be spatially resolved. This characteristic fingerprint of the fiber is permanent and can be used to measure relative displacement or length change along the fiber. Strain in the fiber would result in a spatial shift of the backscatter peaks towards greater distances. This shift or length change can be calculated by applying a cross-correlation algorithm to overlapping sections of a reference measurement and a new measurement section. By shifting this correlation window with the length l_c (correlation length) along the fiber and comparing the reference measurement with a new measurement, displacements caused by strain can be detected and evaluated as length change relative to the reference measurement. The accuracy of the distributed length change measurement and the spatial resolution depend on the chosen correlation length and the degree of backscatter fluctuation along the fiber. The improved spatial resolution and more stable backscatter signal of the OFDR technique considerably increased the precision compared to previously published OTDR results [28]. Fig. 22 (left) shows a series of OFDR measurements of a stepwise strained fiber section at 27 m to 28 m. The strained sections can be located with a spatial resolution of a few cm by evaluating the backscatter increase. Fig. 22 (right) shows the distributed length change evaluation obtained from OFDR data of this PF POF of which the 1 m long section has been strained in steps of 5 mm up to 35 mm. The distributed length change resolution can be better than 1 mm, even at relatively small correlation lengths of 2 m.

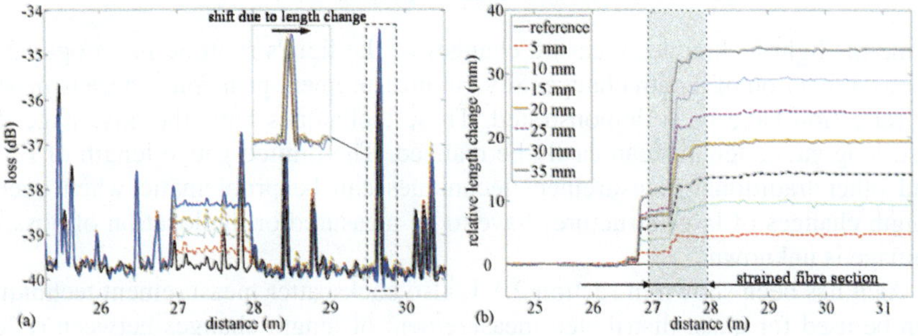

Fig. 22 OFDR measurements of a stepwise strained 1 m long POF section (left) and distributed length change of the same fibre strained in 5 mm steps up to 35 mm (2 m correlation length) (right), from [28]

The accuracy can be improved by correlating longer fiber sections or increasing the measurement time. It is expected that the use of optimized components of the setup will lead to further improved results. Since the characteristic finger print of the fiber is permanent, the correlation technique is insensitive to optical loss along the fiber and the strain signal decrease with time does not lead to measurement inaccuracies. The combination of the two techniques, backscatter increase evaluation and cross-correlation, allows for precise localization of strained fiber sections with cm-resolution and distributed length change measurement along the fiber with a resolution better than 1 mm. Due to the low attenuation and signal dispersion of this fiber type, strain and length change measurements can be conducted with continuously high spatial resolution over several hundreds of meters. The possibility to conduct precise and distributed absolute length change measurements along the fiber is for many applications more interesting than the measurement of local strain levels. Examples can be found in the geotechnical sector or even crack measurement in civil engineering structures where absolute displacement measurement is required.

This development is being continued and will be brought to field application. Although permanent online monitoring of single PMMA or PF POF sensor cables using OTDR is currently not efficient due to the relatively high costs of the interrogation devices, multiplexing solutions or measurement-on-demand approaches can already be economic. The development of suitable interrogation techniques as well as the development of POF cables and integration techniques for example into technical textiles is actively being promoted. The cost of an OFDR system could be reduced if the VNA is replaced by implementing a digital acquisition system [29]. With the expected increase of length change resolution of the combined OFDR and PF POF system, sensor application might not only be found in high-strain measurement niche but might even be an interesting alternative to distributed silica sensor systems for short and medium measurement lengths. The option of easy multiplexing of multiple sensor fibers would increase the cost efficiency of a possible distributed online monitoring system.

2.2 Time-of-Flight Measurement Techniques

Time-of-flight techniques measure changes of the light's runtime in an optical fiber as a function of length change. Several measurement principles in transmission or reflection have been demonstrated. These techniques have the advantage that also long gauge lengths can easily be realized. The limited gauge length of FBGs and other traditional measurement techniques can be problematic when overall length changes of large structures have to be measured or the location of possible damage is unknown.

As it has been shown in section 2.1.1, also backscatter measurement techniques can be used for quasi-distributed measurement of length changes between reflection points in an optical fiber, see Fig. 9. Depending on the used fiber type, the achievable length change resolutions can be well below 1 mm but only static or low dynamic measurement is possible with standard interrogation devices.

The recent development of measurement techniques based on phase shift measurements of a sinusoidally modulated light source allows for precise and dynamic length change measurement. Different designs have been proposed [30,31]. Poisel et al realized an electronic phase shift detector that measures the phase difference between the light waves propagating in a measurement arm and a temperature reference arm using 1 mm PMMA POF [32], Fig. 23.

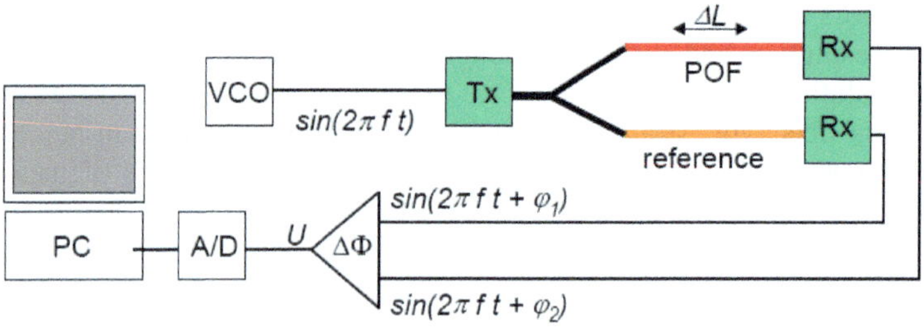

Fig. 23 Schematic of the phase measurement set-up, from [32]

Length changes of 10 μm have easily been detected using this set-up. An application of this technique in transmission to measure the deflection of an aircraft flap model has successfully been shown by Durana et al [32]. Standard PMMA POFs, have been bonded onto opposite surfaces of the flap and the relative phase shift between the fiber at the bottom and the fiber at the top of the flap has been measured during the deflection of the flap, see Fig. 24.

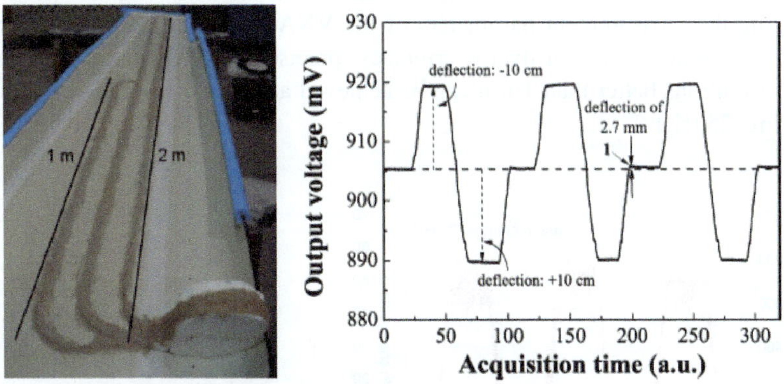

Fig. 24 Aircraft flap with bonded POF sensors (left) and sensor output during deflection of the aircraft flap (right), from [32] (© [2009] IEEE)

The relative length change has been measured with a standard deviation of 7 μm. The phase comparator technique is a cost-effective method when precise and dynamic length change measurement is required. The relatively low instrument costs compensate for the fact that only one sensor can be interrogated per channel.

A recently proposed measurement technique based on the incoherent optical frequency domain reflectometry (OFDR) technique described in section 2.1.2 allows for dynamic and quasi-distributed length change measurement between multiple reflection points in an optical fiber. This technique is based on frequency domain measurement, subsequent time domain filtering, back transformation into the frequency domain and final calculation of updated phase and absolute value information for each reflection point. The measurement principle is presented in detail in [33]. Basically, solving a complex system of equations with the input of only few measurement points in the frequency domain provides precise length change information as well as power change information for each reflection point along the fiber. Any reflecting event in the fiber such as physical contact connectors or open fiber ends can be used as a reference point for simultaneous length change and optical power change evaluation. The gauge length of the single fiber sections can freely be chosen from centimetres to kilometres and theoretically unlimited number of sensor sections can be interrogated.

The presented technique equally works in single-mode and multi-mode silica fibers as well as multi-mode POFs when a light source with a sufficiently broad linewidth is used to prevent interference effects. Only the optical circulator has to be exchanged to adapt to the MM fiber core diameter. Since absolute length changes and optical power changes at *n* reflection points can be calculated from only *n* measurement points in the frequency domain, the measurement repetition rate can be very high. As an example for high-frequency measurement at 2 kHz, a PF POF section, has been alternately strained and released, Fig. 25 (left). By changing the measurement parameters of the VNA and using a system of equations of a higher degree of overdeterminacy, precise length change measurement with resolutions better than 1 μm can be achieved at lower measurement frequencies, Fig. 25 (right).

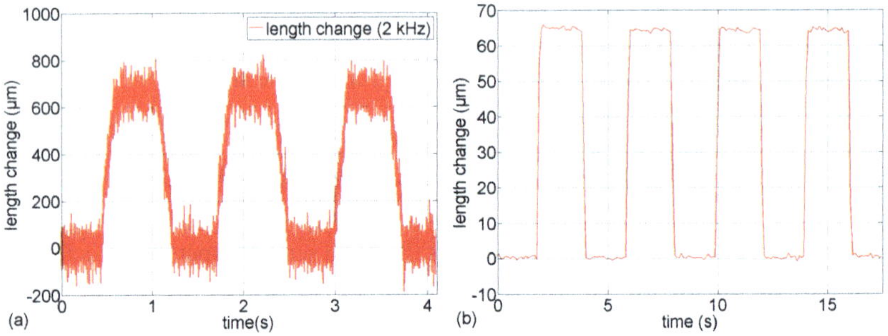

Fig. 25 High-dynamic measurement at 2 kHz with MM POF (left) and high-resolution measurement at 10 Hz with PF POF (right), from [6]

The possibility to also use multi-mode POFs allows for applications where extreme strain is expected. Using this technique, it has recently been shown that strain up to 125 % can be measured in a PF POF cable [6]. Investigations of the mechanical properties of this cable showed that deformation up to 2 % strain are fully elastic and become viscoelastic for strain exceeding 2 %. Care has therefore to be taken when cyclic and dynamic high-strain cyclic processes have to be monitored. The mechanical properties of such a cable could basically be designed and adapted to the requirements by choosing appropriate overcladding and jacketing materials.

This technique has been tested to measure the dynamic deformation of a building under field-like conditions. A two-storey masonry building has been constructed on a seismic shaking table. The building was retrofitted with multifunctional technical textiles comprising various fiber optic sensors for static and dynamic measurement. Three sensor fibers for dynamic OFDR measurement have been installed on the building as indicated in Fig. 26.

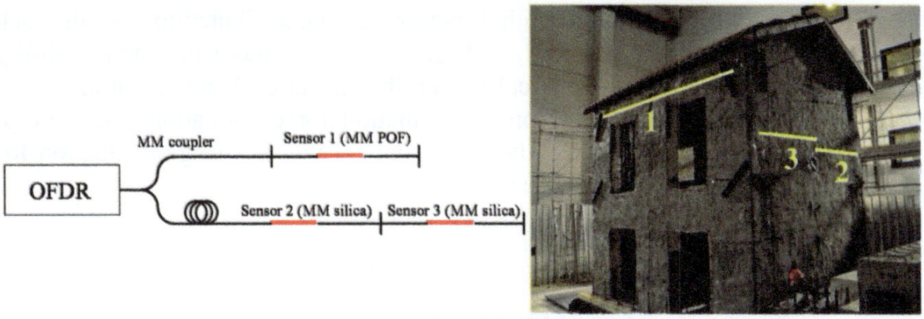

Fig. 26 Schematic of the installed fibers and sensor sections with 4 reflection points in the fiber and masonry building with indications of the locations of the installed sensors 1 (PF POF) and sensor 2 and 3 (MM silica fibers)

Two different fiber types, standard MM silica fibers and a PF POF cable were attached to the locations of interest by gluing or screwing the fibers onto the wall in pre-strained condition. Fig. 26 shows the sensor network comprising silica fibers in one arm and a PF POF in the second arm of a bidirectional coupler. Five independent seismic load tests were conducted with increasing acceleration, each lasting about 45 seconds. The seismic acceleration was in direction of sensor 1 and perpendicular to the wall with the sensors 2 and 3. During the first few seismic loads, several damages have been detected by the sensors, for example at sensor 1 and sensor 3. Fig. 27 shows the measured length change results of all three sensors during the last earthquake test conducted with a measurement repetition rate of 160 Hz.

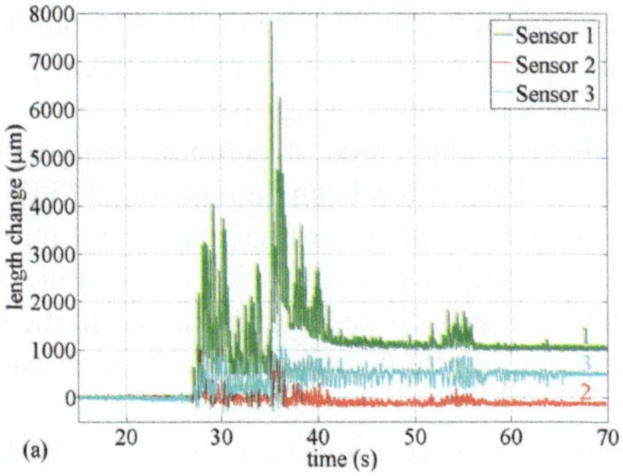

Fig. 27 Length change result of the 3 sensors during the seismic load test (160 Hz measurement repetition rate)

Sensor 1 exhibits the strongest deformation due to its location and existing pre-damage caused by the previous tests. The length change results in Fig. 27 also show a permanent deformation of sensor 1 and 3 originating from cracks in the walls. The relatively strong signal of sensor 3 compared to sensor 2, its permanent length change and oscillation to both directions can be attributed to a small crack perpendicular to sensor 3 that has later been observed in the wall. The possibility of simultaneous evaluation of optical power changes at each reflection or sensor section provides important additional information for deformation and damage analysis of the structure. Fig. 28 shows the optical power change evaluation for each sensor section during the same test.

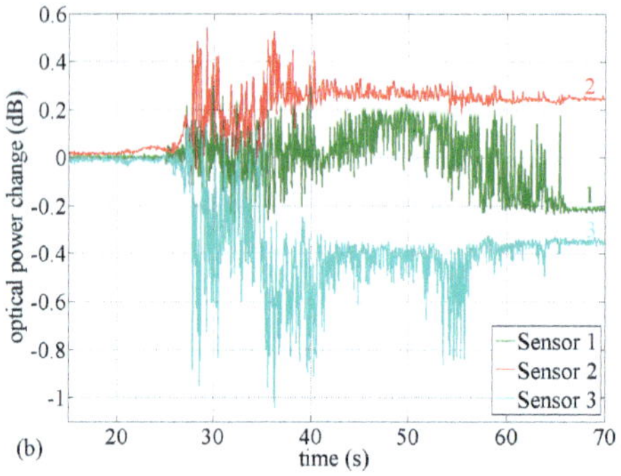

Fig. 28 Optical power change results of the same measurement (27 Hz evaluation)

These data can additionally be used to identify failures in the structure. Sensor 2 shows relatively low power changes mainly due to the deflection of the wall, whereas sensor 3 experiences stronger power changes due to microbends caused by the crack at this sensor.

The results show that two measuremands for each sensor section can be obtained in parallel. The optical power change evaluation can be used to interrogate and multiplex various optical power change measurement principles presented in section 2.4. Also chemical quantities using specially coated fiber sections or fiber ends could for example be implemented. A combined length change and refractive index sensor using this technique has been demonstrated [34].

As for any sensor system, temperature has an impact on the measurement result. The group refractive index changes with temperature can for example be compensated by installing a strain-free fiber in parallel to the strain sensor fiber or by implementing temperature referencing using reflection-based temperature sensors [35].

Time-of-flight measurement techniques are most suitable for long-gauge strain measurement. Fields of application can for example be found in structural surveillance of civil infrastructures like bridges or buildings, in the aeronautic or naval sector or the condition monitoring of wind turbine blades and other industrial structures. The obtained data can be used for damage detection but also for fatigue, creep or load cycle analysis. Due to the dynamic measurement capabilities, also modal analysis can be conducted to detect possible eigenfrequency changes of a structure for early damage detection and interpretation. Such sensor data can considerably contribute to increase safety and reduce costs by optimizing operation parameters and maintenance cycles.

2.3 Interferometric and Single Mode Sensing Techniques

The main reason why the polymer fiber versions of the well-known silica fiber sensor principles have been less studied and applied is the unavailability of appropriate sensor fibers. The advantages of multimode POFs are obvious for multimode fiber links and sensor applications. Single mode silica fibers by contrast, are unrivalled for long-distance data transmission systems. Many sensor principles for high-resolution measurement, such as interferometers, FBGs and Brillouin sensors are based on effects that require single mode operation for optimal results. The unavailability of suitable and acceptable single mode POFs has been the obstacle to benefit from the mechanical advantages of POFs and precise single mode sensing techniques. Until recently, only conventionally produced single mode POFs with extremely high attenuation levels and high cost have been available.

The recent emergence of microstructured POFs (mPOFs) is very promising regarding the possible production of single mode POFs for sensing applications. Microstructured POFs are still a relatively new topic in research. These mPOFs, also referred to as photonic crystal fibers (PCF) or holey fibers, can be produced in many shapes and typically have numerous air holes in parallel to the optical axis, see Fig. 29. This considerably effects the propagation of the light waves and the interaction with the surrounding medium. The light propagation properties can easily be designed including single mode guidance over a wide wavelength range [36].

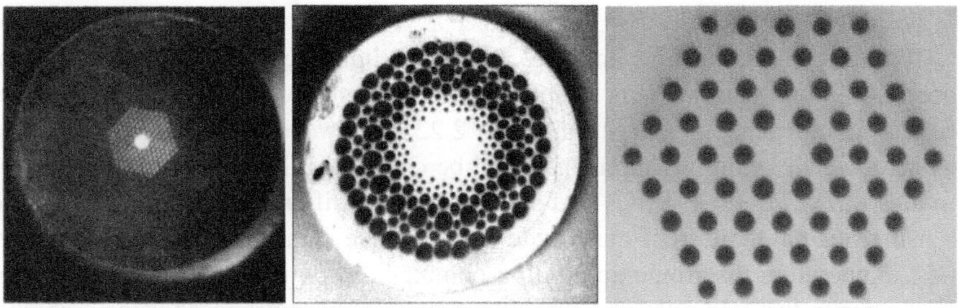

Fig. 29 Examples of microstructured POF from [37,38]

Due to the increased surface area, these fibers show very high sensitivity to gaseous concentrations or liquids and can be specially designed for certain sensing applications.

A big advantage of the mPOF production technique is the easy fabrication of single-mode POFs with relatively low loss of about 1 dB/m [39]. Although still very high compared to multimode fibers, this is much less than reported for conventionally produced single mode POF. With single-mode operation, sensing techniques known to silica fibers can be employed in mPOFs. Interferometric sensing principles such as fiber Bragg gratings (FBGs) or Mach-Zehnder interferometers have been proposed for strain and temperature sensing. Several POF gratings in single mode fibers and microstructured fibers have been presented with the potential for measuring strain exceeding the limits for silica FBGs [40,41,42]. Similar to silica FBGs, widely used in SHM, POF gratings can also be written by UV exposure of the PMMA core. The strain-dependent shift of the resonance wavelength of the grating can be measured in transmission or reflection. Liu et al showed that the strain sensitivity of polymer fiber Bragg gratings is higher than that of silica FBGs and high strain up to 3.61 % can be measured [41], see Fig. 30.

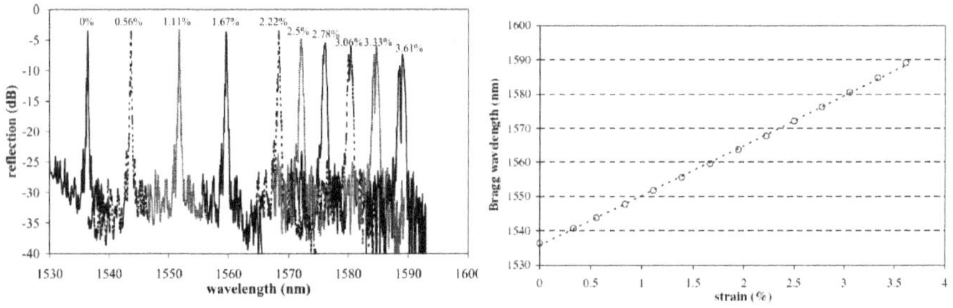

Fig. 30 Reflection spectra of polymer fiber Bragg gratings by the mechanical tensile strain tuning (left) and Bragg wavelengths of polymer fiber Bragg gratings at different tensile strain (right), from [41]

If the fiber is strained beyond 2.22 %, the maximum reflectivity of the spectrum decreases, the spectrum starts to split and the reversibility of the strain tuning becomes time-dependent. For strain up to 2.22 % however, repeatable, linear and hysteresis-free strain measurement could be conducted. Not only the strain sensitivities of PMMA POF FBGs and silica FBGs are different, also the temperature sensitivities have different magnitude and opposite sign. Based on these properties, temperature discrimination with a combined setup has been conducted [43]. Also temperature and relative humidity sensing has been proposed using a combination of POF and silica FBGs [44].

The development of POF FBGs is promising but still at the beginning. Especially long term grating stability is an issue that needs further investigation. Another encouraging development is the development of perfluorinated SM POF. Zhou et al recently produced a SM PF POF using a perform and drawing process with low attenuation of less than 0.2 dB/m in the wavelength range of 1410 nm to 1550 nm and less than 0.5 dB/m for wavelength up to 1610 nm [45]. This is especially interesting for POF FBG development since it has been shown that gratings in a perfluorinated polymer slab are thermally more stable than both, silica fiber gratings and PMMA gratings [46].

Possible fields of application of POF FBGs might be found in high-strain measurement or temperature referencing in combination with silica FGBs.

Also the development of long period gratings (LPGs) in mPOFs is subject to current research. Periodic changes of the refractive index along the fiber have been mechanically imprinted into mPOF resulting in wavelength-depended decoupling of guided modes [47,48], see Fig. 31.

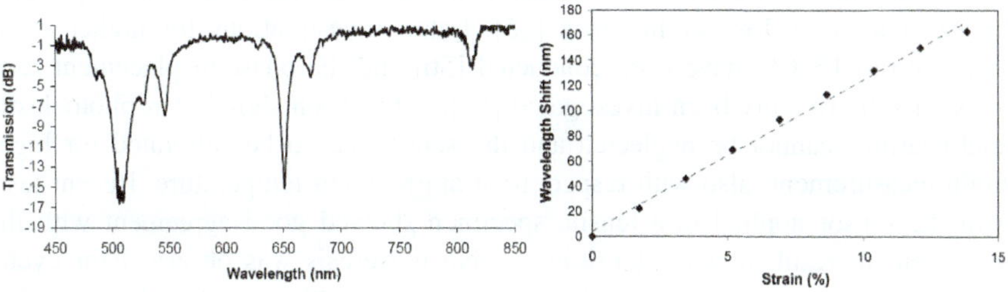

Fig. 31 Transmission spectrum of a mPOF LPG inscribed by heat imprinting [48] (left) and strain results in which the strain was removed rapidly after application [49] (right)

The shift of the transmission minima can be spectrally evaluated and has been used for strain measurement [50,51]. It has been shown that the limit of repeatable strain measurement and the yield limit can be increased by several times compared to silica fibers [52]. Occurring time-dependent viscoelastic effects are related to strain rate and magnitude and are generally small for strain up to 2 % [49,52]. The measurement of higher strain values needs careful calibration and is subject of current research. Recently, the integration of mPOF-LPGs into composite materials has been presented [53] and strain measurement of composite-integrated mPOFs has been conducted [54], see Fig. 32.

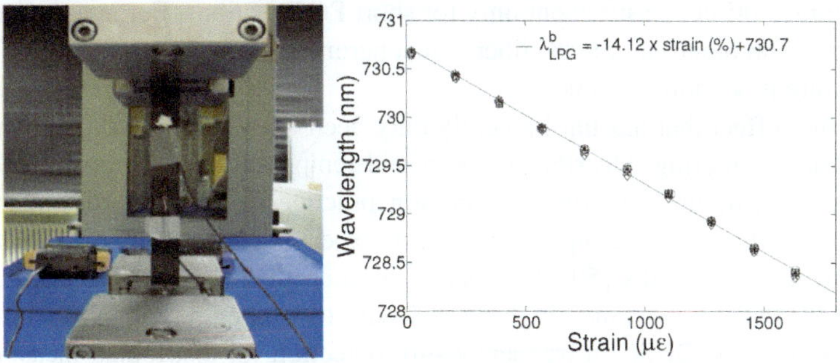

Fig. 32 Carbon fiber reinforced polymer laminated with integrated mPOF-LPG in strain testing machine (left) and sensor response with strain, from [54]

LPGs in microstructured POFs are a promising development for precise high strain measurement but further investigations with respect to relatively strong cross sensitivity to temperature and moisture are required before effectively being used for field applications.

Another development emerging with SM PMMA POFs is interferometry using Mach-Zehnder techniques. The number of detected interference fringes in the visible spectrum is measured as a function of length change of the SM POFs. The strain and temperature sensitivity of SM POF has first been determined by Silva-Lopez et al for a low strain range [55]. Later, investigations for higher strain ranges up to 15.8 % have been conducted [56] and the phase-displacement relations have thoroughly been investigated [57]. It has been shown that photoelastic nonlinearities cannot be neglected and the sensor has to be calibrated for high-strain measurement, also with respect to strain rate and temperature. Recent tests with the sensor applied to a tensile specimen showed good agreement with the measurement result of an extensiometer. No hysteresis was observed for cyclic elongation up to 4 % but the nonlinearity was greater than predicted presumably due to the bonding of the fiber to the specimen [8].

A distributed technique based on swept-wavelength interferometry (SWI), used for high-resolution strain and temperature measurement in SM silica fibers, has recently been demonstrated in multimode PF POFs. Kreger et al showed that SWI can be used for distributed strain measurement of short PF POF sections [58]. Strain resolutions of 3.4 $\mu\varepsilon$ and 0.6°C at a spatial resolution of 20 mm have been achieved with a 2.5 m long gradient index multimode PF POF. This technique measures wavelength shifts in the random but static Rayleigh backscatter signal which is similar to the FBG measurement principle. In single mode silica fibers, very high strain resolution and spatial resolution can be achieved [3]. Due to the strong mode coupling in multimode POFs however, the accuracy quickly deteriorates with increasing fiber lengths. In order to conduct distributed and precise strain measurement in POF over reasonable lengths using SWI, single mode POFs with acceptable attenuation levels have to be developed. SWI is therefore suitable for high resolution measurement only for short POF sections. For length change or strain measurement in longer fibers, incoherent techniques such as OFDR or OTDR might be more suitable.

Another effect that has until recently only been known and used in silica fibers is Brillouin scattering. Distributed strain and temperature measurement based on stimulated Brillouin scattering is common practice using standard silica fibers. Recently, Brillouin scattering has also been experimentally verified in multimode gradient-index PF POFs [59]. Compared to silica fibers, the Brillouin frequency shift in PF POF shows much higher sensitivity to temperature than to strain [60]. Spatially resolved Brillouin frequency shift detection for distributed measurement has not yet been shown. As for the interferometric measurement principles, also Brillouin scattering measurement requires single mode propagation for practical operation. Since POFs in general exhibit very strong mode coupling, only recent low-coupling PF POFs allowed verifying the Brillouin effect in POFs. The very high optical powers required for Brillouin measurement in multimode POFs, the viscoelasticity of the fiber, the strong mode coupling in PF POFs and the strong temperature sensitivity of the fiber are obstacles for application as a distributed strain sensor. Brillouin sensing in PF POFs might rather be used for temperature sensing than for strain measurement. Future developments in this field will show to which extent practical application is possible.

The general success and applicability of the sensing principles presented in this section relies to a great deal on the availability of rugged, low-loss single mode POF. With the availability of such fibers, some of the techniques could match the performance of silica fiber based systems and find application in high-strain measurement.

2.4 Optical Power Change Techniques

The most straightforward and cost-effective technique to detect mechanical impact on the light propagating in optical fibers is direct optical power change measurement in transmission or reflection. Numerous principles have been proposed. Most of them are extrinsic and require some kind of mechanical transducer inducing optical power changes for example due to fiber offset in axial or radial direction or light decoupling due to fiber bends or other means of mechanical impact. These sensors can, after calibration, be relatively precise and are generally low-cost due to the simple design. Basically, all transmission-based sensors and most reflection-based sensors only allow for detection of one sensor per channel, which might reduce the cost advantage and complicates installation when a huge number of locations have to be monitored. Systems based on simple power measurement can generally be designed for high measurement repetition rates and allow for monitoring of dynamic processes.

A typical example of an extrinsic optical loss sensor has been presented by Casalicchio et al for the monitoring of crack widths. Special measurement probes measure the distance of sending and receiving fiber ends as a function of transmitted optical power, see Fig. 33 [61].

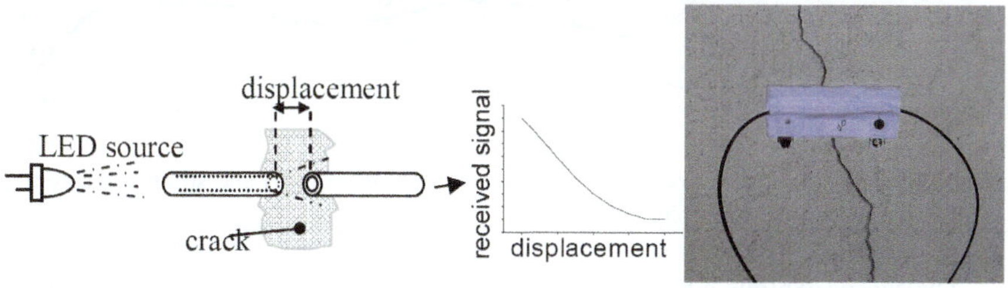

Fig. 33 Measurement principle of the POF sensor and photo of an installed sensor, from [61] (© [2008] IEEE)

The monitoring system has successfully been tested for more than one year measuring the propagation of cracks in a historic monument. Up to 2 μm precision could be achieved in the short term using such a system. Less than 100 μm should be possible for long-term measurements using compensation techniques [62].

A similar technique has been presented in various designs by Kuang et al for static and dynamic measurement [63]. Fig. 25 shows a schematic of the sensor which was used for vibration tests on a free cantilever beam.

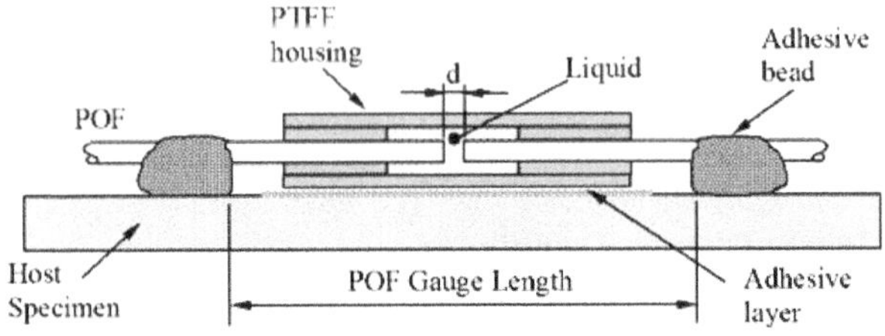

Fig. 34 Schematic drawing of the extrinsic plastic optical fiber sensor, from [63]

Even higher modes of vibration could clearly be detected after an impact-type loading of a composite cantilever beam using this sensor design. High-dynamic loss sensors could therefore also be used for vibration-based damage detection techniques for SHM [63]. A modified version has been adapted for local high strain measurement of a nonwoven geotextile up to 40 % strain [64].

Kuang et al proposed another loss-based measurement principle for curvature and strain measurements by removing a segment of the POF's core and cladding layer [65]. The optical loss along this section is a function of the curvature of the fiber. By bonding such a curved fiber in appropriate orientation to the direction in which the strain is to be measured, precise and repeatable strain measurement can be conducted, see Fig. 35.

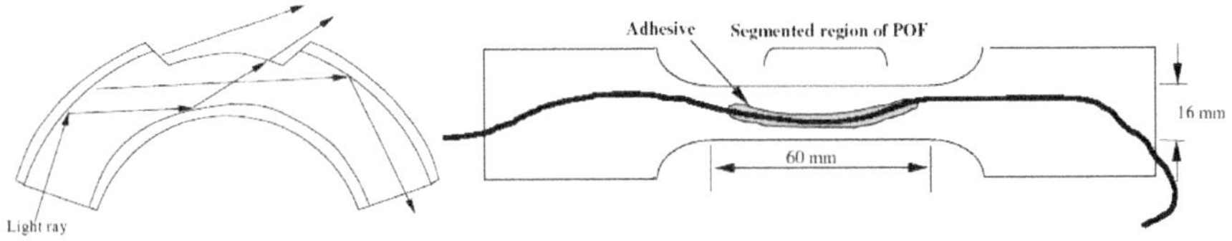

Fig. 35 Schematic of the curved and segmented POF sensor (left) and strain measurement configuration (right), from [65]

The sensor exhibits a highly linear and repeatable response to axial strain up to 1.2 % offering a strain resolution of up to 20 microstrain. Fig. 36 shows the sensor signal for a series of tensile tests.

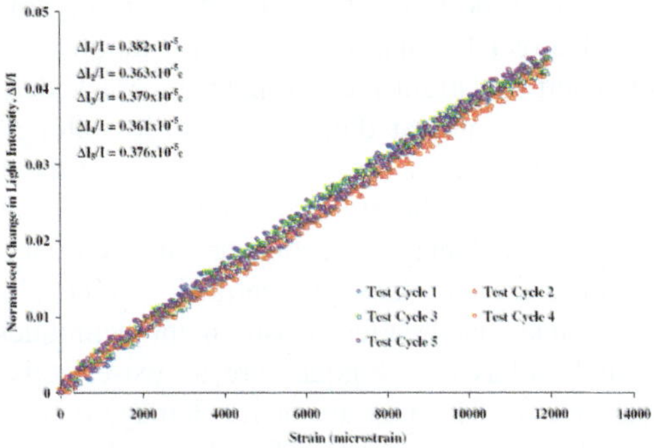

Fig. 36 Plot showing the POF signal response during six tensile loading cycles, from [65]

Also flexural load has been measured with this sensor design. Various other sensor designs for strain- or displacement-induced transmission loss measurement by means of grooved fibers [66] or structural imperfections [67] have been proposed.

Another approach for damage detection is integrated loss measurement along a fiber integrated into or bonded onto a structure. Laboratory tests of transmission loss-based intrinsic sensors to detect cracks and crack evolution in composite laminates [68,69] and concrete beams [70] have been presented. Fig. 37 shows a bare POF directly bonded onto a concrete structure to detect optical loss caused by an opening crack. The extreme local strain at the crack results in cross-section constrictions which induce optical loss in transmission. The authors report that very fine hairline cracks from 0.04 mm width could be detected by transmission loss measurement.

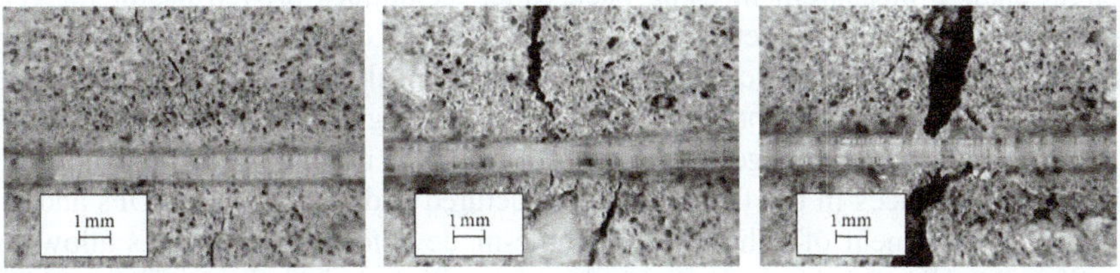

Fig. 37 Photo of a bare sensor fiber and crack propagation of a concrete specimen, from [70]

This application example guarantees the most direct strain transfer from the structure to the light-guiding core of the fiber and shows that measurement sensitivity is strongly related to the sensor application or integration technique. Intermediate layers and mechanically protected cables as shown in fig. 10 reduce the sensitivity for loss-based detection techniques. Direct bonding onto a structure or lamination into a composite structure is more complicated in terms of possible sensor damage but ensures best sensitivity for damage or crack detection. Also Schukar et al showed direct lamination of 500 μm diameter POFs into a glass-fiber composite intended for strain measurement or crack detection [71]. Measurement principles based on integrated optical power loss along the sensor fiber do not provide spatially resolved damage evaluation. Deriving the number or width of occurring cracks or damages is therefore difficult. The application of this sensor type is most useful for early damage detection or damage evolution monitoring of critical regions of a structure. For damage localization and evaluation of the single damaged sections or cracks, backscatter measurement techniques are required.

Generally, optical loss-based techniques are a cost-effective way for precise and dynamic measurement of local strain or for damage detection along a sensor section. Local strain sensors are an option for electrical strain gauges, especially when very high strain is to be measured, electromagnetic compliance is required or corrosion is an issue.

3 Conclusion

The latest development of polymer optical fiber sensors for use in structural health monitoring has been presented. The greatest advantages of POF sensors are their extraordinary strain measurement range, their ruggedness, ease of handling and low cost. POF-based sensors can be employed for a variety of sensing applications although most of the presented sensor systems are not yet commercially available. Extrinsic loss-based sensors can potentially be used for low-cost, precise and dynamic measurement of local strain or deformation. Accumulated loss sensors might find application in early damage detection. Time-of-flight measurement techniques have great potential for the monitoring and surveillance of extended structures. Their dynamic and long-gauge measurement capabilities allow for a multitude of new applications in SHM and industry. Distributed high-strain and length change measurement using backscatter techniques proved useful for geotechnical applications or detection and localization of damage in civil engineering structures. Especially the combination with technical textiles provides low-cost ready-to-install solutions providing health monitoring options. Distributed strain detection and length change measurement up to 500 m length can be conducted. The latest advances in the field of microstructured and single mode POFs and the related development of coherent and single-mode detection techniques allow for applications that have only been employed in silica optical fibers. The dynamic development and expected improvements in the field of sensor fibers as well as measurement and interrogation techniques promise considerable improvement of sensor performance, measurement range and resolution.

As for most other sensor systems, long-term stability, temperature and humidity dependency is an issue that has to be clarified. The viscoelastic behaviour at higher strain has to be investigated for correct interpretation of the measurement results.

Also the application and integration of the sensors into the structures is an important topic. The advantage of being robust and having a low Young's modulus facilitates easy integration and good strain transfer. Direct surface bonding, lamination into composite structures or embedding into concrete can easily be conducted. The integration into technical textiles is a straightforward and cost-effective solution for distributed strain measurement.

Although some of the sensors promise superior performance to existing techniques or open entirely new fields of application in SHM, the key issue for success of the new POF sensor systems is the acceptance by construction companies and the authorities concerned. Therefore, further field testing will be and has to be conducted.

References

1. Thevenaz, L., Facchini, M., Fellay, A., Nikles, M., Robert, P.: Field tests of distributed temperature and strain measurement for smart structures. In: The 4th Pacific Rim Conf. Proc. Lasers and Electro-Optics, CLEO/Pacific Rim, vol. 1, pp. 490–491 (2001)
2. Nöther, N., Wosniok, A., Krebber, K.: A distributed fiber optic sensor system for dike monitoring using Brillouin frequency domain analysis. In: Proc. SPIE, vol. 7003, pp. 700303.1–700303.9 (2008)
3. Froggatt, M., Moore, J.: High-spatial-resolution distributed strain measurement in optical fiber with Rayleigh scatter. Appl. Opt. 37(10), 1735–1740 (1998)
4. Liehr, S., Lenke, P., Krebber, K., Seeger, M., Thiele, E., Metschies, H., Gebreselassie, B., Münich, J.H., Stempniewski, L.: Distributed strain measurement with polymer optical fibers integrated into multifunctional geotextiles. In: Proc. SPIE, vol. 7003, pp. 700302–700302 -15 (2008)
5. Liehr, S., Lenke, P., Wendt, M., Krebber, K., Seeger, M., Thiele, E., Metschies, H., Gebreselassie, B., Münich, J.C.: Polymer Optical Fiber Sensors for Distributed Strain Measurement and Application in Structural Health Monitoring. IEEE Sensors J. 9(11), 1330–1338 (2009)
6. Liehr, S., Krebber, K.: Quasi-distributed and dynamic length change measurement in polymer optical fibers. In: 19th Int. Conf. on Plastic Optical Fibers, Yokohama, Japan (2010)
7. Kuang, K.S.C., Quek, S.T., Koh, C.G., Cantwell, W.J., Scully, P.J.: Plastic Optical Fibre Sensors for Structural Health Monitoring: A Review of Recent Progress. Journal of Sensors, Article ID 312053, 13 (2009)
8. Peters, K.: Polymer optical fiber sensors-a review. Smart Mat. Struct., 20(1),013002, 17 (2011)
9. Koike, Y., Asai, M.: The future of plastic optical fiber. NPG Asia Mater. 1(1), 22–28 (2009)
10. Koike, Y., Koike, K.: Progress in Low-Loss and High-Bandwidth Plastic Optical Fibers. J. of Polymer Sci. Part B Polymer Phys. 49(1), 2–17 (2011)
11. Yoshihara, N.: Low-loss, high-bandwidth fluorinated POF for visible to 1.3-μm wavelengths. In: Opt. Fiber Comm. Conf. and Exhibit, Technical Digest, p. 308 (1998)
12. Liehr, S., Lenke, P., Wendt, M., Krebber, K.: Perfluorinated graded-index polymer optical fibers for distributed measurement of strain. In: Proc. 17th Int. Conf. on Plastic Optical Fibers, Santa Clara, USA (2008)
13. Husdi, I.R., Nakamura, K., Ueha, S.: Sensing characteristics of plastic optical fibres measured by optical time domain reflectometry. Meas. Sci. Technol. 15(8), 1553–1559 (2004)

14. Nakamura, K., Husdi, I.R., Ueha, S.: A distributed strain sensor with the memory effect based on the POF OTDR. In: Proc. SPIE 17th Int. Conf. on Optical Fibre Sensors, vol. 5855, pp. 807–810 (2005)
15. Lenke, P., Krebber, K., Muthig, M., Weigand, F., Thiele, E.: Distributed Strain Measurement Using Polymer Optical Fiber Integrated in Technical Textile to Detect Displacement of Soil. In: Proc. of III ECCOMAS Thematic Conf. on Smart Structures and Materials (2007)
16. Brendel, J.: Optical time-domain reflectometry for POF test and measurement. In: Proc. Int. Conf. on Plastic Optical Fibers, Amsterdam, Netherlands, pp. 45–50 (2001)
17. Lenke, P., Liehr, S., Krebber, K.: Improvements of the distributed strain sensor based on optical time domain reflectometry measurement in polymer optical fibers. In: Proc. 18th Int. Conf. on Plastic Optical Fibers, Santa Clara, USA (2008)
18. Nakashima, H., Takenaka, Y., Mawatari, Y., Orito, K., Yamazaki, T., Tabata, M.: Design of Highly Thermal Resistant Plastic Optical Fibre (POF) as a Step-Index Type Using Chemically Modified Aromatic Polyesters. In: Proc. 19th Int. Conf. on Plastic Optical Fibers, Yokohama, Japan (2010)
19. Liehr, S., Lenke, P., Wendt, M., Krebber, K., Glötzl, R., Schneider-Glötzl, J., Gabino, L., Krywult, L.: Distributed Polymer Optical Fiber Sensors in Geotextiles for Monitoring of Earthwork Structures. In: Proc. of 4th Int. Conf. on Struct. Health Monitoring of Intelligent Infrastructure (SHMII 4), Zurich, Switzerland (2009)
20. Liehr, S., Wendt, M., Krebber, K., Münich, J.C., Stempniewski, L., Metschies, H.: Distributed polymer optical fiber sensors integrated in technical textiles for monitoring of masonry structures. In: Proc. of 4th Int. Conf. on Struct. Health Monitoring of Intelligent Infrastructure (SHMII 4), Zurich, Switzerland (2009)
21. Fukumoto, T., Nakamura, K., Ueha, S.: A POF-based distributed strain sensor for detecting deformation of wood structures. In: Proc. SPIE, 7004, vol. 7004, pp.700469.1–700469.1 (2008)
22. Lenke, P., Wendt, M., Liehr, S., Krebber, K.: Distributed humidity sensing based on Rayleigh scattering in polymer optical fibers. In: Proc. SPIE, vol. 7652, pp. 7653X.1–7653X.4 (2010)
23. Lenke, P., Wendt, M., Liehr, S., Krebber, K.: The Impact of Temperature and Humidity on the Backscatter Profile of PMMA POF. In: Proc. 19th Int. Conf. on Plastic Optical Fibers, Yokohama, Japan (2010)
24. Tanio, N., Koike, Y.: What Is the Most Transparent Polymer? Polymer J. 32(1), 43–50 (2000)
25. Khoe, G.D., Koonen, A.M.J., van Bennekom, P.K., van den Boom, H.P.A., Ng'oma, A.: High Capacity Polymer Optical Fibre Systems. In: Proc. Opt. Comm. ECOC 2002, p. 2 (2002)
26. Technical information sheet, AGCCE Chemical Europe, Ltd
27. Liehr, S., Nöther, N., Krebber, K.: Incoherent optical frequency domain reflectometry and distributed strain detection in polymer optical fibers. Meas. Sci. Technol. 21(1), 017001, 4 (2010)
28. Liehr, S., Wendt, M., Krebber, K.: Distributed strain measurement in perfluorinated polymer optical fibres using optical frequency domain reflectometry. Meas. Sci. Technol. 21(9),094023, 6 (2010)
29. Noether, N.: Distributed fiber sensors in river embankments: Advancing and implementing the Brillouin optical frequency domain analysis. BAM-Dissertationsreihe 64, 1–143 (2010)

30. Doering, H.: High resolution length sensing using PMMA optical fibres and DDS technology. In: Proc. 15th Int. Conf. on Plastic Optical Fibers, pp. 238–241 (2006)
31. Poisel, H.: POF strain sensor using phase measurement techniques. In: Proc. SPIE, vol. 6933, pp. 69330Y–69330Y-5 (2008)
32. Durana, G., Kirchhof, M., Luber, M., de Ocariz, I.S., Poisel, H., Zubia, J., Vazquez, C.: Use of a Novel Fiber Optical Strain Sensor for Monitoring the Vertical Deflection of an Aircraft Flap. IEEE Sensors J. 9(10), 1219–1225 (2009)
33. Liehr, S., Krebber, K.: A novel and quasi-distributed fibre optic displacement sensor for dynamic measurement. Meas. Sci. Technol. 21(7), 075205, 6 (2010)
34. Liehr, S., Krebber, K.: A novel fiber optic technique for quasi-distributed and dynamic measurement of length change and refractive index. In: Proc. SPIE, vol. 7653, 76532V (2010)
35. Chen, J., Huang, X.: Fresnel-reflection-based fiber sensor for on-line measurement of ambient temperature. Opt. Comm. 283(9), 1674–1677 (2010)
36. Large, M.C.J., Poladian, L., Barton, G.W., van Eijkelenborg, M.A.: Microstructured Polymer Optical Fibres. Springer, Berlin (2007)
37. van Eijkelenborg, M.A., Argyros, A., Barton, G., Bassett, I.M., Fellew, M., Henry, G., Issa, N.A., Large, M.C.J., Anos, S., Padden, W., Poladian, L., Zagari, J.: Recent progress in microstructured polymer optical fibre fabrication and characterisation. Opt. Fiber Technol. 9(4), 199–209 (2003)
38. van Eijkelenborg, M.A., Padden, W., Besley, J.A.: Mechanically induced long-period gratings in microstructured polymer fibre. Opt. Commun. 236(1-3), 75–78 (2004)
39. Large, M.C.J., Moran, J., Ye, L.: The role of viscoelastic properties in strain testing using microstructured polymer optical fibres (mPOF). Meas. Sci. Technol. 20(3),034014, 6 (2009)
40. Peng, G.D., Xiong, Z., Chu, P.L.: Photosensitivity and gratings in dyedoped polymer optical fibers. Opt. Fiber Technol. 5(2), 242–251 (1999)
41. Liu, H.Y., Liu, H.B., Peng, G.D.: Tensile strain characterization of polymer optical fibre Bragg gratings. Opt. Commun. 251(1-3), 37–43 (2005)
42. Dobb, H., Webb, D.J., Kalli, K., Argyros, A., Large, M.C.J., van Eijkelenborg, M.A.: Continuous wave ultraviolet light-induced fiber Bragg gratings in few- and single-mode microstructured polymer optical fibers. Opt. Lett. 30(24), 3296–3298 (2005)
43. Liu, H.B., Liu, H.Y., Peng, G.D., Chu, P.L.: Strain and temperature sensor using a combination of polymer and silica fibre Bragg gratings. Opt. Comm. 219(1-6), 139–142 (2003)
44. Zhang, C., Zhang, W., Webb, D.J., Peng, G.D.: Optical fibre temperature and humidity sensor. Electr. Lett. 46(9), 643–644 (2010)
45. Zhou, G., Pun, C.-F.J., Tam, H.-Y., Wong, A.C.L., Lu, C., Wai, P.K.A.: Single-Mode Perfluorinated Polymer Optical Fibers with Refractive Index of 1.34 for Biomedical Applications. Phot. Tech. Lett. 22(2), 106–108 (2010)
46. Liu, H.Y., Peng, G.D., Chu, P.L.: Thermal stability of gratings in PMMA and CYTOP polymer fibers. Opt. Comm. 204(1-6), 151–156 (2002)
47. van Eijkelenborg, M.A., Padden, W., Besley, J.A.: Mechanically induced long-period gratings in microstructured polymer fibre. Opt. Commun. 236(1-3), 75–78 (2004)
48. Hiscocks, M.P., van Eijkelenborg, M.A., Argyros, A., Large, M.C.J.: Stable imprinting of long-period gratings in microstructured polymer optical fibre. Opt. Expr. 14(11), 4644–4649 (2006)

49. Large, M.C.J., Blacket, D., Bunge, C.A.: Microstructured Polymer Optical Fibers Compared to Conventional POF: Novel Properties and Applications. IEEE Sensors J. 10(7), 1213–1217 (2010)
50. Steffen, M., Schukar, M., Witt, J., Krebber, K., Large, M., Argyros, A.: Investigation of MPOF–LPGs for sensing applications. In: Proc. of 18th Int. Conf. on Plastic Optical Fibers, Sydney, Australia (2009)
51. Witt, J., Steffen, M., Schukar, M., Krebber, K.: Investigation of sensing properties of microstructured polymer optical fibers. In: Proc. SPIE, vol. 7714, pp. 77140F–77140F-12 (2010)
52. Large, M.C.J., Moran, J., Ye, L.: The role of viscoelastic properties in strain testing using microstructured polymer optical fibres (mPOF). Meas. Sci. Technol. 20(3), 034014, 6 (2009)
53. de Oliveira, R., Schukar, M., Krebber, K., Michaud, V.: Development of adaptive composites with embedded plastic optical fibres. In: Proc. 3rd Int. Conf. on Recent Advances in Composite Materials, Limoge, France (2010)
54. de Oliveira, R., Schukar, M., Krebber, K., Michaud, V.: Advanced composite materials with embedded POF sensors for structural health monitoring. In: Proc. 19th Int. Conf. on Plastic Optical Fibers, Yokohama, Japan (2010)
55. Silva-Lopez, M., Fender, A., MacPherson, W.N., Barton, J.S., Jones, J.D.C., Zhao, D., Dobb, H., Webb, D.J., Zhang, L., Bennion, I.: Strain and temperature sensitivity of a single-mode polymer optical fiber. Opt. Lett. 30(23), 3129–3131 (2005)
56. Kiesel, S., Peters, K., Hassan, T., Kowalsky, M.: Large deformation infiber polymer optical fiber sensor. IEEE Photon. Technol. Lett. 20(6), 416–418 (2008)
57. Kiesel, S., Peters, K., Hassan, T., Kowalsky, M.: Behaviour of intrinsic polymer optical fibre sensor for large-strain applications. Meas. Sci. Technol. 18(10), 3144–3154 (2007)
58. Kreger, S.T., Sang, A.K., Gifford, D.K., Froggatt, M.E.: Distributed strain and temperature sensing in plastic optical fiber using Rayleigh scatter. In: Proc. SPIE, vol. 7316, pp. 73160A.1–73160A.8 (2009)
59. Mizuno, Y., Nakamura, K.: Experimental study of Brillouin scattering in perfluorinated polymer optical fiber at telecom wavelength. Appl. Phys. Lett. 97(2), 21103 (2010)
60. Mizuno, Y., Nakamura, K.: Potential of Brillouin scattering in polymer optical fiber for strain-insensitive high-accuracy temperature sensing. Opt. Lett. 35(23), 3985–3987 (2010)
61. Perrone, G., Olivero, M., Vallan, A., Carullo, A., Neri, A.: Long Term In- Situ Test of a Low-Cost Fiber-Based Crack Monitoring System. IEEE Sensors, 325–328 (2008)
62. Casalicchio, M.L., Penna, A., Perrone, G.: Optical Fiber Sensors for Long- and Short-Term Crack monitoring. In: IEEE Workshop on EESMS, pp. 87–92 (2009)
63. Kuang, K.S.C., Quek, S.T., Maalej, M.: Assessment of an extrinsic polymer-based optical fibre sensor for structural health monitoring. Meas. Sci. Technol. 15(10), 2133–2141 (2004)
64. Kuang, K.S.C., Quek, S.T., Tan, C.Y., Chew, S.H.: Plastic Optical Fiber Sensors for Measurement of Large Strain in Geotextile materials. Advanced Mat. Research 47-50, 1233–1236 (2008)
65. Kuang, K.S.C., Cantwell, W.J., Scully, P.J.: An evaluation of a novel plastic optical fibre sensor for axial strain and bend measurements. Meas. Sci. Technol. 13(10), 1523–1534 (2002)

66. Chen, Y.C., Xie, W.F., Ke, Y.L., Chen, L.W.: Power loss characteristics of a sensing element based on a grooved polymer optical fiber under elongation. Meas. Sci. Technol. 19(10), 105203, 7 (2008)
67. Babchenko, A., Weinberger, Z., Itzkovich, N., Maryles, J.: Plastic optical fibre with structural imperfections as a displacement sensor. Meas. Sci. Technol. 17(5), 1157–1161 (2006)
68. Takeda, N.: Characterization of microscopic damage in composite laminates and real-time monitoring by embedded optical fiber sensors. Int. J. Fatigue 24(2-4), 281–289 (2002)
69. Wong, Y.M., Scully, P.J., Bartlett, R.J., Kuang, K.S.C., Cantwell, W.J.: Plastic Optical Fibre Sensors for Environmental Monitoring: Biofouling and Strain Applications. Strain 39(3), 115–119 (2003)
70. Kuang, K.S.C., Akmaluddin, Cantwell, W.J., Thomas, C.: Crack detection and vertical deflection monitoring in concrete beams using plastic optical fibre sensors. Meas. Sci. Technol. 14(2), 205–216 (2003)
71. Schukar, M., Grzemba, B., Krebber, K., Luber, M.: Integration technology of POF sensors into composites for structural health monitoring. In: Proc. 18th Int. Conf. on Plastic Optical Fibers, Sydney, Australia (2009)

Optical Fiber Sensors for Structural Health Monitoring

Alayn Loayssa

Universidad Pública de Navarra,
Pamplona, Spain

Abstract. In this chapter the most important fiber optic sensors for structural health monitoring applications are reviewed. Emphasis is placed on sensors that are currently commercially available and have a potential for widespread deployment. Four major sensor types are analyzed: from mature, well-established technologies such as fiber Bragg gratings and interferometric sensors to newer distributed sensor technologies based on Brillouin and Rayleigh scattering effects. For each sensor type their operation is described including its physical fundamentals. Moreover, typical performance specifications as well as application areas are discussed. A descriptive approach is adopted throughout the text so as to facilitate basic understanding of the material to non-experts in the field of photonics.

1 Introduction

Optical fiber technology is greatly responsible for the advent of the information society in which we are living today. From pioneering work in the sixties and seventies (recently awarded with the novel price) to latest developments in ultra-high capacity backbone fiber network and the current trend towards installation of fiber to the home networks, fiber communications has become the veins and arteries through which the blood of our interconnected global village is flowing.

Fig. 1 illustrates the basic structure of an optical fiber, which can be broadly described as a dielectric optical waveguide with cylindrical geometry. Its main constituent parts are the core and the cladding that have a difference in refractive index that leads to the waveguide effect that allows transmission of light through the fiber with extremely low attenuation. There is also some protective outer coating made of acrylate or polyimide materials. Finally, depending on the application, this bare fiber can be surrounded by additional protective layers to form a fiber optic cable. There are many different types of optical fibers depending on the fabrication material and the characteristics of their wave-guiding effect. The predominant material in the fabrication of optical fibers (core and cladding) is silica due to the improved transmission characteristics of the resultant fibers, although plastic fibers are also interesting for their potential for costs reductions. In terms of transmission characteristics optical fibers can be broadly classified as single-mode or multimode depending on the distribution of the optical field in the core.

S.C. Mukhopadhyay (Ed.): New Developments in Sensing Technology for SHM, LNEE 96, pp. 335–358.
springerlink.com

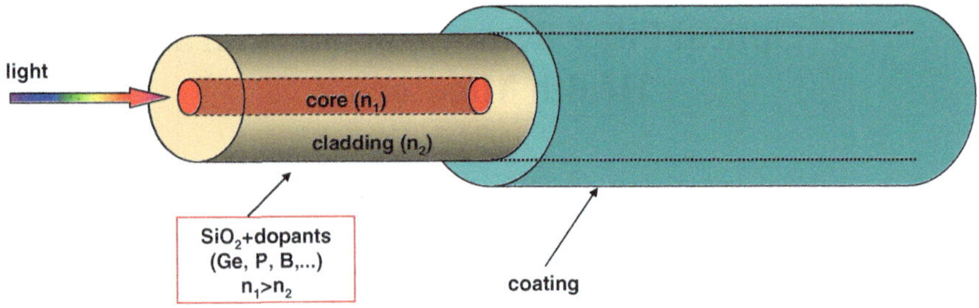

Fig. 1 Structure of an optical fiber

Early in the development of optical fiber technology it was recognized that apart from being an excellent transmission medium for communications due to its low attenuation and large bandwidth, optical fibers could also serve an important role for sensing. In this application the optical fiber is used to transport light to and from an optical transducer that modulates or changes some parameter of light (intensity, spectral content, polarization, phase, etc) in response to some measurand. The transducer can be the optical fiber itself, leading to an intrinsic fiber optic sensor, or some external device, which results in an extrinsic or hybrid sensor [1].

Optical fiber sensors (OFS) are very interesting for structural health monitoring (SHM) applications due to the advantages of this technology compared to conventional sensors. Some of these advantages are inherent to the physical and material characteristics of the optical fibers that made the sensors. For instance, OFS are immune to EM interferences because light propagates in optical fibers within a dielectric material in which interaction with electromagnetic fields can be neglected. This is certainly an asset in many applications where electric motors, generators or transformers are deployed. In addition, the dielectric characteristic of fibers makes them lightning-safe in applications such as wind power generators where the blades must be free from conducting materials. The fact that the transmission of light is confined to the fiber and the absence of electrical currents also makes optical fiber sensors intrinsically safe for deployment in explosive environments. Moreover, the optical fibers are typically made of inert material (mainly silica) resistant to most chemicals and to weathering effects and corrosion. Another important advantage of optical fibers for SHM is their small size with external diameters as small as 125 microns for widely deployed fiber types. This is very important when embedding OFS in order to make sure that the mechanical properties of the host material are not significantly compromised due to the introduction of the fiber [2].

There are also advantages related to the transmission characteristics of the fiber. For example, the light traveling in an optical suffer suffers very low attenuation of its power and this means that large structures can be covered with complex mesh routing of fiber without the need for regeneration of the signal in any active components. The other significant advantage of optical fiber for transmission is their extremely large spectral bandwidth, which leads to the possibility of

propagating light of different wavelengths or colors simultaneously on the same fiber. Each wavelength can be used for the interrogation of a specific sensor in a wavelength-division multiplexing (WDM) scenario. Moreover, at each wavelength light can be pulsed very fast, leading to time-division multiplexing (TDM) schemes. Other possibilities of multiplexing OFS are also available such as coherence-division multiplexing or polarization multiplexing.

Other advantages of OFS are linked to the implementation of the technology itself. There are many situations in which deployment of OFS leads to improved measurements over conventional sensors with simpler installation and maintenance. Moreover, OFS have demonstrated enhanced stability and reliability over time due to some of the characteristics previously discussed. Some OFS can be regarded as direct replacement for conventional sensor alternatives, providing similar measurements, but with additional performance that justifies their use. On the contrary, other types of OFS offer completely novel sensing possibilities that are simply not available with conventional sensors. An example is distributed sensors, which provide the magnitude of certain parameter, e.g. strain or temperature, at every position along an optical fiber. Distributed sensors for structural health monitoring are treated latter in this chapter.

Finally, SHM applications can benefit from the extensive research that has been performed over the years to develop OFS for a very large variety of mechanical, physical and chemical parameters. Nevertheless, the most important measurands for this application are mechanical parameters such as strain, deformation or displacement and some physical parameters such as temperature. Other parameters of interest can be readily derived from these measurands by proper sensor design. For instance, the corrosion of reinforcing steel in concrete structures can be detected by the strain and deformation brought by the large radial pressure exerted on the surrounding material.

In this chapter, we review the most significant OFS for SHM applications. The analysis focuses on the most important sensor types from the point of view of current commercial availability and potential for short-term widespread deployment. Mature, well-established technologies such as fiber Bragg grating (FBG) and interferometric sensors are highlighted first in sections 2 and 3. Then, sections 4 and 5 describe newer distributed sensor technologies based on Brillouin and Rayleigh scattering effects, which are currently having a very significant impact on SHM owing to the enhanced monitoring features that they provide.

2 Fiber Bragg Gratings Sensors

One of the most commercially relevant FOS types is the fiber Bragg grating (FBG), which is finding widespread use as point temperature and strain sensor and a direct substitute for electronic counterparts such as strain gauges. FBG are made by inducing a periodic modulation of the refractive index in the core of an optical fiber. This modulation of the refractive index is made possible by the

photo-sensitivity effect, a nonlinear phenomenon by which the refractive index in the core of a fiber is permanently modified by exposure to ultraviolet radiation. The change Δn of the refractive index depends on the radiation dose, intensity and wavelength. There several techniques that can be used to write gratings on optical fibers such as interferometric methods and phase-mask techniques [3].

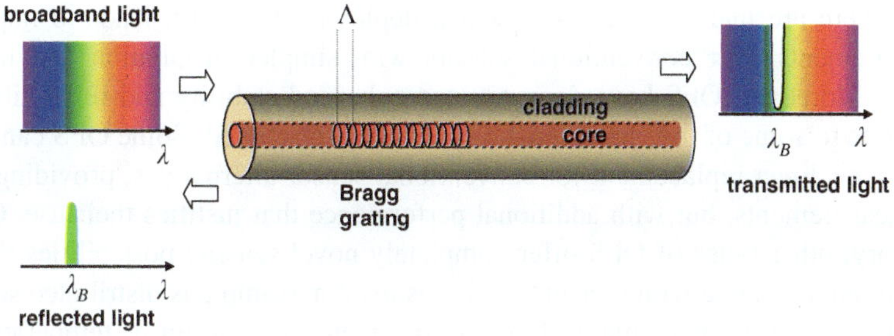

Fig. 2 Uniform fiber Bragg grating as an optical filter for transmission and reflection of light

The simplest and more widely deployed FBG for sensor applications is the uniform FBG (UFBG). This grating can also be regarded as the basic building block of more complex types. In UFBG the modulation of the refractive index has a constant period Λ along the grating length. As schematically depicted in Fig. 2, this device behaves as a wavelength-dependent optical filter for transmission and reflection of light. It is found that overall light around the so-called Bragg grating wavelength λ_B is reflected when the following condition is satisfied:

$$\lambda_B = 2n_{eff}\Lambda \tag{1}$$

with n_{eff} the effective refractive index of the propagating fiber mode. According to basic optics phenomena, part of the light that propagates along the grating is reflected at each refractive index transition. Then, the condition in eq. (1) just conveys the fact that the multiple reflections of light of wavelength λ_B from each grating plane interfere constructively because there is relative 2π phase-shift in their propagation constants. Conversely, if the Bragg condition is not satisfied, the reflected light from each of the subsequent planes becomes progressively out of phase and will eventually cancel out. Only for light around λ_B the weak reflection from each grating plane reinforces itself and leads to a strong reflection. Furthermore, the light that is reflected is removed from the transmitted spectra. Therefore, overall a UFBG behaves as a narrow bandpass filter in reflection and notch filter in transmission. The transmission and reflection spectra can be measured, for instance, using a broadband incident light source or a narrow-band tunable laser. Other types of gratings that are less important for sensor applications are:

long-period gratings, in which light couples into cladding modes, chirped FBG, in which the period of the grating is varied along the length of the grating, or tilted FBG, in which the gratings are written at an angle to the fiber axis.

Sensor applications of UFBG are based on the sensitivity of the Bragg wavelength to strain and temperature. From Eq. (1) the change in λ_B as a function of temperature or strain in the FBG can be derived as [3]:

$$\Delta\lambda_B = 2\left(\Lambda\frac{\partial n_{eff}}{\partial l} + n_{eff}\frac{\partial \Lambda}{\partial l}\right)\Delta l + 2\left(\Lambda\frac{\partial n_{eff}}{\partial T} + n_{eff}\frac{\partial \Lambda}{\partial T}\right)\Delta T \tag{2}$$

where Δl is the change in grating length due to strain. The first term in the expression is related to the strain-optic effect by which a change in strain brings about a variation in the refractive index in the fiber. The second term is simply the grating period change which is proportional to the strain. The third term comes from the thermo-optic effect related to the dependence of refractive index on temperature. Finally, the last term comes from the thermal expansion coefficient of the fiber. The net result of all these variations is that the Bragg wavelength, i.e., the central wavelength of the narrowband filter, depends linearly on strain and temperature over typical ranges of interest of these measurands. The coefficients of this dependence are of the order of 1 pm/με and 10 pm/°C, respectively.

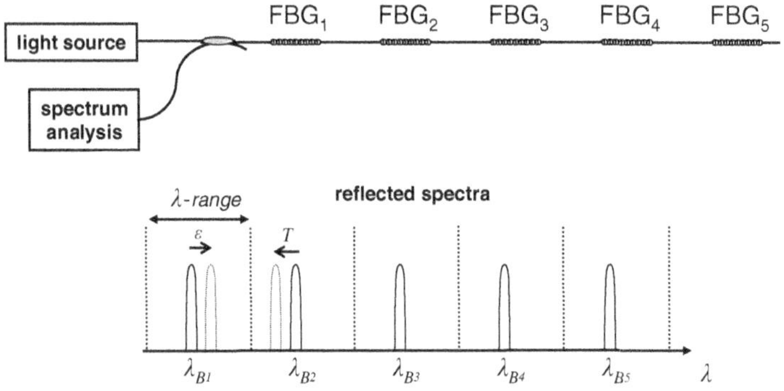

Fig. 3 Wavelength-division multiplexing of FBG sensors

Therefore, from the measurement of the reflection (or transmission) spectrum of a FBG it is possible to measure strain and temperature. This is a robust absolute measurement sensor that does not have the problems with variations in optical attenuation due to transmission or bending losses in the fiber that plague other OFS types. Moreover, having a spectral measurement system means that it is very easy to use WDM: several FBG with different central wavelengths are deployed on the same fiber to simultaneously measure temperature or strain at several locations by measuring the combined reflection spectrum. This concept is schematically depicted in Fig. 3.

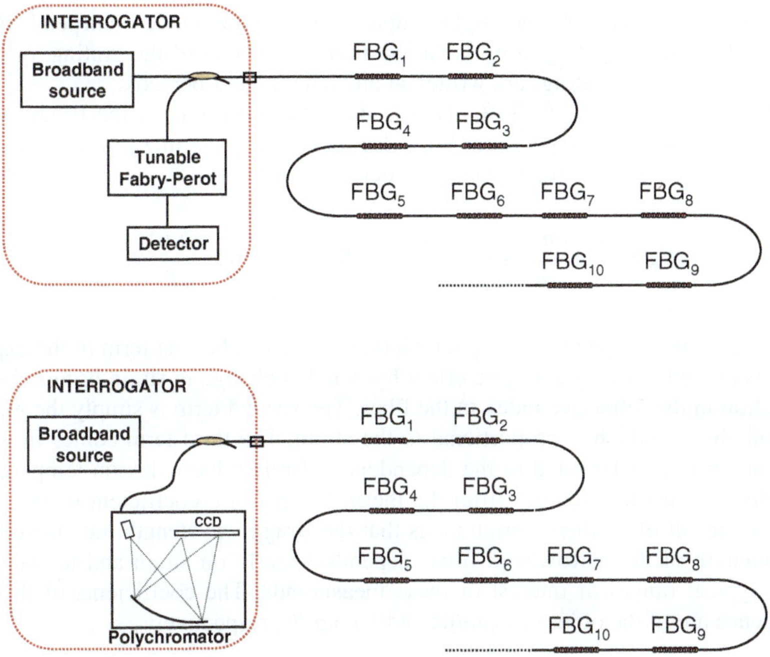

Fig. 4 Experimental setup for FBG interrogators based on (a) tunable filter and (b) polychromators

Multiple methods for the spectral interrogation of wavelength-multiplexed FBG arrays have been proposed in the literature. However, the most widely deployed commercially are based on tunable filters and lasers, and polychromators. Fig. 4 illustrates the basic experimental setups of these systems. Tunable filter schemes rely on the use of a broadband optical source to illuminate an FBG array [4]. The reflected spectrum is analyzed by using a narrow-band scanning tunable filter, e.g., Fabry-Perot, whose output is fed to a detector. An alternative is to use a fast sweeping laser as a light source instead of a broadband source and avoid the use of the tunable filter. This results in an increase of the measurement dynamic range owing to the larger instantaneous power spectral density reaching the detector as well as an enhancement in the spectral range due to the wider wavelength coverage of the tunable laser. In both cases, an electrical signal is detected as a function of time that can be translated to an optical power versus wavelength trace. Polychromator-based interrogators deploy a very similar setup, but by comparison they measure simultaneously the full reflection spectrum of one or more FBGs by using a diffraction grating to spatially project the wavelength components of the incoming light onto a CCD image sensor. In principle interrogators based on tunable filters or lasers tend to have higher wavelength resolution, and hence sensing resolution, than those based on polychromators. However, the latter offer distinct advantages when it comes to performing dynamic measurements because all components in the reflected spectra are measured at the same time.

Commercial interrogators using the techniques just described display wavelength resolution in the pm range, which translates to strain and temperature resolution of the scale of 1 με and 0.1 ºC, respectively. Moreover, dynamic measurements at kHz frequencies are possible. The maximum number of gratings that these systems can interrogate is determined by the total wavelength range of the interrogator divided by the maximum Bragg wavelength shift that the gratings are to accommodate. For instance, using an state-of-the-art interrogator with 80nm wavelength range and using FBG strain sensors with a strain limit of ±2500με and a strain sensitivity around 1pm/με means that a total of 16 grating sensors can be deployed on the same fiber array.

In order to increase the total number of measured FBG, interrogators also provide spatial-division multiplexing (SDM) capabilities in which an optical switch is used to select among several sensor channels; hence multiplying the number of sensors by the number of channels, but also increasing the total measurement time. Another possibility is to combine WDM with TDM as depicted in Fig. 5. In TDM the optical source is pulsed and so that time-of-flight information from the reflection of this pulse from multiple FBGs located at increasing distance can be differentiated even if the gratings wavelengths are partially overlapped. The drawbacks of this method are increased measurement time, which reduce its applicability when dynamic measurements are required, and the need to use gratings with low reflectivity (<5%) to avoid cross-talk arising from multiple reflections [5].

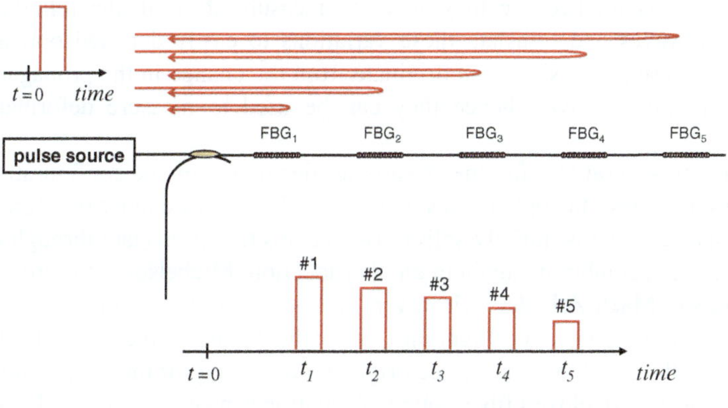

Fig. 5 Time-division multiplexing of FBG sensors

A key issue when deploying FBG sensors to measure strain in SHM applications is that of thermal compensation of the sensors. Indeed, as it is conveyed by eq. (2), FBGs display a cross sensitivity to strain and temperature that makes it impossible to isolate one of these measurands unless additional actions are taken. One possibility to solve this problem is to encapsulate the FBG in passive temperature-compensating packages [6]. These are based on using two materials with different thermal-expansion coefficients so that as the temperature raises the strain is progressively released, compensating the temperature dependence of the Bragg wavelength. Another approximation widely used in practical applications is to use an additional FBG collocated with the FBG strain sensor. This FBG is encapsulated in a strain relief package so that it just measures temperature that serves to de-correlate the measurements of the first grating.

FBG provide direct measurement just of strain and temperature. However, is relatively easy to use these measurements, particularly the strain, in an indirect manner with appropriate mechanical designs that implement other sensors such as accelerometers, inclinometers, displacement meters or pressure meters. Moreover, a number of OFS based on FBG are currently available in the market with multiple options for packaging and for attaching them to the structure to monitor. The latter is particularly important in strain measurements because the reading will be accurate just if there is an effective bonding between sensor and the host material.

3 Interferometric Sensors

Other widely deployed type of point OFS are interferometric sensors. These sensors, as their name implies, are based on the interference of two or more optical waves of the same wavelengths that are added at some position in space. The resulting wave amplitude is determined by the phase difference between the waves. For instance, two interfering waves that are in phase will undergo constructive interference resulting in maximum amplitude, while waves that are out of phase will experience destructive interference and minimum amplitude. Therefore, interferometers are useful because they serve to measure shifts in the relative optical phases of waves and translate these variations to easily detected optical power changes. These phase-shifts can originate from the change in the propagation path length of optical waves, hence they can be used to measure deformation and strain.

There are several interferometer varieties depending on the configuration of the setup used to make the optical waves interfere. In Mach-Zehnder interferometers a single optical wave is initially split in two beams that propagate through different paths before recombining again in another location. Michelson interferometers are analogous to Mach-Zehnders. However, in this case an interference pattern is produced by splitting a beam of light into two paths, bouncing the beams back and recombining them in the same device originally deployed for their separation. Fig. 6 depicts a widely deployed fiber optic deformation sensor based on a Michelson interferometer. Light is injected in an optical fiber and then a fiber optic coupler is use to split light into two optical fibers. One of the fibers is pre-stressed and mechanically attached to the host structure at two positions. The other fiber is laid loose along the same direction. Finally, mirrors are located at the end of both fibers; for instance, by cleaving the fiber tip and coating with reflective material. This sensor measures changes of path imbalance between the two fibers due to the strain of the pre-stressed fiber. Note that this is a point sensor that is bound to the host structure at two specific locations, which separation sets the gauge length of the sensor.

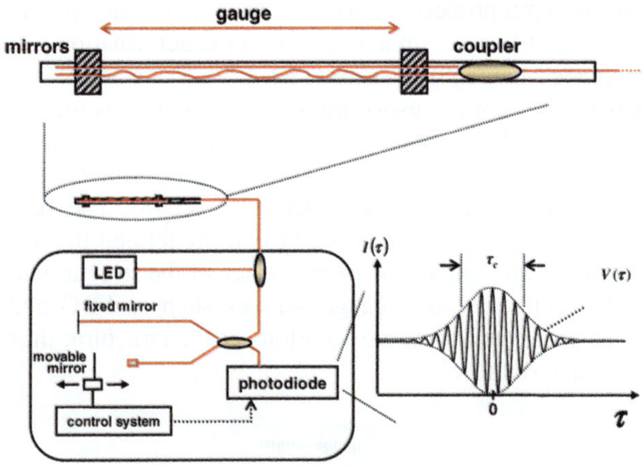

Fig. 6 Long-gauge Michelson interferometric sensor and low-coherence interrogation system

This sensor can be interrogated for instance using low-coherence interferometry. Fig. 6 illustrates the basic experimental setup for this technique. The interrogator is based on another Michelson interferometer that uses a movable mirror to scan the path-length difference. The measurement principle can be analyzed in terms of the theory of two-beam interference for partially coherent light. Temporal coherence is a basic property of light that broadly speaking relates to the degree of similarity of delayed versions of the same wave. It is found that when a light field from a low temporally-coherent light source, e.g. a broadband source such as a light emitting diode (LED), is injected in an optical fiber, then it is spitted to go through two different propagation lengths, and finally it is recombined to make it interfere, the resultant intensity I as a function of the optical path delay τ can be written as [7]:

$$I(\tau) = I_1 + I_2 + 2\sqrt{I_1 I_2}\left|V(\tau)\right| \cos 2\pi v_0 \tau \quad (3)$$

where $I_{1,2}$ the intensities of the waves, v_0 is the center frequency of the light source and V is the temporal coherence function, which gives the degree to which the temporal characteristics of the light from the source match upon certain delay. The temporal self-coherence function can be obtained as the Fourier transform of the power spectral density of the source. The width of V, which is also indicated in the figure, gives the so-called coherence time of the source, τ_c. The inset of Fig. 6 graphically displays eq. (3). Note that the third term on the right hand side of Eq. (3) gives the interference between the two waves and that it is significant just if the relative delay of the two waves is smaller than the coherence time, which is very small for a broadband source. Therefore, when the movable mirror is scanned in the interrogator, an interference fringe is just obtained when the path imbalance between the interfering waves that have propagated along the two Michelsons is close to zero. Using a properly calibrated interrogator, this provides a measurement of the absolute difference in length due to the deformation between the measuring and reference fibers in the sensor.

The Michelson fiber optic sensors are mainly deployed as long-gauge deformation sensors with a resolution and gauge length in the micrometer and the tens of meter range, respectively. This long-gauge makes them suitable to monitor deformation and strain parameters at the structural level [8]. The sensors provide a measurement of the average strain between two predefined points of a structure. Therefore, a global evaluation of the performance of the structure under scrutiny is achieved. On the contrary, short-gauge sensors such as FBG and Fabry-Perots provide information related to single locations at the structure; thus providing information at the material level.

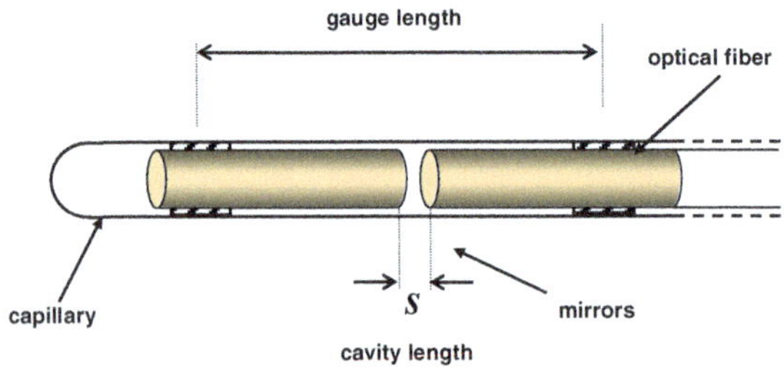

Fig. 7 Extrinsic fiber-optic Fabry-Perot sensor

Fabry-Perot is another type of interferometer that is used in FOS SHM applications. In these interferometers, multiple waves propagate back and forth between two partially reflecting mirrors. Constructive interference occurs if the transmitted beams are in phase, and this corresponds to a high-transmission peak of the interferometer. Fig. 7 depicts a typical fiber optic implementation of an extrinsic Fabry-Perot interferometer (EFPI) sensor. Two endface-cleaved fibers are used as partially reflecting mirrors. These fibers are inserted into an alignment capillary tube with the proper inner diameter and thermally fused at two positions that define the gauge length of the sensor [9].

In general, the response of a Fabry-Perot interferometer is analyzed by considering the multiple reflections of the optical waves between the two mirrors. However, in this case the reflection coefficient of the glass-air interface is small (around 4%) and hence it is necessary to take into account only the initial Fresnel reflection from the glass-air interface at the front of the air gap (reference reflection) and the reflection from the air-glass interface at the far end of the air gap (sensing reflection). Then the intensity of the light I that is coupled back into the fiber is given by:

$$I = A_1^2 + A_2^2 + 2A_1A_2\cos\left(\frac{4\pi s}{\lambda}\right) \quad (4)$$

where A_1 and A_2 are the reflection amplitudes from the reference and sensing reflection, respectively, λ is the operating wavelength and s is the mirror separation, the parameter whose measurement is necessary to extract strain information. There are several interrogation methods for EFPI-based sensors. Notice that derivation of eq. (4) implicitly assumed the use of a coherent light source such as narrow linewidth laser. In this case, measurement of strain relies on detecting changes in the spectral response of the sensor as the gap between the mirrors changes [10]. Other systems rely on the use of low-coherence methods to determine the cavity length. Altogether, Strain sensors based on EFPI provide measurement ranges of few thousand of microstrains and resolutions of the order of tenths of a microstrain.

4 Brillouin Distributed Sensors

Brillouin distributed sensors (BDS) are bound to be a truly disruptive technology in their application to SHM. These sensors have the potential to fulfill the promise of providing a fiber-optic "nerve system" to configure smart materials and structures that can feel the "pain" they are suffering in the form of strain, stress, deformation, delamination, cracks, etc [11]. The main advantages of BDS for this application are related to the distributed nature of the measurements they provide using standard fiber. In contrast to point sensors such as FBG and interferometric sensors, they provide distributed measurements of strain and temperature along every position of the fiber. They measure specifically at points given by the sampling interval, which can be made arbitrarily small, and for each location they give an average value of the measurands integrated over the spatial resolution of the sensor. Therefore, literally hundreds of thousands of measuring positions are possible on a single fiber. Furthermore, a standard singlemode fiber without any modifications is deployed as transducer for strain or temperature. Therefore, the cost per measurement offered by this technology can be very competitive.

In this section the fundamentals of this sensing technology are explained. First, the basics of the Brillouin scattering effect including its dependence on strain are temperature are explained. Then, the focus changes to the description of the techniques that have been devised to harness this nonlinear effect to build viable sensor systems. Here, the working principles and performance parameters of the four main breeds of BDS are discussed. Finally, the latest developments and research lines in the most successful time-domain BDS are reviewed.

4.1 Brillouin Scattering Fundamentals

The Brillouin scattering nonlinear effect is the result of the interaction of optical photons with acoustic phonons in a material [12]. In an optical fiber, spontaneous Brillouin scattering occurs when narrow-band pump light interacts with thermally excited acoustic waves. Due to the acousto-optic effect the acoustic wave generates a periodic perturbation of the refractive index that reflects part of the energy of the pump wave by Bragg diffraction. The reflected light, the Stokes wave, experiences a Doppler shift, the so-called Brillouin frequency shift (BFS), associated to the velocity of the acoustic waves in the fiber. This process can become stimulated Brillouin scattering (SBS) in the presence of an externally-applied conterpropagating Stokes wave with an optical frequency shifted from that of the pump by the BFS. In this case, the counterpropagation of the pump and Stokes waves generates a moving interference pattern that owing to the electrostriction effect induces the acoustic wave that can reflect part of the energy of the pump wave by Bragg diffraction. The reflected light frequency is downshifted by the BFS. Therefore, there is a transfer of energy between the pump and Stokes waves that simultaneously enhances the amplitude of the acoustic waves leading to a stimulation of the process. The net result of this interaction is that as the signals propagate along the fiber, the Stokes wave is amplified whereas the pump losses energy and is attenuated. In terms of spectral response this interaction is characterized by the Brillouin gain coefficient, which has a Lorentzian dependence given by:

$$g_B(\Delta\nu) = g_B \frac{(\Delta\nu_B/2)^2}{\Delta\nu^2 + (\Delta\nu_B/2)^2} \tag{5}$$

with g_B the peak gain coefficient, $\Delta\nu$ the detuning from the center of the Brillouin resonance and $\Delta\nu_B$ the Brillouin linewidth, which is given by the inverse of the phonon lifetime and is of the order of a few tens of MHz. Furthermore, the Brillouin shift is given by:

$$BFS = \frac{2n\upsilon_A}{\lambda_P} \tag{6}$$

where n is the refractive index, υ_A the acoustic velocity and λ_P the wavelength of the pump wave. In silica fibers this shift is around 10.8 GHz at a wavelength of 1550nm.

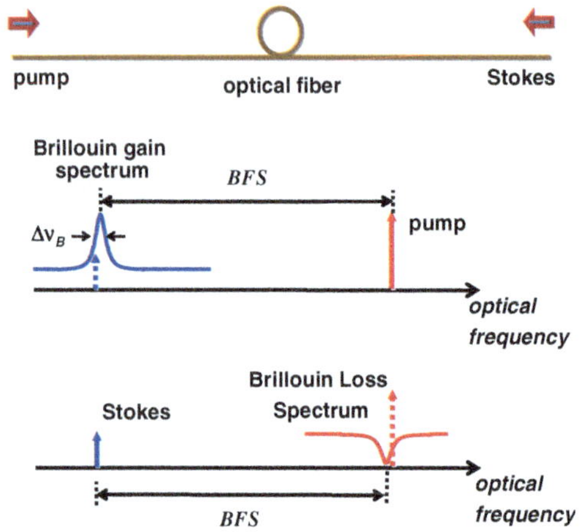

Fig. 8 Basics of the stimulated Brillouin scattering interaction

Therefore, the behavior of the SBS interaction can be summarized as follows. As it is schematically shown in Fig. 8, two related interactions occur: gain and loss. A pump wave injected in an optical fiber generates a Lorentzian Brillouin gain spectrum (BGS) for counterpropagating optical waves (Stokes wave). This BGS is centered at an optical frequency downshifted from that of the pump by the BFS. Simultaneously, the Stokes wave that is being amplified induces a Brillouin loss spectrum (BLS) upshifted in optical frequency also by the BFS.

In its application to sensors the dependence of Brillouin parameters on temperature and strain is exploited. The complete dependence of the BFS on strain can be derived from eq. (6) as [13]:

$$\frac{BFS - BFS_0}{BFS_0} = \left(\frac{1}{n_{eff}} \frac{\partial n_{eff}}{\partial \varepsilon} - \frac{1}{2\rho_1} \frac{\partial \rho_1}{\partial \varepsilon} + \frac{1}{2E_1} \frac{\partial E_1}{\partial \varepsilon} \right) \delta\varepsilon \tag{7}$$

where $\delta\varepsilon$ is the applied strain that generates a change in BFS from a reference value BFS_0 at room temperature and in a loose state of the fiber; n_{eff} is the effective refractive index, ρ_1 is the density and E_1 is the Young's modulus of the fiber. The first term of the right-hand-side summation is determined by the elasto-optic effect, the second is subject to the strain-induced distortion of the fiber and the last term is decided by the strain-induced second-order nonlinearity of the Young's modulus. The latter is found to be the main origin of the strain coefficient of the BFS for silica fibers. Typical values for standard fiber types are around 0.04 MHz/με at 1550nm. Similarly, the dependence of the BFS on temperature is found to have an analogous expression [13]:

$$\frac{BFS - BFS_0}{BFS_0} = \left(\frac{1}{n_{eff}} \frac{\partial n_{eff}}{\partial T} - \frac{1}{2\rho_1} \frac{\partial \rho_1}{\partial T} + \frac{1}{2E_1} \frac{\partial E_1}{\partial T} \right) \delta T \,. \tag{8}$$

In this case, the first term of the summation is related to the thermo-optic effect, the second to the thermal expansion of the fiber and the third to the thermal-induced second-order nonlinearity of Young's modulus. Again the latter is found to be the predominant term. The temperature coefficient of the BFS is of the scale of 1 MHz/ºC for most standard fibers at 1550nm. This value can be slightly modified by thermal stress in the coating of the fiber [14].

4.2 Brillouin Distributed Sensor Configurations

From what has been already explained it is clear that a length of fiber can be used as a sensor by measuring its BGS (or BLS). This can be done by injecting a pump wave from one side of the fiber and a probe wave by the other and registering the gain (or loss) experienced by the latter as their wavelength separation is scanned. Then, the BFS is given by the spectrum peak and it can be translated to a strain and/or temperature value by using the coefficients obtained from a previous calibration of the sensing fiber deployed. However, this system would be measuring the global gain spectrum of the length of fiber, which is the result of the integration of the local gain at each position along the fiber. In order to have spatially-resolved, i.e. distributed, measurements of BFS a mechanism is needed to differentiate contributions to the gain originating from individual locations in the fiber. These can be done in the time, frequency or coherence domains, giving rise to the three main analysis-type BDS: Brillouin optical time-domain analysis (BOTDA), Brillouin optical frequency-domain analysis (BOFDA) and Brillouin coherence-domain analysis (BOCDA).

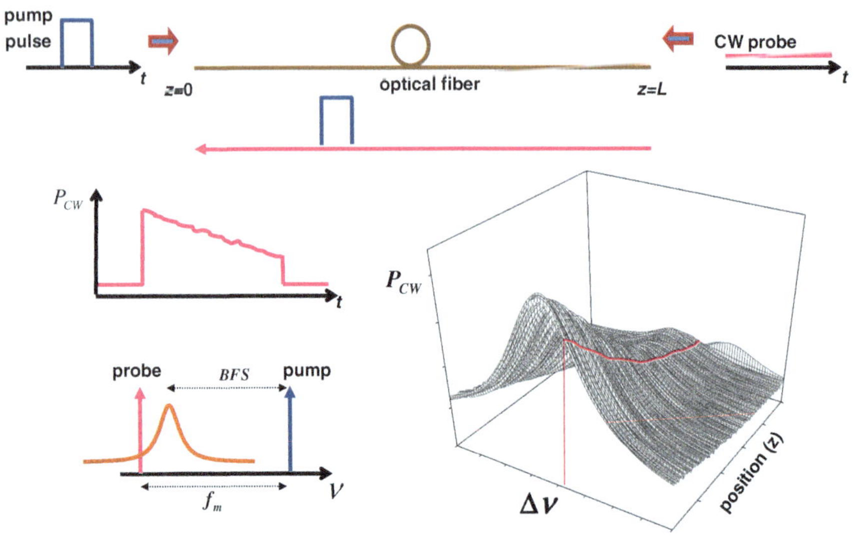

Fig. 9 Fundamentals of BOTDA

BOTDA systems were the first to be developed and probably the BDS type with the greatest potential. BDS really started in a slightly different configuration as a method to quantify distributed optical fiber attenuation alternative to the conventional optical time-domain reflectometry (OTDR) [16]. However, soon its potential for measuring strain [17] and temperature [18] was recognized upon study of the dependence of the Brillouin parameters on these measurands. From this starting point, BOTDA-based BDS research started to thrive with different experiments and setups that sought to enlarge the measurement range and enhance the spatial resolution.

Fig. 9 highlights the fundamentals of the BOTDA system. The basic idea is to mimic OTDR systems by using a pump pulse conterpropagating with a CW probe wave. The pulse propagates along the fiber and at each location imparts Brillouin gain to the probe. This position-dependent gain is measured by a classical time-of-flight method detecting the received probe signal in the time domain. If t_0 is the time when the trailing end of the pump pulse of temporal duration τ enters the fiber, then the probe signal received at $t = t_0 + 2\,z/v$ interacted with the pulse between positions z and $z + u$, where v is the speed of light in the fiber and $u = (\tau / v)/2$ is the interaction length that gives the spatial resolution of the measurement.

For instance, a pulse duration of 10 ns gives a resolution of around 1m. The two factor in the expression for u comes from the fact that the pump pulse and the CW probe wave are conterpropagating. Therefore, the time-depend BOTDA signal can be translated to position-dependent gain by the simple relation $z = (t\text{-}t_0)\cdot v/2$. Then, it is possible to reconstruct the position-dependent Brillouin spectra distributed along the fiber by sweeping the wavelength separation between pump and probe and recording multiple BOTDA time-domain traces, as it is schematically shown in the figure. Finally, strain or temperature is quantified from the BFS measured at each position.

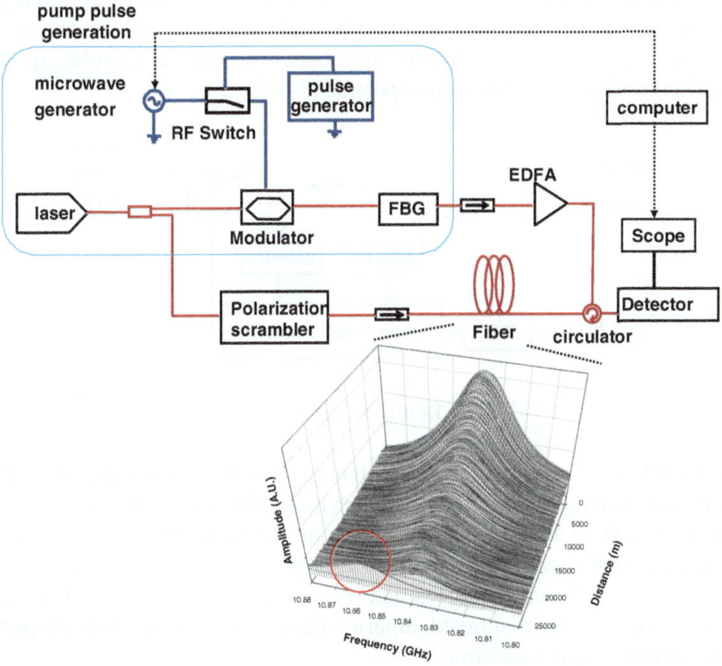

Fig. 10 Optimized experimental setup for BOTDA

A recent optimized experimental setup for the implementation of the BOTDA principle is displayed in Fig. 10. The signal from a single laser is divided in two branches using a fiber coupler. In the upper branch the pump pulses are generated using the RF shaping technique [19]. This is based on generating the pulses in the microwave domain, where it is easier to obtain pulses with good extinction ratio characteristics. The frequency of the microwave pulses is tuned around the BFS of the fiber under test (FUT). Next the pulses drive an optical modulator so as to generate a pulsed sideband that is subsequently used as pump pulse. An optical filter (FBG) is also deployed to remove undesired spectral components before the signal is amplified in an Erbium-doped amplifier (EDFA) and launched into the fiber under test (FUT). In the lower branch the laser signal is directly used as probe wave after a polarization scrambling procedure that compensates polarization effects in the Brillouin interaction. The inset in Fig. 10 displays an example distributed measurement of Brillouin spectra using this system.

The BOFDA principle is completely analogous to that of the BOTDA, but the time-frequency duality is exploited [20]. Its basic experimental setup is outlined in Fig. 11. Here, instead of pulsing the pump it is sinusoidaly modulated. This causes the probe signal to also acquire a sinusoidal modulation originating from SBS interaction. Then, the probe signal is photodetected and its relative relationship to the original signal in terms of amplitude and phase-shift is recorded. Hence, a complex transfer function can be measured by sweeping the modulation frequency. A temporal pulse response similar to that of the BOTDA is finally obtaining by means of an inverse Fourier transformation. Again this process is repeated while scanning the wavelength separation between pump and probe signals to get the required position-resolved gain spectra.

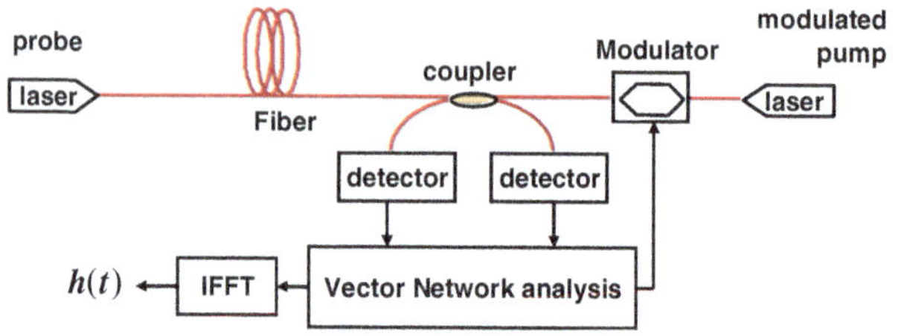

Fig. 11 BOFDA experimental setup

The BOFDA scheme offers some potential advantages over BOTDA. The costs of the experimental setups can be somewhat smaller due to the narrow-bandwidth operation of system as it works just with tone-modulated signals. In principle this also increases the measurement signal-to-noise ratio (SNR) as the instantaneous detection bandwidth can be very small. Nevertheless, demonstrated BOTDA systems have consistently displayed superior performance than BOFDA particularly in terms of data acquisition time.

The final variety of analysis-type BDS is the BOCDA. This technique controls the relative coherence between the pump and probe waves so as to localize the effective SBS interaction at a specific position along the fiber [21]. The principle of the technique is outlined in Fig. 12. The pump and probe lightwaves are modulated in frequency sinusoidaly with a frequency f_m and counterpropagated. This causes that only at certain locations in the fiber the frequency separation between the two waves remains constant over time. These are the correlation peaks at which the beat between pump and probe wave is narrower and hence maximum efficiency in the Brillouin gain imparted to the probe is achieved. At the rest of locations there is a variation in the relative frequency that leads to a reduction in the effective SBS gain imparted to the probe wave at those locations. In actual measurements the delay and modulation frequency is adjusted so that there is a single correlation peak within the length of sensing fiber. Therefore, the gain experienced by the probe after crossing the fiber comes mainly from the position of the correlation peak. Moreover, sweeping the wavelength separation between pump and probe in the usual way the full BGS at that location is recovered. In order to measure other locations of the fiber it is necessary to modify the modulation frequency or the relative delay between pump and probe.

The spatial resolution Δz of the measurement with BOCDA sensors is given by:

$$\Delta z = \frac{V_g \Delta v_B}{\pi f_m \Delta f_m} \tag{9}$$

Where V_g is the group velocity and Δf_m is the peak frequency deviation of the optical FM modulation. Resolutions in the centimeter range have been comfortably demonstrated with this technique even with dynamic measurements [22]. The measurement range d_m is given by the separation of two correlation peaks because, as it was previously mentioned, it is necessary that a single correlation peak exists within the fiber in order to avoid ambiguities:

$$d_m = \frac{V_g}{2f_m} \tag{10}$$

Notice that Δz and d_m are not independent of each other. Increasing the spatial resolution requires reducing the measurement range. In fact the number of effective sensing points N along a fiber is given by [23]:

$$N \equiv \frac{d_m}{\Delta z} = \frac{\pi \Delta f_m}{\Delta v_B} \tag{11}$$

N around 1000 can be achieved using realistic modulation parameters, although different enhancements have been proposed to increase this number. This limitation in the measurement range for a given spatial resolution, together with the increased measurement time required to scan all positions in a fiber, are the main drawbacks of BOCDA systems compared to BOTDA. On the other hand its main asset is the extremely high spatial resolution that it provides.

BOTDA, BOFDA and BOCDA are analysis-type BDS that use an external wave to probe the SBS gain provided by a pump wave. An alternative method is the Brillouin optical time-domain reflectometry (BOTDR) that just launches a pulsed pump wave into the fiber and measures the backscattered spontaneous Brillouin scattering in a single-ended configuration [24]. Fig. 13 depicts a typical configuration for a BOTDR system [25]. A narrow laser is divided in two branches by a fiber-optic coupler. In one of the branches it is pulsed using an optical modulator, amplified and launched into a length of singlemode fiber. Then, as the pulse propagates along the fiber spontaneous Brillouin scattering is generated that travels back to the detector. This backscattered signal is coherently detected in a wideband photo-receiver using the other laser branch as local oscillator; thus generating an RF beat. The variation of the frequency of this RF signal over time can be translated to a variation of BFS along the fiber following the same principle that was previously explained for BOTDA. In practical experimental setups, the instantaneous frequency of the detected RF signal can be measured by an electrical heterodyne receiver followed by analog-to-digital conversion and data analysis.

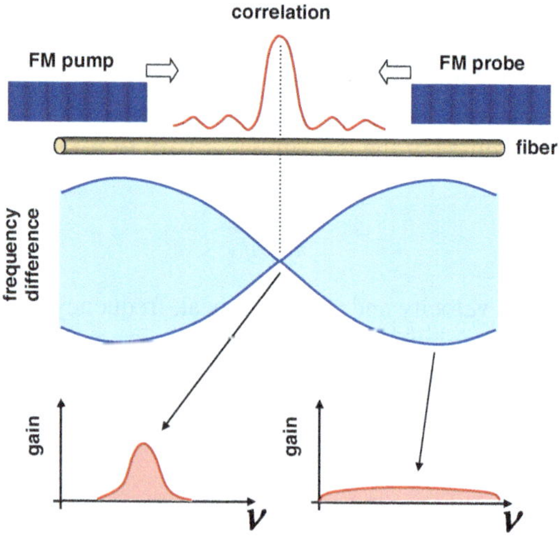

Fig. 12 Fundamentals of BOCDA measurements

The main advantage of the BOTDR sensor concept is it single-ended configuration that is very convenient for the instrumentation of large structures, e.g. pipelines, in which analysis-type sensor deployment is complicated by the need to access both ends of the test fiber. However, the price to pay for this convenience is a reduction of the SNR of the measurements because the spontaneous Brillouin scattering signal is very weak. Therefore, massive averaging is required to obtain meaningful measurements, which increases the measurement time. On the contrary, in analysis BDS the Brillouin interaction is stimulated by the use of an externally-injected probe signal and thus the measurement performance is significantly enhanced.

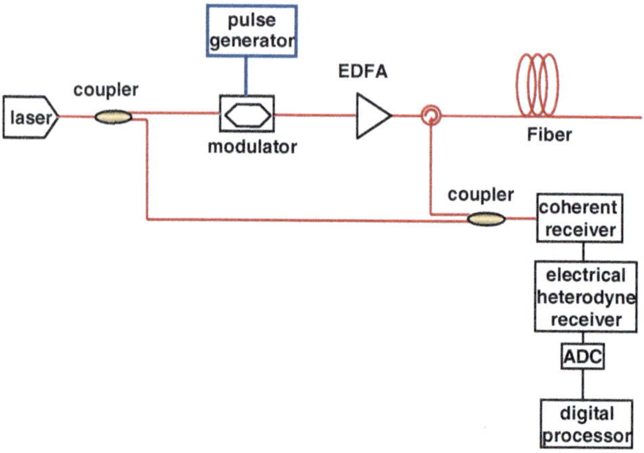

Fig. 13 BOTDR experimental setup

There are a handful of commercial BDS systems currently in the market. Most deploy basic BOTDA with typically 1-m spatial resolution and around 1-MHz BFS resolution, which according to the coefficients in Eqs. (7-8) translates to resolutions of the strain and temperature of the scale of 10με and 1°C, respectively. The measurement range extends up to tens of kilometers. BOTDR systems with comparable resolution performance but increased measurement time and reduced dynamic range are also available.

4.3 Enhanced BOTDA Setups

The most successful BDS sensor type to date is the BOTDA. This is the concept that has been the object of the most intense research effort in the last two decades because of is potential for performance, simplicity and its similarity to the well-established OTDR technology. Recently, research in BOTDA has been directed mainly in two lines: enhancing the spatial resolution and extending the sensor range. In the standard configuration of a BOTDA sensor the spatial resolution is limited to around 1 m. This limitation stems from the broadening of the BGS as the pump pulse duration is reduced. Indeed, the effective BGS is the convolution of pulse spectrum and the Lorentzian Brillouin linewidth. The latter is of the order of a few tens of MHz as determined by the acoustic lifetime of phonons in the fiber ($\tau_A \approx 10$ ns). For long pulses (reduced spatial resolution) this convolution approximately equals the intrinsic Brillouin spectrum. On the contrary, as the pulse width approaches the duration of the acoustic lifetime the pulse spectrum broadens over the natural Lorentzian linewidth and increasingly determines the final BGS linewidth. The BGS is measured in the presence of noise. Hence, the narrower the final spectra, the better the precision in the determination of the peak of the BGS and thus of the strain and temperature in the fiber. Therefore, for a given precision and measurement time the pulse duration has to exceed a duration of around 10ns in most setups (≈ 1-m spatial resolution).

Solutions to enhance the resolution over the acoustic lifetime limit have been proposed. They are based on the observation that pre-excitation of the acoustic wave in the Brillouin interaction can overcome the BGS broadening effect [26]. The basic idea is to have Brillouin interaction before the arrival of the pump pulse. This can be achieved by the presence of pre-existing CW pump and Stokes signals. In this way, upon arrival of the pulse, it can reflect on the pre-existing grating without the need to generate its own interaction. Therefore, the interaction spectrum experienced by the pump wave is defined by the natural Brillouin linewidth and not by the convolution of the pump spectrum and Lorentzian profile. This principle has been exploited in several configurations. For instance, using a pulse over a CW pump pedestal [27] or introducing a "dark pulse" [28], i.e., a temporal suppression of an otherwise continuous pump wave. More recently an improved physical explanation for the acoustic wave pre-excitation has been developed that has lead to an optimized setup based on using optical phase-shift instead of optical intensity pulses [29].

The other direction of improvement of BOTDA is expanding the range of the sensor so that large structures can be monitored. This effort is driven by applications such as the instrumentation of km-length pipelines and railways. The main practical problems in BOTDA setups when the length of the sensing fiber increases are fiber attenuation and nonlinear and nonlocal effects. Range is limited because of the attenuation of the pump pulse as it propagates along the fiber. When the pulse is small the gain of the probe wave is buried in detection noise and more averaging is demanded to obtain significant measurements; hence, greatly increasing the measurement time. In principle, this could be mitigated by increasing the injected pump power. However, the maximum pump power is limited by the appearance of other nonlinear effect such as modulation instability [30]. Solutions to this limitation have been proposed using for instance optical pulse coding to increase the measurement signal-to-noise ratio [31]. Other option is deploying optical amplification to compensate fiber attenuation. Raman amplification is particularly suitable for this purpose because the sensing fiber itself is used as amplification medium [32]. Furthermore, with Raman amplification the gain is distributed along the fiber, thus preventing the existence of locations in the fiber with high power that could lead to the manifestation of detrimental nonlinear effects.

The other significant limitation to long-range BOTDA sensing is nonlocal effects. Nonlocal effects refer to the fact that local measurements of Brillouin gain depend on the interaction at every preceding locations. This originates from the depletion of the pump pulse by the CW probe as it propagates along the fiber. Ideally, as the pump pulse travels to a given measurement location it is just affected by the attenuation of the fiber. However, with the probe wave present there is Brillouin interaction at all proceeding locations with energy been transferred from pump to probe. This depletion of the pump is wavelength-dependent, thus it distorts the measured gain spectra because the Brillouin gain depends on the pump power. Altogether, this introduces a systematic error in the measurement that is larger as the end of the fiber under test is approached. Techniques to compensate this effect have been also proposed. An obvious solution is to lower the power of the probe wave. However, this results in a reduction of the received SNR. Other proposals rely on measuring the pulse energy loss to compensate the measured spectra or to numerically reconstruct the unknown BFS profile to fit the measurement data [33].

Another important topic of recent research in BDS is how to decouple the temperature and strain measurements. The problem is similar to that found in FBG: the BFS jointly depends on strain and temperature. An obvious solution is to use two fibers, with one "loose" fiber dedicated just to measure temperature. Other approaches rely on using fiber with multiple acoustic modes [34].

5 Rayleigh Distributed Sensors

The last method of distributed sensing that is also commercially available is based on Rayleigh scattering in an optical fiber. This effect originates from random fluctuations of the index of refraction in the core and it manifests as a small distributed reflection of the power of the optical signals that propagate along the optical fiber. The reflected signal as a function of location is a random but static property of each particular fiber. Furthermore, the random fluctuations of the index of refraction that lead to the distributed reflection of optical waves can be modeled as a long, weak Bragg grating with a random variation of amplitude and phase along the grating length. The fundamentals of the Rayleigh measurement technique lie precisely in this Bragg grating analogy. As it was discussed in section 2, changes in environmental parameters such as strain and temperature modify the period of the grating and the index of refraction; thus changing the local resonant wavelength.

Fig. 14 schematically displays the setup required to implement this sensing concept. It is basically an optical frequency domain reflectometer (OFDR) [35]. Light from a narrow-linewidth tunable laser is split into two paths by an optical coupler. The measurement path directs the signal to a fiber under test and uses an additional fiber coupler to recover the backscatter signal. This signal is recombined with the signal from the reference path and detected. A polarization beam splitter and two separate detectors are deployed to provide polarization-independent measurements [36]. In addition, a polarization controller is located in the reference path to ensure that the reference local oscillator optical signal is evenly distributed between the two orthogonal polarizations of the beam splitter.

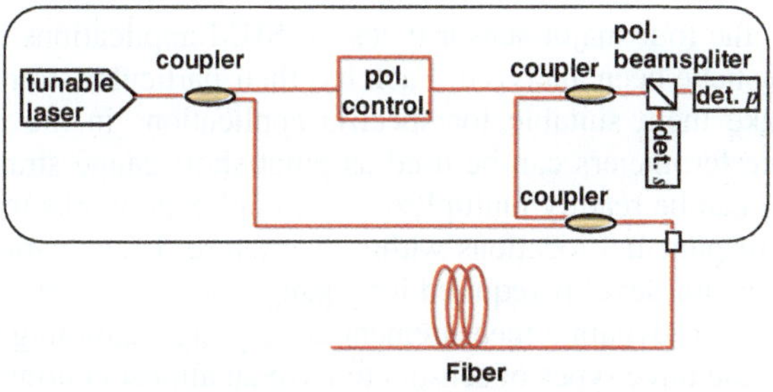

Fig. 14 Distributed Rayleigh sensing setup

This single-frequency interferometric setup can measure the complex reflection transfer function of the sensing fiber and obtain the time response of Rayleigh reflections by means of Fourier transformation. The spatial resolution Δz and the maximum measurement length Lmax are given by [37]:

$$\Delta z = \frac{c}{2n_g \Delta f} \qquad L_{\max} = \frac{c}{4n_g \delta f} \tag{12}$$

where n_g is the group index in the fiber, c the speed of light and Δf is the bandwidth of the wavelength sweep and δf is the optical frequency step.

The procedure to perform measurements of strain or temperature with this system starts by measuring and storing the Rayleigh backscattering of a given fiber in some reference state, e.g. ambient temperature and "loose" state. Next, upon strain or temperature change, the new Rayleigh response of the fiber is compared to the reference state signature. This is done by breaking the data for the full length of the fiber into small spatial intervals. Then, for each interval the measured and the reference time-domain data are Fourier transformed into the optical frequency domain and the spectral shift of the "local Bragg grating" is calculated by cross-correlation [38]. Therefore, the total number of measurement points is the total length of the gratings divided by the spatial interval. This can not be arbitrarily high because the SNR of the cross-correlation depends on the number of data points in each interval. The wavelength shift of the backscatter pattern due to a temperature or strain change along the fiber is identical to the response of a fiber Bragg grating sensor given in eq. (2).

Commercial distributed sensing systems based on Rayleigh OFDR provide centimeter-scale spatial resolution in lengths of fiber of around hundreds of meters with micrometer or tenth-of-degree resolutions in the measurement of strain or temperature, respectively.

6 Conclusion

In this chapter, the four major sensor types for SHM applications in terms of current availability have been analyzed. Each has their particular strengths and weaknesses that make them suitable for specific applications in the field. FBG and Fabry-Perot interferometers can be used as point short-gauge strain sensors. Particularly, FBGs can be readily multiplexed in complex networks to evaluate strain at a multitude of punctual locations within a structure. If evaluation of integrated strain at the structural level is required long-gauge interferometric sensors are also available. Moreover, dynamic measurement at very high sampling frequencies are possible with these three types of sensors to have an almost continuous monitoring of the response of the area of interest under variable conditions. On the other hand, distributed Brillouin and Rayleigh sensors main asset is the reduced cost they provide per sensing point. The sensing range can be larger in BDS, but Rayleigh distributed sensors have the potential to provide higher spatial resolution and dynamic measurements with greater frequencies.

References

[1] López-Higuera, J.M.: Handbook of Optical Fibre Sensing Technology. Wiley, Chichester (2002)

[2] Kuang, K.S.C., Cantwell, W.J.: Use of conventional optical fibers and fiber Bragg gratings for damage detection in advanced composite structures: A review. Appl. Mech. Rev. 56, 493 (2003)

[3] Othonos, A., Kalli, K.: Fiber Bragg Gratings: Fundamentals and Applications in Telecommunications and Sensing. Artech House Publishers, Boston (1999)

[4] Kersey, A.D., Berkoff, T.A., Morey, W.W.: Multiplexed Fiber Bragg Grating Strain Sensor System with a Fiber Fabry-Perot Wavelength Filter. Opt. Lett. 18, 1370–1372 (1993)

[5] Morey, W.W., Dumphy, J.R., Meltz, G.: Multiplexing Fiber Bragg Grating Sensors. In: Proc. of SPIE, vol. 1586, pp. 216–224 (1991)
[6] Yoffe, G.W., Peter, A., Krug, F., Ouellette, Thorncraft, D.A.: Passive temperature-compensating package for optical fiber gratings. Appl. Opt. 34, 6859–6861 (1995)
[7] Saleh, B.E.A., Teich, M.C.: Fundamentals of Photonics. Wiley Interscience, Hoboken (2007)
[8] Glisic, B., Inaudi, D.: Fibre Optic Methods for Structural Health Monitoring. Wiley Interscience, Hoboken (2008)
[9] Murphy, K.A., et al.: EFPI sensor manufacturing and applications. In: Proc. Smart Structures and Materials 1996: Industrial and Commercial Applications, San Diego, pp. 476–482 (1996)
[10] Chena, J., Chena, D., Genga, J., Li, J., Caia, H., Fanga, Z.: Stabilization of optical Fabry–Perot sensor by active feedback control of diode laser. Sensors and Actuators A 148, 376–380 (2008)
[11] Hotate, K.: Fiber Optic Nerve Systems for Smart Materials and Smart Structures. Optical Sensors, OSA Technical Digest (CD) (Optical Society of America paper SWB2) (2010)
[12] Agrawal, G.: Nonlinear Fiber Optics. Academic Press, London (2006)
[13] Zou, W., He, Z., Hotate, K.: Investigation of Strain- and Temperature-Dependences of Brillouin Frequency Shifts in GeO2-Doped Optical Fibers. J. Lightwave Technol. 26, 1854–1861 (2008)
[14] Kurashima, T., Tateda, M.: Thermal effects on the Brillouin frequency shift in jacketed optical silica fibers. Appl. Opt. 29, 2219–2222 (1990)
[15] Nikles, M., Thevenaz, L., Robert, P.A.: Brillouin Gain Spectrum Characterization in Single-Mode Optical Fibers. J. Lightwave Technol. 15, 1842–1851 (1997)
[16] Horiguchi, T., Tateda, M.: Optical-fiber-attenuation investigation using stimulated Brillouin scattering between a pulse and a continuous wave. Opt. Lett. 14, 408–410 (1989)
[17] Horiguchi, T., Kurashima, T., Tateda, M.: A technique to measure distributed strain in optical fibers. IEEE Photon. Technol. Lett. 2, 352–354 (1990)
[18] Kurashima, T., Horiguchi, T., Tateda, M.: Distributed-temperature sensing using stimulated Brillouin scattering in optical silica fibers. Opt. Lett. 15, 1038–1040 (1990)
[19] Zornoza, A., Olier, D., Sagues, M., Loayssa, A.: Brillouin distributed sensor using RF shaping of pump pulses. Meas. Sci. Technol. (2010), doi:10.1088/0957-0233/21/9/094021
[20] Garus, D., Krebber, K., Schliep, F., Gogolla, T.: Distributed sensing technique based on Brillouin optical-fiber frequency-domain analysis. Opt. Lett. 21, 1402–1404 (1996)
[21] Hotate, K., Hasegawa, T.: Measurement of Brillouin Gain spectrum distribution along an Optical Fiber Using a Correlation-Based Technique – Proposal, experiment and simulation. IEICE Trans. Electron. E83C, 405–412 (2000)
[22] Hotate, K., Tanaka, M.: Distributed Fiber Brillouin Strain sensing with 1-cm spatial resolution by correlation-based continous-wave technique. IEEE Photon. Technol. Lett. 14, 179–181 (2002)
[23] Song, K.-Y., Hotate, K.: Enlargement of Measurement Range in a Brillouin Optical Correlation Domain Analysis System Using Double Lock-in Amplifiers and a Single-Sideband Modulator. IEEE Photon. Technol. Lett. 18, 499–501 (2006)
[24] Shimizu, K., Horiguchi, T., Koyamada, Y., Kurashima, T.: Coherent self-heterodyne detection of spontaneously Brillouin-scattered light waves in a single mode fiber. Opt. Lett. 18, 185–187 (1993)

[25] Alahbabi, M., Cho, Y.T., Newson, T.P.: 100 Km distributed temperature sensor based on coherent detection of spontaneous Brillouin backscatter. Meas. Sci. Technol. 15, 1544–1547 (2004)
[26] Bao, X., Brown, A., DeMerchant, M., Smith, J.: Characterization of the Brillouin-loss spectrum of single-mode fibers by use of very short (10-ns) pulses. Opt. Lett. 24, 510–512 (1999)
[27] Kalosha, V.P., Ponomarev, E.A., Chen, L., Bao, X.: How to obtain high spectral resolution of SBS-based distributed sensing by using nanosecond pulses. Opt. Express 14, 2071–2078 (2006)
[28] Brown, A.W., Colpitts, B.G., Brown, K.: Dark-Pulse Brillouin Optical Time-Domain Sensor With 20-mm Spatial Resolution. J. Lightwave Technol. 25, 381–386 (2007)
[29] Foaleng, S.M., Tur, M., Beugnot, J.-C., Thévenaz, L.: High Spatial and Spectral Resolution Long-Range Sensing Using Brillouin Echoes. J. Lightwave Technol. 28, 2993–3003 (2010)
[30] Alasia, D., Herraez, M.G., Abrardi, L., Martin-Lopez, S., Thévenaz, L.: Detrimental effect of modulation instability on distributed optical fiber sensors using stimulated Brillouin scattering. In: 17th International Conference on Optical Fibre Sensors, pp. 587–590 (2005)
[31] Soto, M.A., Bolognini, G., Di Pasquale, F.: Analysis of pulse modulation format in coded BOTDA sensors. Opt. Express 18, 14878–14892 (2010)
[32] Zornoza, A., Pérez-Herrera, R.A., Elosúa, C., Diaz, S., Bariain, C., Loayssa, A., Lopez-Amo, M.: Long-range hybrid network with point and distributed Brillouin sensors using Raman amplification. Opt. Express 18, 9531–9541 (2010)
[33] Minardo, A., Bernini, R., Zegni, L., Thevenaz, L., Briffod, F.: A reconstruction technique for long-range stimulated Brillouin scattering distributed fibre-optic sensors: experimental results. Meas. Sci. Technol. 16, 900–908 (2005)
[34] Zou, L., Bao, X., Shahraam Afshar, V., Chen, L.: Dependence of the Brillouin frequency shift on strain and temperature in a photonic crystal fiber. Opt. Lett. 29, 1485–1487 (2004)
[35] Glombitza, U., Brinkmeyer, E.: Coherent Frequency-Domain Reflectometry for Characterization of Single-Mode Integrated-Optical Waveguides. J. Lightwave Technol. 11, 1377–1384 (1993)
[36] Soller, B.J., Wolfe, M., Froggatt, M.E.: Polarization resolved measurement of Rayleigh backscatter in fiber-optic components. In: Proceedings Optical Fiber Communications Conference 2005, paper NWD3 (2005)
[37] Soller, B.J., Gifford, D.K., Wolfe, M.S., Froggatt, M.E.: High resolution optical frequency domain reflectometry for characterization of components and assemblies. Opt. Express 13, 666–674 (2005)
[38] Froggatt, M., Moore, J.: High-Spatial-Resolution Distributed Strain Measurement in Optical Fiber with Rayleigh Scatter. Appl. Opt. 37, 1735–1740 (1998)

Sensors Systems, Especially Fibre Optic Sensors in Structural Monitoring Applications in Concrete: An Overview

S.K.T. Grattan[1], S.E. Taylor[1], P.M.A. Basheer[1], T. Sun[2], and K.T.V. Grattan[2]

[1] School of Planning, Architecture & Civil Engineering
The Queen's University of Belfast Belfast BT9 5AG United Kingdom
[2] School of Informatics and School of Engineering & Mathematical Sciences
City University London Northampton Square London EC1V 0HB United Kingdom
k.t.v.grattan@city.ac.uk

1 Background

Reinforced concrete is the most popular construction material in the world due to its flexibility to make different complicated shapes, yet providing strength, long service life and structural integrity. However, a major issue for reinforced concrete structures is the corrosion of the reinforcement bars (rebars) when exposed to aggressive environmental conditions, such as those in marine or urban environments. The corrosion is normally caused by the ingress of chlorides, as in the case of marine environment, or carbon dioxide, as in the case of urban environment; the latter causes a reduction in the alkalinity of concrete through a process called carbonation and steel loses the protection provided by the concrete. Corrosion products (rust) occupy many times the volume of the original steel and as a consequence the integrity of the structure is severely compromised and occasionally leads to a catastrophic structural failure. Therefore, it is highly desirable to obtain information about factors which initiate the corrosion and the rate of corrosion once it has already started, both of which will help civil engineers to manage their reinforced concrete structures in a cost-effective manner.

Why is all this important? We implicitly depend, in a modern society, on the quality and utility of the structures that surround us; for our homes, our commerce and our leisure. They must be fit for purpose and safe. In addition, the construction industry worldwide is of multibillion dollar value – in the UK alone it represents some 6-8% of GDP and annual growth rates of up to 12% have been achieved in recent years. The figures of major developed countries are similar and typically the construction industry represents some 5% of GDP [Grattan et al, 2006a]. Concrete structures are very widely used across the world today and rely upon the use of rebars to provide strength and structural integrity [Basheer et al, 2006a]. However, the corrosion of rebars can lead to the creation of waste materials (corrosion products known commonly as rust) which occupy many times the volume of the original steel [Ervin et al, 2006 and Grattan et al, 2007]. The effect of this is to severely compromise the integrity of the structure

S.C. Mukhopadhyay (Ed.): New Developments in Sensing Technology for SHM, LNEE 96, pp. 359–425.
springerlink.com

– occasionally leading to a catastrophic structural failure. Thus it is important to identify the onset of corrosion before it leads to the deterioration of the structure. Figures such as £600million in the UK alone are being spent in just one year to repair concrete structures in the UK alone [Grattan et al, 2007] – a figure multiplied many times over worldwide.

There are many limitations in current practice in the determination of both the probability and the rate of corrosion of rebars in reinforced concrete structures [Leng et al, 2006; McPolin et al, 2005; Majumder et al, 2008]. For example, non-destructive tests for the identification of both the probability and the rate of corrosion are influenced by environmental conditions of the concrete. Alternatively, the owner is reliant on the corrosion waste products becoming visible on the concrete surface, this usually represents a point where excessive corrosion has occurred and costly repairs are inevitable. It is clearly desirable to have a system capable of monitoring the changing condition of the steel which will indicate problems in advance of this stage of excessive corrosion but it is also beneficial to have a system that is both passive and compatible with the structure by not weakening it through installation or on-going presence and use. These will all lead to significant cost savings for the sector which could then be reinvested into new-build and further development.

The research reported in this Chapter presents an overview of current techniques and a report of the success of an innovative approach to monitoring the progress of corrosion of rebars: using fibre optic sensors (FOS) for pH monitoring and also the use of fibre optic strain sensors. This aspect is focused into two main areas supporting the theme of better structural health monitoring: the first being the development of optical fibre based pH sensors for the monitoring of changes in concrete due to chemical processes occurring, such as carbonation, with the second being the development of optical fibre strain sensors to measure quantitatively changes in steel reinforcement bars due to corrosion. The development, performance and detailed evaluation of the sensors in the laboratory were examined. A comparison is made with the results from conventional techniques which are currently employed in the field but many of which are destructive or not suited for retrofitting. Conclusions on the suitability of the fibre optic sensors for longer-term monitoring of reinforced concrete structures for corrosion are drawn.

2 Corrosion of Steel in Reinforced Concrete Structures

Concrete is a mixture of aggregate, cement, water, air (entrained during mixing or purposely added) and often other additional binders and admixtures. The ratios of these components affect all properties of concrete, such as rheology, dimensional stability, microstructure, mechanical properties (including strength characteristics), transport properties and durability characteristics, as outlined by other researchers [Popovics, 1998, Neville, 1996 and Newman and Choo, 2003]. The aggregate takes up the majority of the volume occupied and, except for water in most countries, is the least expensive component. It is generally inert and does not normally cause any adverse reactions within the concrete, however where they are of a lesser quality they can lead to alkali aggregate reactions, where some aggregates react with the alkali hydroxides in concrete, causing expansion and cracking over a period of many years. The cement paste is used to bind the aggregates. The water is of a minimum specification to ensure low levels of contaminants [BS EN 1008], which otherwise could adversely affect the setting and hardened properties of the concrete. Hardened concrete is inherently weak in tension and steel reinforcement is placed in the tension zones of a structure to carry the tensile forces. It is also used as a means of controlling cracking in concrete.

Corrosion of steel embedded in concrete, due to issues such as carbonation (chemical reaction between carbon dioxide and hydrated cement phases in concrete, resulting in the formation of calcium carbonate) and the ingress of chlorides, is a major source of financial burden for the construction industry and has been considered by many to be the number one durability problem to infrastructure [Schiessl, 1988]. In the United States alone corrosion costs a total of nearly $300 billion per year according to Koch et al, (2001). This report stated that corroding structures which can be repaired, without the need to replace the whole structure account for over $100 billion per year.

Sensors should be designed to provide information prior to the initiation of corrosion so to take appropriate measures to prevent further damage. Corrosion is commonly defined as a destructive interaction between a material and its environment. In this instance the corrosion referred to is that of the oxidisation of the steel reinforcement due to a chemical reaction within the concrete. The mechanisms of corrosion of steel in concrete are elaborated below and Figure 1 shows how corrosion can lead to an increase in localised volume of the metal, which in turn can then lead to cracking of the concrete.

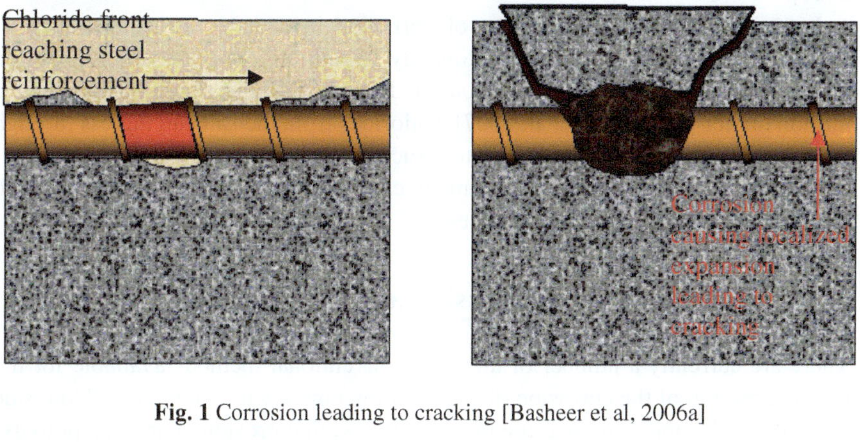

Fig. 1 Corrosion leading to cracking [Basheer et al, 2006a]

The ability to monitor the expansion of the steel due to corrosion and the factors that cause this initiation accurately and without destructive methods will prove vital in:

(i) Cost reduction - Corrosion of steel embedded in concrete is a major source of financial burden for the management of infrastructure due to huge cost in repairing and maintaining deteriorating structures and bringing them back to service. Reducing this cost by identifying corrosion early in the life of a structure contributes to reducing the labour needed for undertaking repairs, avoiding structural failures (and any possible related litigation) and reducing indirect costs from disruption to infrastructure, e.g. traffic delays.

(ii) Increasing the safety of the structures – early detection of any weaknesses can prevent total failure of a structure.

(iii) Extending the lifetime of structures - use of such sensors can enable preventative action at an earlier stage in the decay process.

(iv) Providing data from inaccessible areas - e.g. from sub-sea structures – as the sensors are embedded they can be interrogated at any point after construction.

(v) Reducing unplanned shutdown – achieved by adequate warning which enables a scheduled maintenance programme.

The majority of the expenditure on instrumentation during the total construction process is in the construction phase. These are usually removed or not expected to survive longer than the completion of the construction. FOS offer the advantage of being embedded and thereby allowing access to critical data right from the earliest stages of construction and through the life cycle of the structure. This is a clear financial benefit to industry and can improve both the quality and accuracy of the results of structural health monitoring [Fuhr and Spammer, 1998; Tennyson et al, 2001].

Impacting directly on the onset of corrosion in concrete structures, such as marine and bridge structures, approximately 15 million tonnes of salt is spread on main roads each year in the US alone and in the UK the figure has reached 2 million tonnes [Hammond et al, 2007]. Chlorides from the salt can ingress through the concrete in a reinforced concrete structure and cause corrosion of the steel reinforcement. The natural environment can enact upon the structure through chemical, biological or physical processes.

3 Characterisation of Corrosion and Its Causes

There are currently a number of different conventional methods available for the characterisation of the corrosion of steel reinforcement within concrete. Alongside this there is the ability to measure the causes of such corrosion in an attempt to use data to prevent corrosion from occurring. Each of the following methods has its own advantages and limitations. Most structures rely on a maintenance schedule through the use of the conventional methods as outlined below, along with visual inspection [Bungey et al, 2006 and Broomfield, 2007].

3.1 Carbonation Depth Measurement

A number of methods that are available are reviewed below.

(i) Indicator spray

The pH of a concrete can be determined through the use of an indicator spray, using a 1% phenolphthalein in 70% ethyl alcohol solution [RILEM CPC 18, 1988]. This is sprayed on a freshly broken surface of concrete. The phenolphthalein indicator solution demarcates concrete above a pH of approximately 9.5 with a pink colour and that below this pH stays with no colour change. Therefore, the depth to the pink colouration from the surface is measured at several locations on the freshly broken surface of concrete and an average value is reported as the depth of carbonation. The principle of this test is that the pH value changes in concrete during carbonation from around 13 to less than 9 and the region that is being carbonated can be determined with this test. However, it is known that the passive layer on steel breaks down at around a pH of 11, so the phenolphthalein test is not entirely adequate to determine the onset of corrosion due to carbonation. This indicator is only of use after there has already been a substantial decrease in pH, at which stage the corrosion may have damaged the structure. For most practical cases, the phenolphthalein test is regarded as a reliable technique, which is low cost and simple to use. However, on occasions some aggregates can make the colour change more difficult to observe due to their own colour [Richardson, 2002].

(ii) Thermo-gravimetric analysis

Thermo-gravimetric analysis (TGA) relies on the change in the weight of a sample when it is heated [Villain and Platret, 2006]. To ensure the accuracy of such a reading there is need for control on the weight, the temperature and the temperature change involved in the process. As the temperature is raised the weight is constantly monitored and therefore a plot of temperature against weight can be made. The powdered concrete is heated at a known rate and each chemical component is characterised by the temperature at which it decomposes. The carbonated phases dissociate at around 650°C and the carbon dioxide emissions lead to a weight loss. This data can then be used to relate the weight loss to the degree of carbonation of the concrete, as well as the determination of other parameters.

(iii) Acid digestion

The chemical analysis of cementitious material can be carried out in a number of different ways. Acid digestion relies on wet chemistry techniques. From research carried out by Moller [1995] it is possible to digest a sample with hydrochloric acid and determine the number of moles of carbon dioxide given off. This is carried out in a closed container and the increase in pressure is used to estimate the carbon dioxide released. Potentiometric titration is then carried out on the solution that remains, after filtering, to determine the calcium oxide content. The degree of carbonation of the sample is then found from the relationship shown in Equation 1

$$\text{Carbonation} = (\text{released } CO_2)/(\text{measured CaO}) \quad (1)$$

The steps involved in this process are labour intensive and require costly specialist laboratory equipment. As a result it is regarded as being a slow and complicated process for carbonation assessment.

(iv) X-ray diffraction

Crystalline materials, i.e. those consisting of a regularly ordered lattice of atoms or molecules, produce a characteristic diffraction pattern when an x-ray beam is incident upon it. This pattern is then compared on a computer database of standard crystal structures for identification of the species [Ramachandran, 1995]. As a result carbonation can be detected in concrete samples when subjected to x-ray diffraction, due to the crystalline nature of calcium carbonate. It has been discussed by others as being a process of qualitative benefit rather than specifying the level of carbonation [Moller, 1995]. The identification of each peak produced in the diffraction pattern and the quantification of each species requires not only extremely expensive equipment but also extremely skilled personnel with the knowledge of both the technique and the crystal structure of minerals present in the material.

(v) Water digestion

Dust samples obtained from a concrete under investigation can be added to a known volume of distilled water and the water soluble solids can be extracted over time. This solution can then be tested for a pH level which is indicative of the level within the sample [McPolin, 2007]. In order to obtain reliable readings, the test needs to be carried out in a laboratory under controlled environment. Otherwise, variations in temperature during digestion could vary the pH values. It has been shown by McPolin et al [2005] that there is a variation to be expected between the pH readings reported depending on the ratio of distilled water added to the quantity of concrete dust used at the digestion phase. In the application to carbonation measurements in concrete samples however such differences are not of great significance [Rasanen and Penttala, 2004]. Providing the ratio is kept constant for all depths investigated then the effect will be nullified. Also there is an interest in the trend through the depth of a sample as opposed to the exact pH measured.

3.2 Chloride Content Determination - Overview

Several methods of chloride extraction are detailed, both acid and water digestion after which the quantitative analyses methods are described. This provides an insight into the processes required to determine accurately the chloride content from a concrete dust sample.

(i) Acid digestion

This technique is used to release not only the dissolvable chloride ions but to release the bound chloride ions as well, through exposure to a harsh acidic environment [Climent et al, 1999]. Powder samples are taken and then added to nitric acid, which can also be heated and stirred to add to the effect. This leads to the chloride ions being released into the solution, which can then be quantified using chemical titration, as discussed in the next sub-section. In a way similar to that of the determination of the carbonation profile, dust samples are collected from different depths and analysed to obtain a chloride profile. If determination of the chloride content which initiated the corrosion is required, only a single sample needs to be taken at the reinforcement level to determine the chloride content [Bungey et al, 2006].

(ii) Water digestion

As stated in the previous section, chloride ions can be extracted using water digestion as well. This involves mixing the dust sample with a solvent, such as water, and measuring the amount of chloride passing into solution [Glass et al, 1996]. This is known as the water soluble chlorides. The end result will be dependent on some of the variables used during this process, for example the ratio of dust to water used, the mixing time and the mixing method. As a result these must be tightly controlled for cross-comparison purposes.

3.3 Quantitative Methods for the Determination of the Chloride Content

The chloride content in the solution which was obtained either by acid digestion or by water digestion can be determined using laboratory methods, such as chemical titration, or semi-quantitative methods, for example the Quantab strip. These methods are elaborated below.

(i) Chemical titration

Titration can be broken into two main sections, viz. Volhard and potentiometric titration.

Volhard titration is a back titration which relies on visual indicator determining the end point. An excess of silver nitrate is added to the extracted solution to produce a silver nitrate precipitate, which can be filtered off. The number of nitrate ions released is the same as that of the chloride ions that were originally present in the sample. Ammonium iron (III) sulphate is usually added at this stage to act as an indicator. The solution is then titrated against a known solution of ammonium thiocyanate, which leads to the creation of silver thiocyanate. Any additional thiocyanate over and above what is needed for the complete conversion of ammonium thiocyanate to silver thiocyanate produces a red-brown complex when in combination with the silver nitrate, indicating the end of the titration. The precision of the test will rely heavily on the experience and skill level of the user [Nilsson, 1996].

Potentiometric titration can also be used to determine the level of chlorides found in an extracted solution. In this method the voltage across the analyte (the solution containing chloride ions) is measured between a reference and indicator electrode. A silver nitrate solution is, once again, used as a titrant, together with a silver electrode to monitor the potential of the extraction solution. There is a risk of interference from the presence of other ions, such as bromide and iodide, and where this is expected then a chloride specific electrode must be used. The voltage is recorded as levels of the titrant are added and so the voltage is provided as a function of the presence of the ions. Once the potential stabilises and is constant then it is known that the process is completed. This is then correlated to the chloride concentration.

The potentiometric titration is a more simplistic than the Volhard technique, due to the ability to process multiple samples at the same time through the use of automatic titration equipment. Due to this automation there is also less of a reliance on the operator for the accuracy. Neither however can be used as a field test and must be carried out within a controlled laboratory environment [McPolin, 2005].

(ii) Use of ion selective electrode

Specific ion electrodes can be expensive but can provide an accurate measure of the ionic content in the solution. They work on the principle that the potential that is measured in a solution is proportional to the concentration of chloride ions in that solution. Once the ion selective electrode has been calibrated it is possible to obtain direct value of the concentration. A drawback of this method is the requirement to re-calibrate frequently to remove the effect of any drift caused by scale formation on the electrode. Bamforth [1997] reported that there is also a dependence on temperature that needs to be accounted for while using the ion selective electrodes. Despite these issues it remains one of the most simple and rapid methods available for the determination of chloride content in the lab and field.

(iii) Quantab strip method

Quantab strips are a moderately accurate testing method which can be performed quickly. They rely on powdered samples being digested in nitric acid, which is then neutralised by the addition of sodium carbonate to remove any opportunity for the high acidity to interfere with the determination of a chloride level [Deeks and Hao, 2004]. The Quantab chloride titrator is made up of silver dichromate impregnated in a capillary column within a thin plastic strip. The strip is placed into the filtered solution containing chloride ions, which allows the fluid to rise through the capillary column. When the chloride reacts with the silver dichromate this produces a colour change, from brown to white. As a commercial product a calibration chart will have been provided by the manufacturer and the result can then be read off. It is known that the readings can be affected through the presence of additional ions and can even be thrown off by certain types of aggregates. It is however of benefit where a fast result is required to provide an indication of the chloride levels [Bungey et al, 2006].

4 Techniques Used to Determine the Extent of Corrosion Damage

The extent of corrosion damage can be measured using different levels of sophistication and the reliability of each depends on numerous factors. One of the simplest methods is visual inspection, but if a quantitative estimate of the damage is required, various non-destructive tests need to be carried out. Some of the most commonly used methods are discussed briefly in this section, along with a description of factors which could influence the measurements.

4.1 Visual Inspection

Visual inspection is usually the first step in any investigation. The main aim of such an inspection is to provide initial feedback on the issues being faced and an estimate of their extent [Broomfield, 2007]. Through the use of digital photography and concise note taking these details can be of great benefit to the engineer, even if not present in person at the structure. The obvious limitation of such an inspection is also the same as the potential advantage. A skilled operative can determine issues and be able to provide an invaluable report, whereas a less experienced operative can fail to notice subtle indicators to structural defects. The ability to establish whether cracks, spalling and even rust products are present is vital to determining the monitoring and testing requirements of any structure.

Due to the similar nature of some of the on-surface characteristics it is often impossible for the engineer to determine the exact cause of the issue. It should however be possible to identify the most appropriate course of action to be taken. As a result it becomes vital that the engineer properly documents the findings so that there is clarity for future engineers involved in the process. In some instances the use of binoculars or even telescopes may be required for such an inspection; such can be the level of difficulty in gaining access to the region of interest

[Bungey et al, 2006]. Cost is a key factor in the determination as to how often a visual inspection will be carried out. The cost associated with sending out a suitably experienced engineer to conduct an inspection can be significant, given the sheer scale of infrastructure such as bridges and how long an adequate inspection would take.

4.2 Half-Cell Potential Measurement

The half-cell potential measurement is used to assess the probability of the corrosion of reinforcement within concrete and is commonly used where reinforcement corrosion is already suspected. As ions move through the concrete between the anode and cathode there is an accompanying electric potential field surrounding the bar that is corroding. With the half cell method it is possible to measure this free corrosion potential and determine the voltage difference between the steel and a reference half-cell which is in contact with the concrete surface through a high-impedance voltmeter [Broomfield, 2007]. The half-cell potentials, therefore, represent the ease with which the atoms of iron will give up their electrons and enter the solution as positive ions. Figure 2 shows a simplified schematic of this technique:

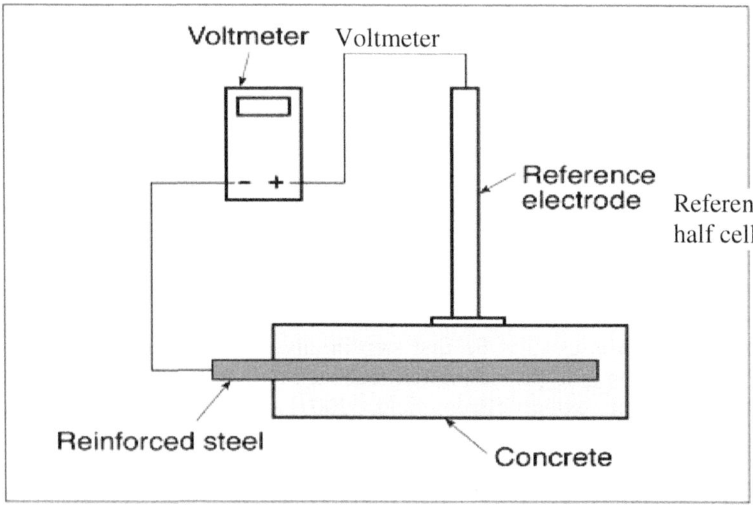

Fig. 2 Schematic diagram of half-cell technique [Nawy, 2008]

A standard reference electrode in a suitable electrolyte (known as the half-cell of an electrical circuit) is placed on the concrete surface, this electrode would normally be copper and the electrolyte would be copper sulphate, and makes contact to the concrete surface through a porous plug and a moistened sponge. The electrical circuit is completed when the reference half-cell is connected to the steel embedded in the concrete [Nawy, 2008].

The corrosion potential is associated with the severity of steel corrosion. As a result of terminal connections the half-cell reports negative voltages and the more negative a value the greater the tendency to lose its electrons, i.e. to corrode. Where the reinforcement is entirely embedded within the structure being investigated there is the need to break away the cover concrete to allow for the electrical circuit to be completed. The measurement of half-cell potentials using this test requires a good contact between the reference half-cell and the concrete surface because the potential of any metal in contact with concrete is a function of a number of variables, e.g. surface quality. It is also vital that the surface is sufficiently moist to allow the circuit to be complete. It is regarded as being sufficiently moist if the measured potential does not change by more than ±20mV in a 5 minute period [ASTM, 1991]. There are also limitations when the surface is actually too wet because this can lead to increasingly negative potentials and may provide a misleading high probability of corrosion of the steel. If the bar is corroding then the excess electrons in the bar will tend to flow to the half-cell placed on the surface and the more of the electrons there are the higher the probability of corrosion [Malhotra and Carino, 2004].

Knowledge of the potential does not provide information on the amount of corrosion, it is possible however to map the potential and identify possible corrosion sites. The half-cell test will ultimately provide an indication to the user of the regions that require further investigation, by giving an indication of the likelihood of corrosion occurring. It can also be extremely useful in confirming that there has been a return of the passive layer protecting the steel reinforcement following repairs and maintenance [Bungey et al, 2006 and Broomfield, 2007].

The process of half-cell potential measurement has been made all the more complicated by the increasingly common use of corrosion inhibitors which can influence the readings obtained and need to be accounted for. These inhibitors can cause the negative potential to reduce due to their own anodic/cathodic status. The industry guidelines [ASTM, 1991] states that the half-cell potential method should not be used in conjunction with epoxy coated and galvanised reinforcement bars. Even a dense cover of concrete will affect the results obtained, due to the readings becoming similar with the increase in cover regardless of what is actually happening internally. An increase in chloride ion concentration will cause a significant shift in the corrosion potential to larger negative values [Elsener, 2001].

Half-cell potential measurements can only be used to determine the probability of corrosion activity taking place at the time of the reading. [Gu and Beaudoin, 1998]. ASTM C876 gives the following guidance for interpreting the readings from half-cell measurements:

→ Potential more positive than -200mV there is a high likelihood that no corrosion is occurring at the time of measurement
→ Potential more negative than -350mV there is a very high likelihood that there is active corrosion
→ The corrosion activity is deemed to be uncertain when in between -200 and -350mV

However, in the NDT special technical session from Rilem [2002] contrasting guidance was provided. Rather than relying on an absolute value of potential for determination of corrosion hazard, greater consideration must be given to the interpretation of the results. As there is a potential for a number of the concrete properties to affect the reported value, such as moisture content, temperature etc, it is proposed that there are different corrosion indicating values for different structures. Rather than focusing solely on the potential level there is a need to determine the potential differences between active and passive areas.

There are limitations to the use of the half cell technique:

(i) poor surface contact caused by a failure to remove adequately any contaminants before use can provide misleading readings,
(ii) cracked concrete can distort the current path,
(iii) the presence of other metals and stray currents can distort the readings,
(iv) There is also a potential for repairs to create conditions where the readings can no longer be regarded as meaningful, through alterations in the alkalinity and resistivity of the pore solution.

4.3 Resistivity Measurements (Wenner 4-probe)

The Wenner **4-probe** system measures the electrical resistance of the concrete, which can be directly related to the possible rate of corrosion of steel embedded in it. Traditionally the resistivity readings are used in tandem with the half-cell tests. Electrical resistance of the concrete controls the ease with which ions can migrate between anode and cathode [Malhotra and Carino, 2004] due to the fact that corrosion is an electrochemical process. It operates under the principle that there are 4 equally spaced electrodes, as shown in Figure 3, in an equally spaced array referred to as the Wenner configuration. The spacing that is used is required to be larger than that of the maximum size of the aggregate used. There is then a constant low frequency alternating electrical current passed between the two outer probes and at the same time a measurement made of the electrical potential between the inner pair. As in the case of half-cell apparatus, there is a need to ensure that good electrical contact is established between the electrodes and the surface of concrete. This is normally achieved by wetting the wooden plugs attached to tip of the electrodes.

Resistivity is the electrical resistance of a unit volume of material and is determined through the following equation:

$$\rho = \frac{RA}{L} \tag{2}$$

where ρ is the resistivity (ohm-cm), R is resistance (Ohms), A the area (cm^2) and L the length (cm). Therefore the resistivity from the Wenner probe system is found by:

$$\rho = \frac{2\pi s V}{I} \quad (3)$$

where 's' is the spacing between the probes (cm), V is the voltage (Volts) and I the current (Amps).

This measurement can only indicate the capacity of the concrete to allow corrosion, not actually pinpoint corrosion itself or indicate if it has started. There is a dependence on the surface conditions for the accuracy of the results and moisture conditions have been shown to have a large impact on the readings [COST 509, 1997]. The ambient temperature also has a large effect on results, as the temperature decreases the resistivity readings will increase.

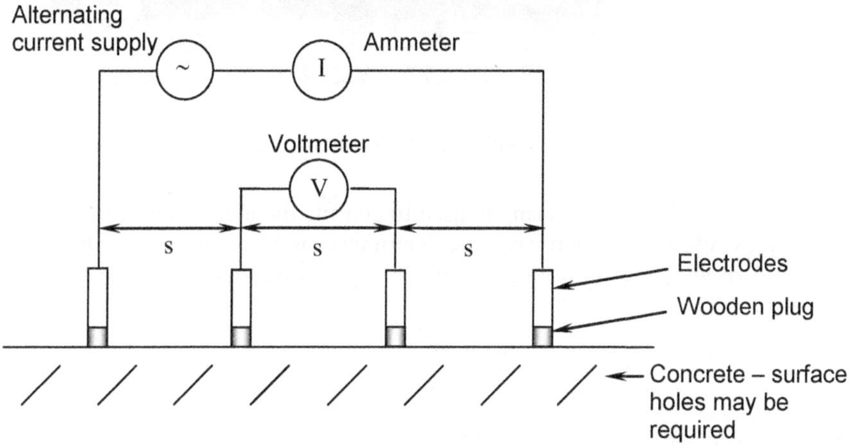

Fig. 3 Schematic of Wenner 4 probe resistivity meter [Glass et al, 2000]

The figures obtained from the 4-probe method have been defined by Bungey [1989] as follows:

- >20kΩcm - there is a low likelihood of significant corrosion
- Between 10 and 20 kΩcm - there is a low to moderate likelihood of corrosion
- Between 5 and 10 kΩcm - there is a high likelihood of corrosion
- <5kΩcm - there is a very high likelihood of corrosion

4.4 Linear Polarisation Resistance (LPR)

The LPR measurement determines the corrosion rate using electrolytic test cells. An external current is applied to the cell, polarising the steel and then monitoring the effect on the reference electrode potential (Figure 4). Usually conductive foam is soaked in water and used to enhance the contact with the concrete surface [Broomfield, 2007].

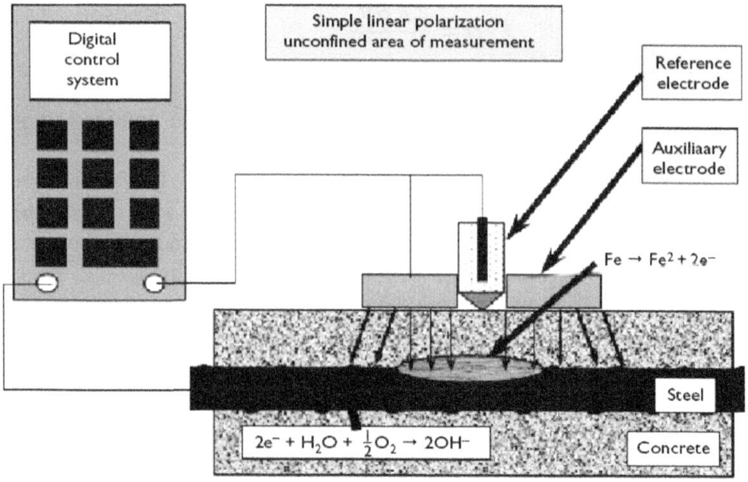

Fig. 4 schematic diagram of LPR with unconfined measurement area [Broomfield, 2007]

In some instances a guard ring is used to confine the area of impressed current and thereby allow for a more accurate determination of the area of reinforcement being polarised. The polarization resistance (R_p) can be found from the following equation:

$$R_p = \frac{\Delta E}{\Delta i} \tag{4}$$

where ΔE is the change in voltage (V) and Δi is the change in applied current (A).

It can also be shown that the corrosion rate is related to the polarization resistance by the following equation:

$$i_{corr} = \frac{B}{R_p} \tag{5}$$

where i_{corr} is the corrosion current density (ampere/cm^2) and B is a constant (in Volts).

It has been suggested that the following be used as guidelines figures for the LPR method [Malhotra and Carino, 2004;Bungey et al, 2006]:

- <0.1μA/cm^2 – negligible corrosion risk
- 0.1→0.5 – low corrosion risk
- 0.5→1 – moderate corrosion risk
- >1 – high corrosion risk

The LPR method is known to be limited by temperature, relative humidity and other effects, all of which leads to an uncertainty about the value of the constant B that should be used [Millard et al, 2001]. It can also be quite a slow process requiring lengthy periods to ensure stability and can mean that premature measurements are possible where equilibrium has not been reached. The assumption is made that any corrosion is occurring uniformly across the whole area being measured across. Furthermore, the instantaneous corrosion rate being measured may not be reflective of the typical corrosion rate. Andrade and Alonso [2001] suggest that confining the current using a guard ring method can overcome this difficulty.

5 The Need for Managing Structural Health through Better Sensor Systems

5.1 Limitations of Existing Methods of Assessing the Causes and Extent of Corrosion of Steel in Concrete

As has been detailed above there are a number of factors which can lead to the degradation of a concrete structure. It is also clear that assessing the conditions involved is not a simplistic task, a number of the factors are interlinked and either retarding or accelerating the corrosion process dependent on the condition of the other. There is also a clear issue when attempting to even make such a measurement that the interpretation of the readings provided can be themselves altered depending on the conditions experienced at the time and there are no simple conclusions that can be drawn based solely on one set of results.

Examples of the limitations with current techniques are:

- Current techniques rely on analysis of the effects of corrosion and look to demonstrate the probability of likelihood of a particular event.
- All of the techniques and testing methods, as described in this chapter, require the user of the equipment to be at the site in question and able to access the area(s) of the structure where it is deemed to be important to perform these measurements.
- They are also reliant on the skill of the visual observer of the structure in question to determine what (if any) further action is required in terms of monitoring.
- The use of metallic components which will themselves corrode and degrade when subjected to a harsh environment.
- The user of the technology is required to have a good working knowledge of how the system works in order to ensure the quality of the readings and thereby the results.

5.2 Opportunities Provided by New Types of Sensors – Use of Fibre Optic Techniques

It is for the above scenario that sensors are being developed to attempt to bring clarity to the parameters of importance and to attempt to remove the uncertainty in measurement. The ability to provide a reading that is quantitatively related to a particular chemical species or to provide strain readings from within the structure at the level of the reinforcement can give a greater level of confidence to the user. By being able to be more specific on what exactly is happening within the structure will therefore be a step forward. To be able to then develop these sensors into a network that provides an array of readings from a series of targeted regions will be the ideal end point of their overall research in this sphere.

The sensors as researched in this work are strain and pH detection through the use of fibre optic principles. Such sensors offer a number of advantages over conventional sensors as well as the conventional methods employed to investigate these parameters [Grattan and Sun, 2000; Al-Azzawi, 2007].

- FOS are lightweight, cheap, easy to install, EMI immune and robust.
- There are other methods such as x-ray imaging available but these require the removal of some of the structure under investigation. This has the potential to damage the structure or even leave it more susceptible to corrosion. The FOS can be embedded and therefore do not require the removal of samples.
- Current tests, such as spraying a pH indicator onto a freshly broken concrete to determine the likelihood of corrosion, rely on these failures to have occurred in the structure before any measurement can be made. FOS can produce results from the moment they are installed and, providing they are suitably packaged for the harsh conditions, can be used to provide information at any stage in the life cycle of the structure. Such measurements can then be reported to the customer at regular intervals and any anomalies can be easily noted.
- There is the ability to write the sensors in a series and attach them so that operational time on site is minimal. Results can be read out from any point and provide details across a number of key areas in the structure.
- FOS have no associated human error with them, the hardware is attached and results downloaded. This can be achieved as the sensing element is fixed and not susceptible to human error.

As well as fibre optic sensors, electrical resistance sensors, which are commonly used in industry, have been investigated in this research. They have been known to be a cost-effective and robust method of determining strain, moisture movement and internal changes in concrete for a number of years [Benmokrane et al, 2006]. The electrical sensors used in this research were Electrical Resistance Strain Gauges (ERSGs), which were compared with the fibre optic sensors used.

Through the development of such sensors there can be a more comprehensive analysis of the influence and interdependence of the key parameters, such as chlorides, pH changes or strain levels, thereby leading to more informed engineering decisions by the end user community. As described above, there are the two main sections in the corrosion cycle that are of interest, namely the initiation period and the active corrosion phase. During this first stage sensors can assist in providing the user with data otherwise unavailable, which can be used to introduce a more tailored maintenance schedule. There are clear cost benefits to this approach as well as the reduction in duration of closure of the structure, which in itself can be of tremendous financial benefit. There will also be the ability to monitor during the active corrosion stage and to make repair or replacement decisions in a more informed manner. This will lead to a dramatic improvement in the service life prediction of the structure. To be able to assess the requirement for repairs/replacement better will lead to not only financial benefits similar to those during the initiation phase but also will lead to an increased health and safety level for infrastructure as well as both public and expert confidence.

6 Sensor Methods of Monitoring Reinforced Concrete Structures

6.1 Sensor Technology

A sensor can most easily be described as a device capable of reliably and repeatedly monitoring a physical, chemical or biological process. This is usually seen as a change in a parameter of the sensor and this change can then be related through communication to a further device, which in turn reports this either as a measured parameter or signal [Grattan and Meggitt, 1999]. Sensors are used in almost all walks of life in the 21st Century. Their use ranges from household appliances, e.g. kettles, to extremely high technology applications, e.g. in space stations. Novel sensors are continually being developed and researched in a range of industries to provide feedback to engineers on the status of a parameter of interest in a specific region. Without their use many activities and devices would become impossible or even too dangerous to be completed. Sensors can play a key role in providing vital data and information to the engineers looking to maintain and monitor civil infrastructure and within this context the developments in both sensor systems and structural health monitoring methodologies are reviewed in this chapter.

6.2 Types of Sensors for Structural Monitoring

It is important at the outset to distinguish between 'Structural Health Monitoring' and 'Structural Monitoring' as two distinct aspects of the monitoring of structures. 'Structural Health Monitoring' is taken here as meaning the monitoring of the condition of structures for their durability whereas 'Structural Monitoring' is monitoring methods which are used to estimate the structural capacity. Both types are reviewed in this chapter as the research carried out has been in both areas.

Presently there are two different types of sensors available which are making an impact on structural monitoring applications and they are Fibre Optic Sensors (FOS) and Electrical Sensors (ES).

FOS, though not necessarily a recent development themselves, are the more recent addition to this particular sector and aim to capitalize on the advantageous characteristics of fibre optic cable, e.g. small size, light weight and immunity to electromagnetic wave interference due to the use of light for sensing and signal transmission [Grattan and Sun, 2000]. To develop a fibre optic sensor system, a light source, some optical fibre, a sensing element or transducer and a detector are usually required [Grattan and Meggitt, 1999]. The sensor/transducer modulates a particular parameter of the optical system, e.g. intensity, wavelength, polarisation, phase, etc. when a target measurand changes and this causes the change in the optical signal received by the detector. Typically the light will be reflected back along the fibre, as shown in Figure 5, however there are sensors where the light passes through and is then connected to a detector.

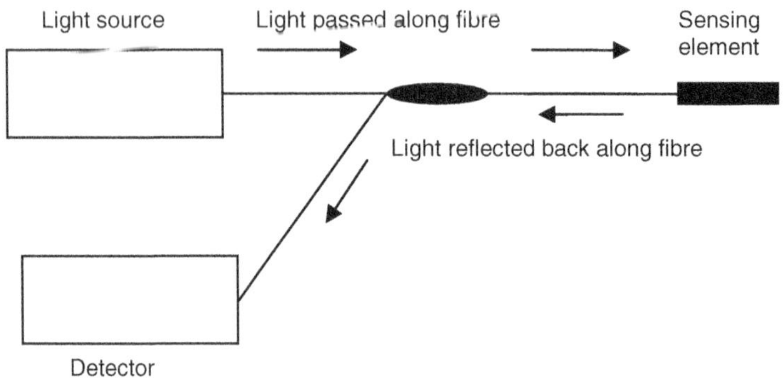

Fig. 5 Schematic diagram of a typical fibre optic sensor system [Grattan and Meggitt, 1999]

Strain and temperature sensing, for example, can be achieved through the use of FOS, providing Structural Monitoring as defined earlier. Both types of sensor have been used in extensive field testing around the world [Gebremichael et al, 2005; Tennyson et al, 2001; Mufti, 2003] and have shown themselves to be comparable, and in some cases, superior to other available techniques. The advantages of such FOS sensors, namely their immunity to EMI, lightweight components, robust but flexible nature, not requiring lengthy surface preparation and their inert nature, especially in the context of concrete monitoring, have been demonstrated. There are also factors which have been shown to restrict their more common use and replacement of existing technologies, such as the cost of the sensors and equipment to interrogate them, once they have been fractured they are not easily repaired, a temperature/strain interdependence requiring corrective actions to be taken and the lack of current standards available regulating their installation and use. Sensors for these parameters are currently commercially available and are being used in a number of applications including Structural Monitoring. Research has also been carried out into the development of pH and chloride sensors, relying on a number of different FOS based techniques to carry out Structural Health Monitoring [Fuhr et al, 1997; Tang and Wang, 2007; Xie et al, 2004]. Absorbance based sensing (e.g. sol-gel sensors) relies on electromagnetic radiation being absorbed by the material and relating the reduction in optical power to the amount of the material under investigation. Fluorescence techniques use the optical phenomenon where absorbed light creates a molecular excitation and as a result the material re-emits light at a different wavelength. Long Period Grating and Fibre Bragg Grating sensing for durability measurements rely on the interaction of a coating with that which is being measured and either a resulting change in refractive index or contraction/expansion of the coating material respectively. Again the sensors have been shown to have positive qualities, such as those described previously as well as being able to provide specific measurement details for a parameter rather than returning a general measurement which does not pinpoint the causes or effects. However, they have been shown to have durability issues, especially within the highly alkaline concrete environment, leading to difficulty in performing a reliable calibration and also bringing into question their longevity. It has been commented that a service life for a sensor should be in the region of 25 years [Hannon, 2007] and to date this has not been deemed possible with such sensors. Further research must be carried out into their high pH durability and packaging issues addressed.

Electrical sensors have the advantage of years of being used in the field, having shown themselves to be of benefit through being reliable, robust and cost-effective [Bungey et al, 2006]. There are, however, limitations with their use and, as a result, FOS are gradually being accepted as a replacement for electrical sensors [KTV Grattan et al, 2007]. For example, their susceptibility to electromagnetic radiation or the fundamental issue of their corrodible metallic structure and hence potentially leading to reported values being altered. The most commonly used electrical sensor within this field is the Electrical Resistance Strain Gauge (ERSG). ERSG are a well established monitoring technique and benefit from numerous trials and research in the field having been reported [P Robins et al, 2001]. The advantages in their use are clear in that they are robust, if well protected can have a long lifetime, if their cabling is fractured they can potentially be repaired relatively easily and they exhibit a fast response to changing conditions. There are however disadvantages also, as already stated they can corrode, a high level of engineer skill and experience is required to ensure their proper fitting, a flattened region of that which is being measured is required and different techniques are required when attaching to different materials. Embedded electrode sensors (such as covercrete electrode array sensors, anode ladder system and multi-ring electrode moisture sensor) can be used for Structural Health Monitoring applications, providing vital feedback on parameters such as moisture, chlorides and carbonation within the concrete [Basheer et al, 2006a].These sensors work on the principle of measuring the resistance between a pair of electrodes at different covercrete depths and calculating their ratio relative to the initial resistance level [McCarter et al, 2001]. They benefit from the advantages of being embedded within the concrete and thereby able to give the user a direct measurement from within the region of interest, they have been extensively field tested and shown to be reliable and also providing timely data. There are however disadvantages, such as their non-specific reporting from within the concrete requiring further testing to determine the precise issue as well as their susceptibility to temperature variations [McCarter et al, 1995].

The following sections provide further specific details on both of these sensor groups, including their advantages and disadvantages to the user specifically in regard to structural monitoring and structural health monitoring.

7 Fibre Optics in Sensor Applications

7.1 Basic Principles of Fibre Optics

Fibre optic cabling has found its way into many different applications, such as telecommunication, medical devices and structural monitoring. They are of great benefit in these applications as they have extremely low propagation losses and are highly flexible [Al-Azzawi, 2007]. The cross section of a typical fibre optic cable is shown in Figure 6:

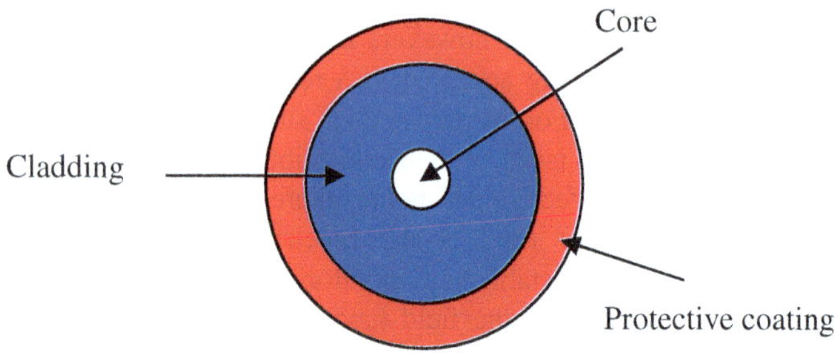

Fig. 6 Cross-section of a fibre

The central zone is called the core and the zone immediately surrounding it is the cladding. The cladding is of a slightly lower refractive index (referred to by the letter 'n' in equations) than that of the core and this difference is to ensure that the loss of light across the boundary is minimised due to the conditions of Total Internal Reflection (TIR) being satisfied. The outer zone in Figure 6 is the protective coating that is present in most traditional uses of fibre cabling. This is a coating on the fibre to provide increased protection, strength and resistance to the effects of the environment on the core and cladding. As fibre is often laid in harsh environment, e.g. underground tunnels or on sea-bed, etc, there is a need for such a level of protection to minimise the environmental damage to the fibre. When compared to more traditional 'wire' methods, such as the use of copper wire in telecommunications, this is one disadvantage of fibre optic cable. For the standard wires soldering is possible to re-attach the ends, whereas for fibre *fusion splicing* is usually required, which is not as simple or readily mobile a process to carry out [Al-Azzawi, 2007].

Optical fibres are most commonly made from fused silica glass (SiO_2) and can have a diameter similar to that of a human hair, in the order of 10s of microns. Silica fibre with an appropriate dopant, such as germanium, has the advantage of lower losses, even over very long distances, and displays higher durability than its plastic counterpart. Alternatively, plastic fibres have greater flexibility, are more resistant to inorganic chemical attack and allow greater light collection compared to silica fibre [Grahn et al, 2002].

There are different types of fibre optic cables widely available and they can generally be divided into two main categories: 1) single mode and 2) multimode. Single mode fibres confine the light to a very small diameter of fibre core (typically ~5-10μm) and only one ray of light (one electro-magnetic mode) may propagate [Muller, 2002]. In general single mode is less prone to losses than multimode as the light takes the most direct route through the length of the fibre. Multimode fibre typically has a core that is between 50 and 100μm, most commonly being one of the following three sizes; 50, 62.5 or 100μm. Multimode fibre, though typically suffering greater losses, is able to carry much higher power than the single mode. The number of modes that can propagate is dependent on the numerical aperture of the fibre, its core diameter and the transmitting wavelength. Bragg gratings, which were used in this research, tend to be written into single mode fibre as multimode leads to multiple Bragg wavelengths being returned with the potential for confusion [Zhan et al, 2006].

The principles underpinning the operation of fibre optic cable is governed by Snell's Law and is not discussed here – fuller discussion can be seen in a number of textbooks such as Grattan and Meggitt [1995], Udd et al [2007].

7.2 Writing Fibre Bragg Gratings (FBGs) in Optical Fibres

Photosensitivity is the term used to describe the reaction observed when certain materials are exposed to photons. This applies also to fibre optic cable: it means that when the fibre core is exposed to strong Ultraviolet (UV) radiation the refractive index of the core is modified [Grote and Venghaus, 2001]. This affords the possibility of creating a series of changes in refractive index along the cable, leading to a Fibre Bragg Grating (FBG), as discussed in detail by Grattan and Meggitt [2000]. The Bragg grating is so named due to the similarity in the behaviour with the interaction of x-rays and lattice planes in crystals as originally observed by Lawrence Bragg [Measures, 2001].

Since their first discovery the methods used to create FBGs has evolved in attempts to increase various positive characteristics of the grating itself (e.g. reflectivity or speed of writing). The most well known methods for FBG creation are phase-mask techniques, point-by-point writing and the free-space interferometric technique [Grattan and Meggitt 2000] – of these the phase-mask technique is most commonly used in sensor applications.

A phase mask is a series of grooves with a specifically designed spacing between them (Figure 7). It is fabricated so that the plus and minus first order diffraction obtains the majority of the energy, whilst minimising that of the zeroth order and those beyond the first. Both the FBG and the similar Long Period Gratings (LPG) work on the principle that an ultraviolet (UV) laser shining on a coating-stripped photosensitive fibre using a phase/amplitude mask can induce refractive index modulation of the fibre core [Meltz et al, 1989]. The mask used for FBG creation is called a 'Phase Mask' and that for LPG creation is called an 'Amplitude Mask'.

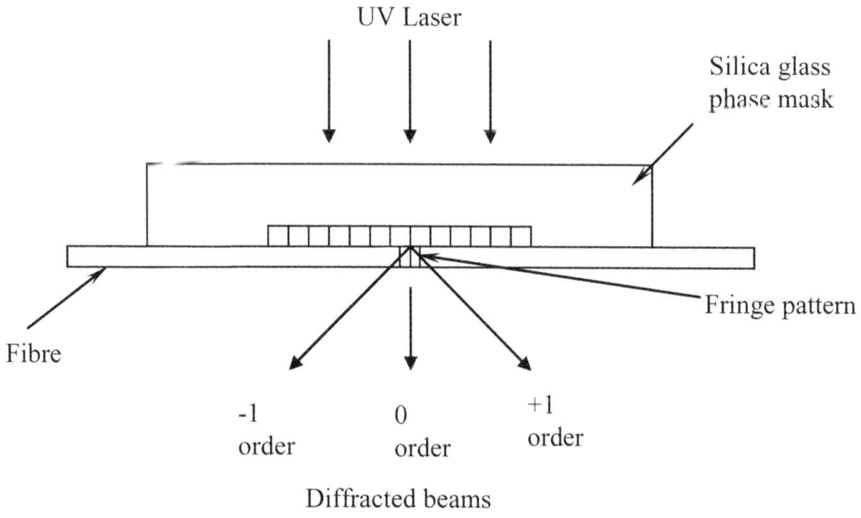

Fig. 7 Schematic of FBG writing setup [Al-Azzawi, 2007]

As shown above, the UV laser beam is diffracted after passing through the phase mask and the diffractive beams of ±1 order combine to create an interference pattern, which is then imprinted onto a photosensitive fibre placed behind the phase mask.

The way that light then behaves when it reaches this modified section of the fibre is dictated by the spacing between each refractive index interface and the effective refractive index of the fibre core as dictated by Equation 6 [Grattan & Sun, 2000]. For an FBG this modulation has a period of ~1μm whereas for an LPG this can vary from ~100μm to 1mm.

$$\lambda = 2n_{eff}\Lambda \tag{6}$$

where n_{eff} is the effective refractive index of the core and Λ is the period of the FBG.

Each individual phase mask will have a wavelength of grating that will be created relative to its spacings and so can only be used to produce this particular grating. The period of the grating can be determined by the period of the phase mask being used for the fabrication:

$$\text{Period of the imprinted grating} = \Lambda_{mask} / 2 \tag{7}$$

where Λ_{mask} is the period of the phase mask.

This allows the creation of a region of fibre with a predetermined Bragg wavelength and can lead to sensors in series all reporting from different environmental conditions and not interfering with one another due to the use of Wavelength Division Multiplexing (WDM) technique. To create a sensor with a different wavelength, a phase mask with a different Λ_{mask} would be required. The use of a phase mask does not put any increased specification requirements on the light source (laser) being used. The only requirement is good spatial coherence and an Excimer laser is normally used during the grating writing process as they offer high repetition rates and a large energy per pulse [Othonos and Kalli, 1999].

FBGs rely on the coupling of the forward propagating mode and the backward counter propagating mode from the grating, the period of which will be determined as shown above.

Changes in the environment surrounding the grating induce changes in either the effective refractive index of an FBG or the grating period, thus causing a grating wavelength shift. Due to the repeatability of these sensors, it is possible to provide calibration information for comparison of results. For a bare FBG, generally the wavelength to strain relation would be in the region of 1.2pm/$\mu\varepsilon$ and for temperature 10.8pm/^{o}C in the 1520-1570nm range [Ren et al, 2006].

For stability with temperature changes, the fibre should be annealed after the grating has been written. If a grating is written into a hydrogen-loaded fibre, thermal annealing can release trapped gas; otherwise it would increase the average refractive index of the fibre and temporarily shift the grating peaks to longer wavelengths. Annealing can also remove those sites which could be unstable over longer periods, to prevent future issues with the grating. The process of annealing can enhance the Bragg grating's ability to deal with higher levels of environmental temperatures. If annealing for this purpose, it is recommended that the temperature for annealing is 50°C higher than the operating temperature that they are subjected to. It has also been suggested by Gebremichael et al [2005] that for some specific purposes the annealing process is performed whilst in an Argon atmosphere, thereby preventing the degradation of the acrylite coating. As the temperatures approach the glass transition temperature of the fibre (for silica ~1050°C) there is a total erasure of the induced refractive index changes. It is possible, however, to create gratings using different materials as the core of fibre.

Of particular relevance for structural monitoring is that changes in the refractive index should last at least twenty five years in normal circumstances but it has recently been suggested by Brönnimann et al [2006] that the operational lifetime of a FBG could be as long as fifty years if it has been correctly installed. Pal [2004] has carried out more detailed model lifetime predictions for FOS gratings and has determined these at various temperatures. The determination is based upon the reflectivity and the shift in the Bragg wavelength. It was found that a grating with an initial reflectivity of 99% reduces to 97% in 100°C and 70% in 200°C for a period of 100 years. However, at 300°C only 8% reflectivity would remain after 100 years. The Bragg wavelength is predicted to shift by 0.22nm over 100 years at 100°C, increasing to 0.6nm for 200°C and 1.5nm for 300°C.

7.3 Use of FBGs in Sensor Applications – Strain Transfer

There are a number of factors that will affect the strain transfer in FBGs when they are used for structural strain measurements. The key factors are:

1) Length of sensor – if it is too short (<35mm) it becomes difficult to embed and the data can be affected by any inhomogeneous properties of the host material. If it is too long (>45mm) then it can be easily damaged or moved.
2) The thickness of the adhesive used to bond the measurand and FOS – if this is too thick then there may be no strain transferred, whereas if it is too thin then it can de-bond under very low strains.
3) Young's modulus of the adhesive – this parameter should be as high as possible to maximise the strain transfer.

The maximum strain transfer occurs when the interlayer thickness is minimal and the sensor length is maximised. G-D Zhou et al [2006] recommend that the length of the sensor be greater than 35mm and less than 45mm.

These sensors detect both temperature and normal strain and there is a need to distinguish the two effects. The strain variation results from an increase of the period (Λ) during the higher stress and the temperature causing thermal expansion of the fibre material, which increases the period. For both of these parameters it is not the light intensity that is the observed parameter but the shift in the wavelength. This distinction can be achieved in a number of ways and the simplest way is to have two sensors side by side, one attached to the sample to pick up strain and temperature and the other not attached to allow for only temperature variation. Majumder et al [2008] have detailed more fully the various ways in which this compensation can be achieved.

The strain values detected by a standard FBG are usually up to a maximum of 3k-5kμε, however some, such as Zhou et al [2006], have demonstrated methods to increase this. In their paper an FBG was developed that was able to measure up to 100kμε but at a cost of reduced resolution. The FBG was attached to a small spring that effectively took on a proportion of the strain and thereby reduced the value of strain being transferred to the FBG.

7.4 FBGs in Sensor Multiplexing Applications

The nature of the grating sensors means that they are suitable for multiplexing (interrogating results from more than one sensor point at a time). Multiplexing can have a number of different formats, either serial – all in the one length of fibre or parallel – in different fibres but using the same light source and interrogation system. Multiplexing is not possible with the other electrical methods of analysis available, e.g. Electrical Resistance Strain Gauges (ERSGs) [Measures, 2001].

The following are the key multiplexing techniques:

(i) Time Division Multiplexing (TDM): Short pulses of light are sent down the fibre and the different gratings, within the length being interrogated, are differentiated by the timings of the returned signals. To ensure that this is possible the detector must be time-gated and synchronised. The limited scanning frequency is an issue for this technique, reducing the ability to deal with dynamic signals.

(ii) Wavelength Division Multiplexing (WDM): Each grating within the length of fibre is written at a different wavelength and therefore the response in that wavelength region can be clearly distinguished from the others. As a result each FBG is effectively assigned a particular section of the broadband light being channelled through the fibre core. This can lead to issue of overlapping where the gratings are written too close to one another and their operating conditions cause them to alter towards one another.

(iii) Coherence Division Multiplexing (CDM): pairs of gratings are used with different spacings and the reflections are interrogated with a Michelson interferometer to separate their returns in the coherence domain.

(iv) Frequency Division Multiplexing (FDM): Each sensor operates with a signal that is modulated at a different frequency and, by using different bandpass filters, it is possible to ensure that only the specific signal for each sensor actually reaches it.

(v) Spatial Division Multiplexing (SDM): Each sensor is individually attached by means of a switching system.

FBGs have found a number of uses since their discovery including in the telecommunication industry (for dense wavelength division demultiplexing), monitoring civil structures (bridges, dams, buildings, etc), remote sensing (power cables, oil wells, pipelines etc) as well as more conventional strain, temperature and pressure sensing. In most applications they are able to benefit from their ability to provide relevant data regardless of intensity drifts or any losses associated with the fibre optic cabling in use. A market overview recently reported that the FBG market size was somewhere between 15 and 35 million US Dollars per year [Mendez, 2007]. As part of the overview a growth of 15-25% annually was predicted. It was however pointed out that there are a number of factors still to be fully resolved before the widespread acceptance of FBG technology can be expected. This includes the preconceived idea of the fragility of fibre optic cable, the associated costs of interrogating the sensors and the need for manufacturers to provide sensing solutions rather than a generic sensor.

7.5 Long Period Gratings (LPGs)

LPGs are created by similar refractive index perturbations in the fibre core as an FBG and are typically of the order of 30mm in length [James and Tatam, 2003]. For LPGs, the period is many times larger than the wavelength in the fibre and greater than that of FBGs, ranging usually between 100μm to 1mm, due to the use of an amplitude mask rather than a phase mask during writing. The LPG works on the principle of coupling the propagating core mode (the light that is travelling though the central core of the fibre) and the co-propagating cladding mode (light that has been allowed to cross into the cladding region) as opposed to relying on the backscattered signal. LPGs can also be referred to as 'Evanescent wave sensors', as a fraction of the radiation in the fibre extends a short distance from the core into the cladding. The intensity of this light will decay exponentially as the distance from the interface between the core and cladding increases [Grattan and Meggitt, 1999; James and Tatam, 2003]. These gratings have been used in a number of sensor applications but not to the extent that FBGs are used today and are not discussed further here.

7.6 Optical Absorbance Sensors

Absorbance based sensing relies on the absorption of electromagnetic radiation by the material and the resulting reduction in optical power can be related to the amount of absorbing material in the beam path. I_0 and I represent the optical intensity before and after absorption respectively. These can then be related to the absorbance of the absorber, A, by the following equation:

$$A = \log_{10} \frac{I_o}{I} = \varepsilon l C \qquad (8)$$

This is better known as the Beer-Lambert law, where l is the optical path length, C is the absorber concentration and ε is the molar absorptivity.

7.7 Fluorescence Based Sensors

Fluorescence is an optical phenomenon that occurs when light absorbed by a material creates a molecular excitation which causes the material to re-emit light as a different wavelength. For fluorescence based sensors the incident radiation will be at a shorter wavelength than that which is emitted and the gap between these two is called the *Stokes Shift*. The influence of the localised environment on the material will lead to a change in the fluorescence properties, which can be calibrated for use as a sensor.

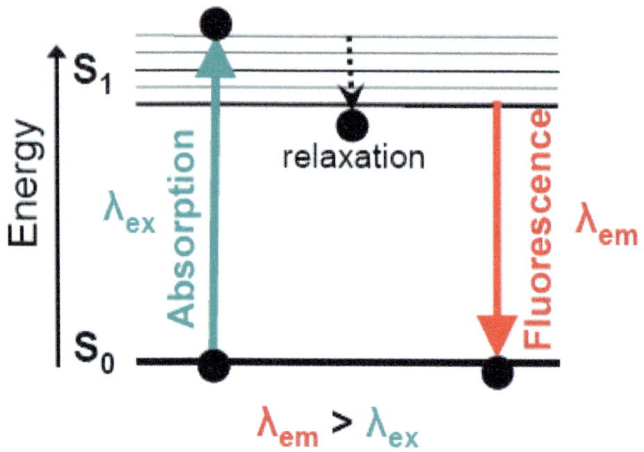

Fig. 8 Diagrammatic representation of fluorescence [Campbell, 1997]

In fluorescence based fibre optic sensing light is transmitted through the fibre in the same fashion as other techniques; however, on reaching the sensing region fluorescence occurs and this wavelength shifted light is emitted and returns to a detector via a second fibre (in many instances more than one fibre is used for collection) [Collins et al,1998]. Fluorescent sensors can be used via a number of methods, such as intensity shifts, wavelength changes or decay lifetime [Grattan and Meggitt, 1999]. The light source must be specifically chosen to ensure fluorescence occurs, due to the nature of the process the wavelength is specific to the chemical being used. The most popular light sources are LEDs due to their low power requirements, long lifetimes and low heat generation. Fluorescence sensing is then underpinned by the principle of the linear relationship between the intensity of the fluorescence and the concentration of the chemical species being investigated. In some cases the chemical species itself can be used to provide the fluorescence but in others there is a need to use an additional fluorescent dye. It is then possible to calibrate a sensor on the quenching of the fluorescence of a specific dye in the presence of the chemical species being investigated [Geddes, 2000; Huber et al, 1999; Huber et al, 2001].

A positive advantage of the use of the fluorescence technique is that of the specific wavelengths involved meaning that there is less likely to be cross interference with another chemical species and so results are regarded as reliable. It is also advisable that the Stokes Shift be as large as possible to ensure that the fluorescent response and the incident light are not allowed to overlap.

As above there is the potential to create a Fibre Optic Sensor (FOS) using one of several techniques but there are numerous different potential approaches to form and use a chemical sensor. A few of the more common examples are listed below:

(i) where the fibre actually makes contact with the analytical medium - In this case the measurement is one of the fluorescence or absorptivity of the medium, which then corresponds to the concentration. The problem here is selectivity; this becomes harder as all of the chemical species in the medium may interact with or damage the fibre.

(ii) where a transducer is used, or in other words an optically active indicator - These can be designed to be specific to the target analyte. This will usually be attached in some formation on the fibre tip.

(iii) using porous glass fibre sensing.

8 Electrical Sensors

8.1 Electrical Resistance Strain Gauge (ERSG)

These are the most commonly used electrical sensors in civil engineering applications. ERSGs work on the basis that their electrical resistance varies in proportion to the amount of strain applied to the device. As a result if the device is attached to a structure in a way that means it experiences the same deformation then the resistance measured can be related to the strain level experienced by the structure. It will normally consist of a fine wire arranged in a grid pattern (schematic shown in Figure 9 and a picture in Figure 10) in an attempt to minimise the size but yet maximise the resistance [Sabnis, 1999]. This pattern is then bonded to a backing, which then in turn is attached to the sample for testing. The backing is mainly intended as an aid to handling, gives support to the wires and ensures a more accurate alignment. Similarly for any method being employed for strain testing it is vital that the sensor or gauge is attached correctly to allow the strain to be properly transferred. The first practical application of the technique was demonstrated by Simmons and Ruge in the late 1930s [Doyle, 2004]. Due to their lightweight and relatively low cost a large number of gauges can be used to investigate the behaviour of a structure. Remote reporting of strain levels can be easily achieved as well as the recording of their output [Sabnis, 1999]. They also demonstrate a good linearity in response to the strain levels applied and sensitivity as small as 1 micro-strain.

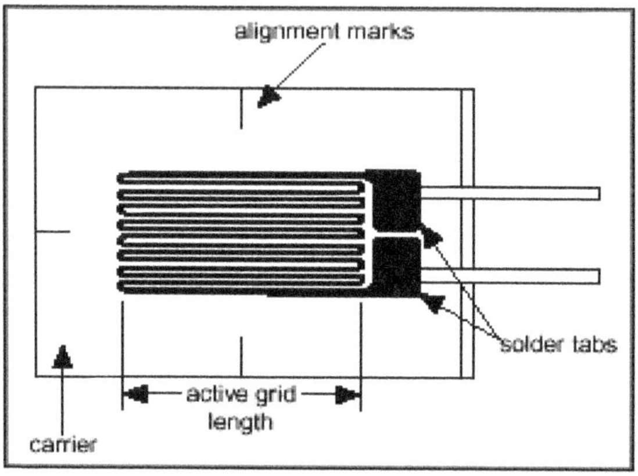

Fig. 9 Electrical Resistance Strain Gauge layout

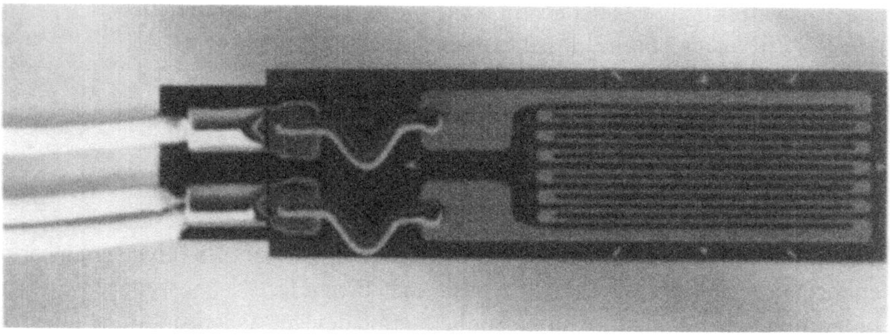

Fig. 10 Picture of ERSG [Sabnis, 1999]

ERSGs are susceptible to temperature effects and Electro Magnetic Interference (EMI), they are metallic and thereby liable to corrode, they require careful surface preparation to ensure strain transfer and hence accurate readings and therefore rely on the skill level of the engineer performing their installation [Benmokrane et al, 2006]. The main issue that is faced is that of the temperature effects. Both the gauge and that which is being measured can be affected by this. As a result self-compensated gauges have been produced, which have been shown to have little apparent alteration in changing temperature conditions. These sensors however have a very narrow range of application in terms of temperature and specimen material [Doyle, 2004]. FOS demonstrate a linearity in response over many orders of magnitude, they are flexible and have a higher temperature tolerance [Othonos and Kalli, 1999]. It has also been shown by Tennyson et al [2001] that when embedded in concrete the FOS are more durable than the ERS, which are more susceptible to chemical damages.

8.2 Covercrete Electrode Array Sensors

The Covercrete Electrode Array (CEA), which was developed by McCarter et al at Heriot-Watt University, Edinburgh [McCarter and Brousseau, 1990; McCarter et al, 1995], provides the engineer with real-time data and feedback on the condition of the covercrete and the spatial distribution of cover-zone properties. They give an insight into the water, ionic and moisture movement through the concrete. The anode-ladder-system, described in this section, can also be used for monitoring the electrical properties of the concrete at various depths from the exposed surface. The CEA however benefits from a greater degree of flexibility and can be used for multiple applications [Basheer et al, 2006a].

To create a CEA, 10 electrode pairs are mounted on a Perspex former, as shown in Figure 11, and this in turn can be attached to the reinforcement. The electrodes are positioned such that they are at different depths from the concrete surface and thereby can provide an insight into the internal behaviour by depth of the concrete. They are made of stainless steel and have a diameter of 1.2mm. All cabling coming from the CEA is channelled out and away from the exposed surface. As a result of the potential for temperature alterations causing misleading readings thermistors are also mounted on the same former so that resistances measured can be corrected for temperature variations.

The electrical resistance between pairs of electrodes is influenced by the resistance of the aggregate and the cement matrix in concrete as well as that of the pore solution within concrete [McCarter et al, 2001]. For any given concrete and degree of hydration of the cement, the pore solution resistance influences the resistance measured between the pairs of electrodes. Therefore, if there is any change in moisture content or chloride content in concrete, this can be assessed by measuring the change in electrical resistance between the pairs of electrodes. In addition, any changes in cement hydration or the structure of hydrated cement paste also will change the electrical resistance for a given concrete [Basheer et al, 2006a]. Through the use of a ratio, relative to the initial resistance value, a term

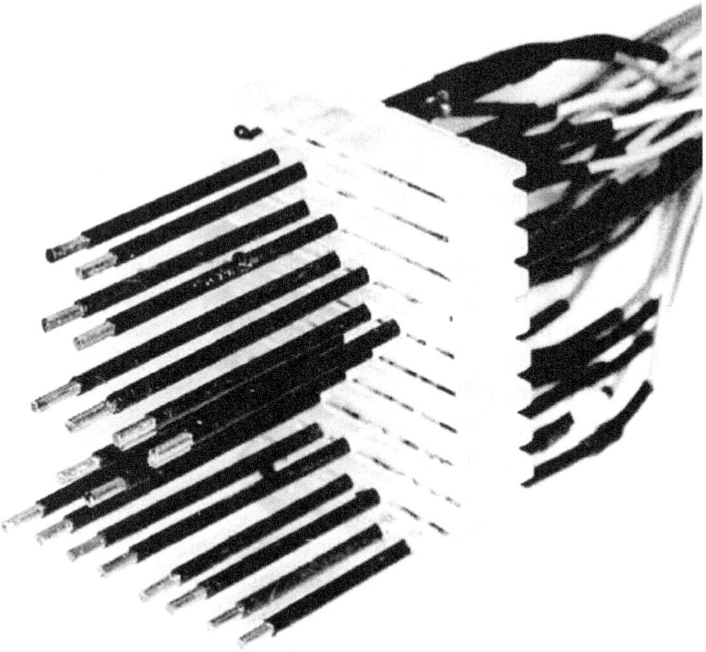

Fig. 11 The Covercrete Electrode Array (CEA) [McCarter et al, 2001]

can be derived which allows for quantification of the movement of water (or other such species). This resistance ratio will decrease as the water moves into the region of the CEA as there will be an increase in the conductance of the pore solution [McCarter et al, 1996]. This resistance should decrease up until the point where the water has passed beyond the region of the CEA at which stage a constant ratio should be reported. As would be expected the plotting of this ratio will provide an indication of the rate of water movement through the sample, where a steep gradient points to a faster movement and a more gentle gradient points to a slower movement, McCarter et al [1995]. CEAs have been extensively field tested by their developers and found to work well [McCarter et al, 1995].

In addition to the use of a CEA it is possible to embed the probes separately at the different depths and not treat them as a single sensing unit [Basheer et al, 2006a]. These electrodes will be covered with a water proof heat shrink tubing along the whole length, except for a central 10mm long region. They will also be allowed to protrude from the side of the slab with the heat shrink material removed and a connection to a conductivity meter established. This will then yield a conductance measurement between each pair of electrodes at the depths in question.

The above arrangement was used to study the ingress of chloride solution by McPolin [2005] and the advance of carbonation front by Basher et al [2006a]. The carbonation front can be identified only if the moisture content is uniformly distributed within the concrete because for a given moisture content the change in resistance is caused by the change in structure of the hydrated cement paste. However, it may be noted that any change in structure due to carbonation could result in an associated change in moisture content and, hence, monitoring carbonation using electrical resistance is not straightforward.

(i) Anode-Ladder system

The anode-ladder system (Figure 12) has been in worldwide use since the early 1990s providing data on the corrosion risk to new concrete structures [Raupach and Schießl, 2001; Schießl and Raupach, 1992; McCarter et al, 2005]. It gives an indication of the depth of the critical chloride content required to initiate reinforcement corrosion. The user is then in possession of an estimated timeframe

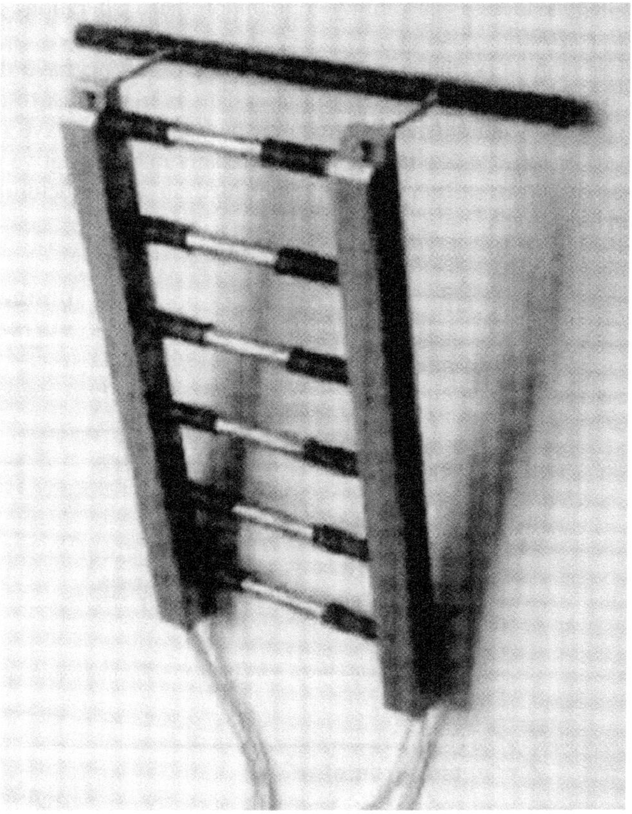

Fig. 12 The anode-ladder system installed to monitor the corrosion risk of the reinforcement [Raupach and Schießl, 2001]

for the start of corrosion in their structure and so can plan to take preventative action and avoid the corrosion initiating in the structure. Such preventative measures are usually significantly lower than the costs of repairs after corrosion has occurred [Raupach and Schießl, 1997]. The sensor measures the potential and electrical resistance in its localised environment and can thereby point to parameters influencing corrosion, such as humidity, oxygen availability and even corrosion behaviour after depassivation.

The electrodes that are embedded are a piece of black steel (anode) and a noble metal (cathode), as shown in Figure 13. As stated previously, the highly alkaline environment within concrete ensures that both the electrodes which are embedded will not corrode initially and the electrical current that is able to pass between them will be negligibly low. If one of the causes of depassivation should occur, such as an increase in the chloride levels or carbonation, then there will be no such protection for the anode and this will lead to an electron flow between the black steel and the noble metal, which can then be measured. Critically it has been established that the metal chosen for the anode shows no significant difference in corrosion behaviour to reinforcing steel. As a result if these electrodes are placed at varying depths there is an ability to monitor these alterations through the concrete [Naus, 2000].

The key advantage of this sensor system is the ability to have data to hand before any corrosion has actually taken place. This is in contrast to a number of the other available technologies that require the corrosion to have initiated and may therefore be too late for any meaningful repairs or preventative action to be taken. They do however need to be embedded in the structure during the construction phase and cannot be retro-fitted.

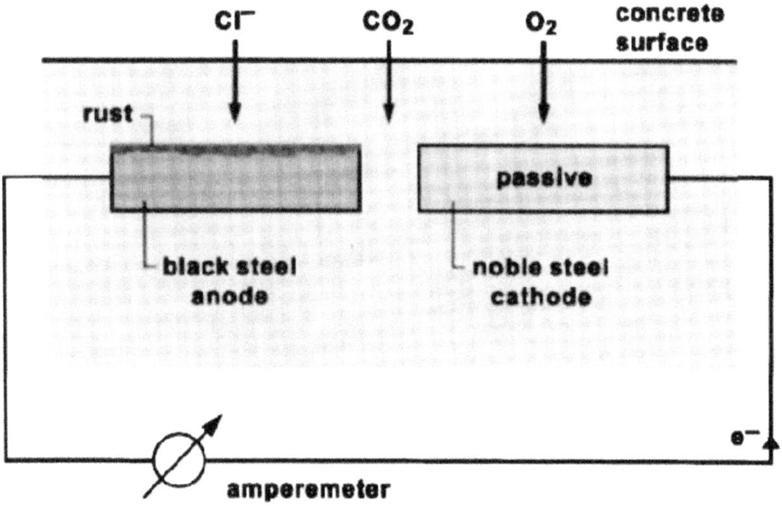

Fig. 13 Macrocell consisting of a black steel anode and noble metal cathode [Raupach and Schießl, 2001]

(ii) Multi-ring electrode moisture sensor

After depassivation of the steel reinforcement has commenced the major factor influencing the corrosion rate is the availability of moisture. If the concrete is very dry then it will exhibit a high level of electrolytic resistance and as a result low rates of corrosion. In an attempt to measure this electrolytic resistance multi-ring electrodes can be embedded [Dhir and Jones, 1996]. Alternating noble metal and insulating rings are vertically sleeved onto a PVC rod, so that readings are taken perpendicular to the concrete surface [Sakai et al, 1995]. The multi-ring electrode is embedded such that the upper ring is 2.5mm from the concrete surface, the thickness of the layer of non-conducting material, and the resistance between consecutive rings are measured using an AC Ohmmeter. The data produced allows for the derivation of a profile (see Figure 14). They have the advantage of being able to be embedded during either the construction phase or else after construction during repairs, for example [Dhir and Jones, 1996]. Data can also be of benefit in the assessment of the success or failure of a coating or surface treatment that may have been applied. They are however susceptible to cracks developing in between

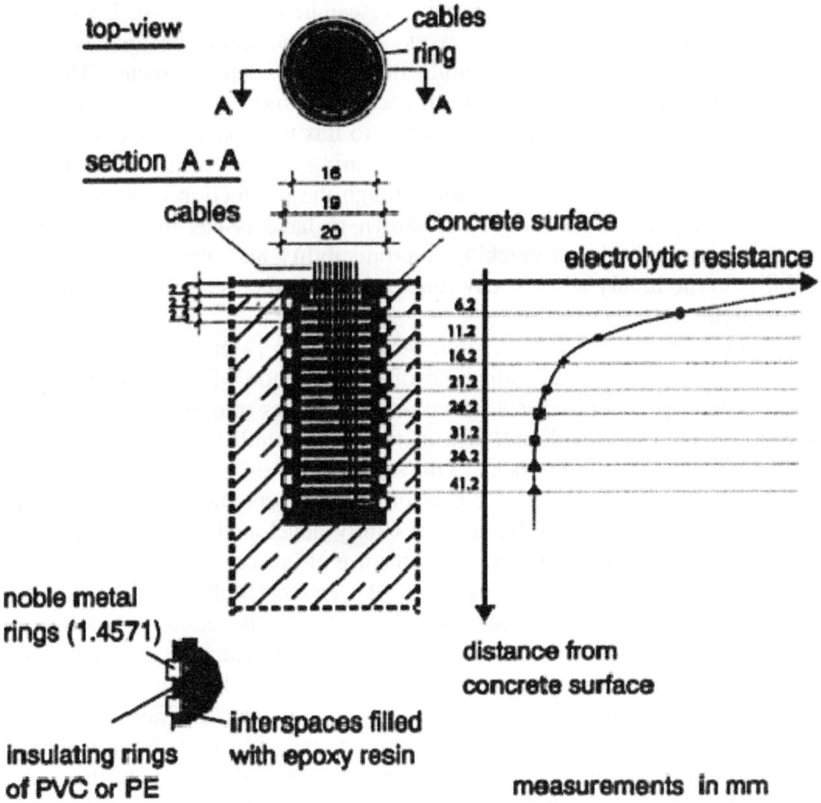

Fig. 14 Schematic representation of the multi-ring electrode and a qualitative diagram of measured values [Sakai et al, 1995]

the PVC and concrete leading to a preferential channel for water to ingress, negating the readings and actually being harmful to the structure being monitored [McCarter et al, 2001].

9 Meeting Today's Needs for Better Monitoring of Structures

The ideal solution for monitoring both durability and structural properties of concrete is the installation of the sensors at the time of construction and therefore providing an insight into the parameters of interest from the outset. Through routinely monitoring such a structure, data can begin to be collated and stored for future reference and provide invaluable information to those who would seek to predict the longer term performance of the structure. Both the electrical and fibre optic sensors described in this chapter can be seen to be developed with this goal in mind, seeking to provide such vital and timely reporting. The challenge has been, and continues to be, the step of moving a sensor system from the laboratory and into the field.

To more fully equip structural engineers new, more innovative and industrially acceptable, approaches are always being researched and developed, such as the optical fibre approach taken in this work. Fibre optic strain sensors have already shown their ability to work within the concrete environment. This work concentrates on developing their use to encompass more than the return of strain levels applied to the reinforcement. Tied in to this they have been developed and refined to add to the structural health monitoring aspects of a sensor system by determining the initiation of corrosion through the production of waste products. Sol-gel based pH sensors have been shown to have issues in their fabrication through shrinkage induced cracking, reproducibility and also through a lack of durability in the highly alkaline environment. Both aspects are investigated within this research.

The development of the fibre optic strain sensors [Merzbacher et al 1998] is needed to provide a clearer indication of the initiation of the corrosive process within concrete. Electrical resistance strain gauges require a high level of protection to be embedded and, also as they are metallic, are not thought to be appropriate for such measurements. This sensor can then provide an early warning mechanism for the creation of corrosion by-products through the increase in localised volume. Added to this a successfully developed fibre system could be used to cover a large structural area with the use of just one single fibre.

Previous work into the development of pH sensors [Badini et al 1989, Basheer et al 2005] has raised limitations which must first be addressed before their potential for use within the concrete environment can be explored further. Electrode based systems will provide feedback on the chloride and carbonation processes that lead to reinforcement corrosion but they are non-specific, may require the corrosion to have already started and therefore require additional testing to be carried out to provide the user with timely data. This further stage of testing will not only take up further time and cost, they can also in some instances be harmful to the structure and may even leave the region more susceptible to the initial issue.

An effective optical fibre sensor network based structural health monitoring system, combined with those researched here, could provide an effective solution to the prevention of structural decay utilising the particular advantages of fibre optic techniques to create a sensor system network well suited to large structures and multiple (non-identical) sensor devices. FOS produce wavelength-encoded signals which are not susceptible to instrumental drift and allow multiplexing of multiple sensors on a single fibre, in addition to possessing the many advantages demonstrated by the use of optical fibres as the basis of measurement systems. Given the issues discussed and weaknesses highlighted above of conventional technologies, optical fibre sensors have shown real promise for on-line monitoring, potentially to offer superior performance over or to complement their currently employed counterparts due to their effectively unlimited sensing length and the ability to withstand harsh environments over a wide temperature range, without electromagnetic interference or damage from corrosion.

The essential issues identified to be researched, given the above information and the need for effective multipurpose sensor systems, are the development and evaluation of an effective optical fibre based strain sensor system for determining the impact of corrosion and acting as a forewarning of the corrosive process having commenced and the development of a pH sensor capable of enduring the high alkalinity found within concrete, whilst being able to report accurate and repeatable pH data to the engineer.

9.1 Carbonation in Concrete and pH Changes

Carbonation is a critical problem of environmental degradation, arising from the absorption of atmospheric carbon dioxide and leading to the reduction of the pH level in concrete. This in turn leads to a loss of passivity of the steel reinforcement and structural cracking due to the formation and expansion of the waste products arising from the rusting of the reinforcement. All this arises from a reaction between the carbon dioxide and alkalis in the pore solution of the cement paste. Thus while carbonation does not itself cause deterioration, it is important to monitor it as a precursor to an environment which allows deterioration to take place [McPolin et al, 2005]. Although there are other corrosion mechanisms e.g. due to the ingress of chlorides, carbonation is the main mechanism seen in urban areas which are often rich in CO_2.

10 Fiber Optic pH Sensing for Concrete Structures

10.1 Prior Research on Fiber Optic pH Sensors

As has been discussed, both conventional electrical techniques and fiber optic sensors (the focus of this work) are widely available for a range of sensor applications. It is valuable to reiterate that fiber optic sensors have enormous potential for structural monitoring: they offer advantages over electrical systems in a number of ways, namely that they are small and lightweight, non-electrical in operation and are immune to electromagnetic interference: the fibers are inert to degradation and there is considerable potential for multiplexing of a number of sensors on a single network, thereby reducing system complexity. Progress on the development of fiber optic sensors, particularly for structural monitoring and emphasizing success in physical sensor development (particularly both strain and temperature monitoring), has been reported by some of the authors and others [McPolin et al, 2005, KTV Grattan et al 2005, KTV Grattan et al 2006a, SKT Grattan et al 2007]. That work has reviewed the background to such sensors in some detail (and thus it is not reproduced here) but the designs of the chemical sensors developed thus far had not proved to be adequately reproducible for long term use in this type of demanding application – thus this fuller study and the development of a better design and sensor fabrication strategy was required. This was envisaged to ensure that durable and sufficiently accurate sensors for monitoring concrete could be manufactured, reproducibly and reliably. Sol-gel based sensors, one of the approaches in this work, were considered in some detail in that prior research [McPolin et al, 2005] but a major issue not adequately addressed in much of the previous work was overcoming the cracking of the sol gel during the fabrication stages and obtaining a better solution to this problem has been a focus of this work to create a hard-wearing, yet operational sensor. Further, achieving adequate durability of a probe specifically designed for applications to longer term monitoring in structural concrete and also able to sustain the very high pH were other key issues: the probe would be required to tolerate the harsh conditions of the concrete environment but yet be sufficiently absorbent to chemicals from the localized environment to indicate the pH change through an indicator color change.

10.2 Aims and Objectives of the FOS Systems Reported

In order to deal with the above requirements, a suitable pH monitoring method that is both non-destructive and provides timely information to the user to give information on the condition of the concrete is needed. In this work, these issues are addressed through a series of experiments which have the aim of demonstrating and thus evaluating the performance of operational pH sensor devices and obtaining working data on their operation with actual concrete samples under known conditions. The approach taken has been to evaluate the design and comparable performance characteristics of a number of different pH sensor systems, outlined in detail below, that have been determined from experimental and laboratory-based testing on concrete samples, following from an initial evaluation of and comparison of their performance with standard laboratory-based pH measuring methods.

Thus in summary the series of tests carried out was designed

- to achieve the carbonation of cement mortar samples in an accelerated fashion and in a known and reproducible way
- thus to use these samples to test the sensors developed to monitor the effect of changes in the high pH range
- to do so through the determination of the pH level of the near surface mortar extracted from the samples subjected to accelerated carbonation.

In order to evaluate and contrast the performance of the different pH sensor systems considered, a series of cross-comparison tests was carried out.

10.3 Four Different FOS-Based Approaches to pH Sensing

This was carried out on the samples prepared under controlled conditions (as discussed in detail below) were evaluated:

- Sensor A: a sol-gel based sensor containing an appropriate colorimetric indicator for the pH region under study,
- Sensor B: a commercially available fiber optic pH sensing disc – a disc with an entrapped indicator dye relying on the absorption of light for its measurements (but not specified for use in these hazardous conditions) and using thymol blue as the indicator material
- Sensor C: the fluorescence-based sensor using a proprietary indicator
- Sensor D: alongside this, the 'standard' laboratory pH test unit based on a glass electrode was used for cross-calibration.

To do so, representative samples of cement mortar were prepared and subjected to a known accelerated carbonation process (to alter the pH and thus to provide a basis for measurement) and it is these samples which were used for the subsequent monitoring tests.

(i) Sample preparation

The testing of the pH probes was using samples of cement mortar: creating cubes of 100mm side. The mix proportions used for these cubes were selected to be a cement-to-sand ratio of 0.25 and a water to cement ratio of 0.5.

A total of 6 cubes was created for the testing regime where 3 cubes were to be crushed to provide the 28 day strength measurement (using conventional laboratory based techniques) to ensure the quality and representative nature of the samples and 3 additional cubes were set aside for the dust drilling process which would provide the material from which the pH solutions for testing were created. All samples were de-moulded the day after casting and placed in water at 20°C for a further 3 days to ensure that there is sufficient time to allow hydration. Once removed from the water the samples were wrapped in polythene sheeting and placed in a controlled environment of 20°C and 55% relative humidity for a period of 14 days. After this the sides of the cubes were painted with an epoxy paint with one side left unpainted to allow for the ingress of carbon dioxide later in the testing regime. For a further 14 days the cubes were heated at 50°C to remove the moisture, as it is known that carbonation is critically affected by moisture levels, being optimised between 55 and 65% relative humidity.

(ii) Sample treatment

After being heated, the samples were drilled and the dust sample created was carefully collected, with drilling being carried out at two different depths, 5mm and 10mm, on the unpainted cube surface using a 20mm diameter drill bit. The dust created was immediately stored in an air-tight, clean container to prevent sample loss or any potential contamination. Further, for reference, a relative humidity measurement was taken using standard instrumentation at both depths and data were recorded.

Each hole that had been drilled was then filled again with cement mortar of the same mix proportions as originally used to create the samples. Once this had been allowed to harden the samples were placed in a carbonation chamber where the environment settings were 20°C, 65% humidity and 5% carbon dioxide (to create known and standard test conditions). The dust that had been collected from the drilling process was then split with a proportion being used for thermal analysis measurements with the remainder being used for water digestion testing, following the recommendations of Rasanen and Penttala [2004]. The details of those tests are beyond the scope of this investigation but they confirmed the representative nature of the samples used.

10.4 Sensor Design and Use Issues

A number of different sensor designs was created (Sensors A – C discussed above) with the broad details of these designs discussed below. The generic design of the sensors used is shown in Figure 15 where the active element at the sensor 'head' is addressed by light from a suitable broadband light source through a fibre bundle and (in the case of Sensors A and B) a change in the absorption spectrum is recorded. For Sensor C the fluorescence spectrum (seen against a 'zero light' background) through the use of excitation from a carefully chosen LED emitting at a wavelength overlapping with a major absorption feature is recorded – in each case sampling the intensity at known, key wavelengths in the spectrum and using the intensity change as discussed as being representative of the pH. In all cases this change was calibrated against the pH of a known set of buffer solutions in the range pH 9 to 13. In all cases the silica fiber bundle (Ocean Optics RF200) was used and (except for Sensor C) a commercial light source (Ocean Optics LS-1) was employed in conjunction with the spectrometer (Ocean Optics USB2000).

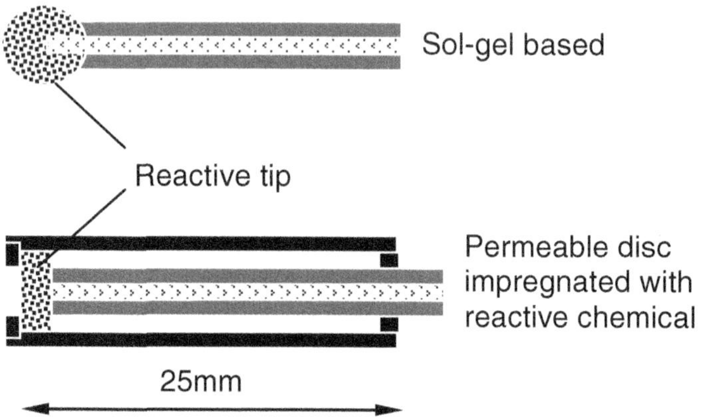

Fig. 15 Generic design of fiber based pH sensors

(i) Sensor A – sol-gel sensor developed for this application

Building on prior work on sol-gel based sensor design [McPolin, 2005] the key requirement was that a durable and sufficiently accurate sensor for monitoring concrete could be fabricated, reproducibly and reliably. The essential theoretical background to the absorption determination that correlates with the pH monitoring is discussed in some detail in that paper and not reproduced here. Overcoming the problem of cracking of the sol gel during the fabrication and achieving the resulting durability of the probe were critical issues to create a sensor to tolerate the harsh conditions of the concrete environment. For the very high pH environment in which it was to work, the approach taken in this work was to focus first on the sol-gel manufacturing process and to conduct a series of experiments that would enable a satisfactory sol-gel with an encapsulated indicator dye to be produced. This then could be incorporated into the distal end of a fibre optic probe (Figure 15), to make measurements in concrete samples.

(a) Sol-gel fabrication

Thus a critical aspect of the research was the 'recipe' for a suitable durable, non-cracking sol-gel and to achieve an optimization of the key parameters in the fabrication process was required. To do so a number of tests and evaluations were carried out over a period of several months and only key details are reproduced below. Arising from that, the following were identified as the specific details of the optimum features of the fabrication process, determined from the results of the sol-gel manufacturing process:

- The heating time required for the sol-gel solution with 2ml of GPTMS (Glycidoxypropyltrimethoxysilan) to allow the creation of the sol-gel was determined as 30minutes at 80°C.
- Coverings were required for the drying and heating stages of the process to control the evaporation process which formed the gel (for the smaller samples no covering was found to be required).
- The sample size for use with the probe tip was created from 250μl solutions dispensed to be heated and dried.
- An optimised mixing technique based on all of the investigated factors was then derived and used.

(b) Indicator Dye

A critical aspect of the fiber optic probe design is the selection of a suitable indicator to measure the very high pH present in concrete samples. A limited number of indicators is available for this region and for the indicators selected, it was important first to confirm the chemical stability of the indicator in the sol-gel formation process. Cresol red and thymol blue (which were able to cover the pH range in question) were selected and their stability to the environment was established through a series of tests, not reported in detail here. Confident of their stability, the sol-gels into which the indicator was incorporated were moulded into millimetre-sized samples to fit the distal end of the sensor in the base of a small test tube, yielding a specimen as shown in Figure 16.

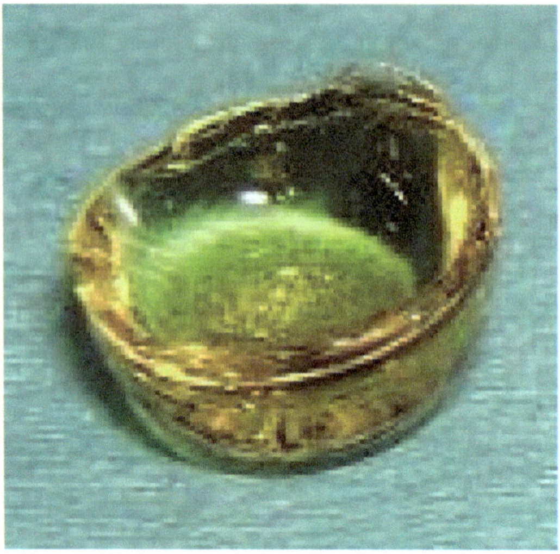

Fig. 16 Photograph showing the sol-gel specimen after hardening, approximately 2.5mm in diameter

(c) Evaluation of the performance of the sol-gel sensor: calibration against buffer solutions

The samples created were calibrated using a series of buffer solutions of high pH – ranging from pH 9 to a maximum value of pH13. The response of the sensor to these different levels of pH was investigated and the results are as reported below. It was found that the samples did survive well the high pH solutions with no indication of any deleterious effects even after prolonged exposure – this had extended to 24 months at the time of writing. To create a visual check, sol-gels containing the same indicator (cresol red) from the same batch had been placed separately in a pH12 and in a pH13 solution. A colour difference between the two samples that was visible to the naked eye was seen. The sol-gels were used attached to a fibre optic bundle allowing light to be transmitted to a spectrometer to examine the spectral detail of the optical spectrum produced, using the set up shown in Figure 15. The samples had been prepared with a view to durability – thus a long response time (well suited to the evaluation of very slowly changing civil structures) was tolerable to achieve the durability required that allowed a lifetime (from above) extending to many years. Samples were left for at least 12 hours to allow for stabilization of the colour change to occur and spectra were recorded and examined to note the spectral differences between them, as shown in Figure 16. Of the two candidate indicator materials, the thymol blue sol-gel sample showed a single peak and there was an overlap in the spectra for pH 10 and pH12, meaning that potential use of this sensor for pH measurement in this region was more limited due to the more limited spectral differences being generated.

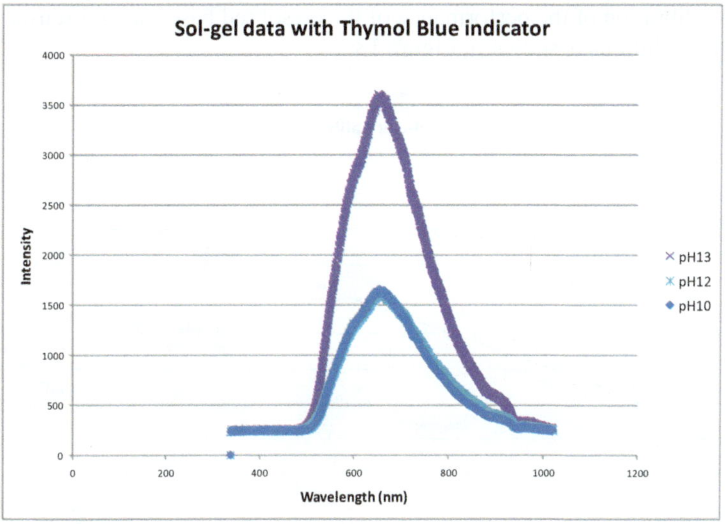

Fig. 16 Sol-gel spectrum after being in the three different pH levels with thymol blue indicator

In light of this, an alternative indicator was sought and incorporated and as can be seen from Figure 17, the spectrum of cresol red showed two peaks allowing for a pH measurement to be obtained through a ratio-based approach (of the ratios of the intensities of the two major peaks shown). This is particularly valuable as it allows for compensation for any other optical losses within the system e.g. fibre bending and when examined in detail, this was found to be a repeatable and thus appropriate approach to the measurement. Thus in subsequent work, cresol red was taken as the indicator of choice for the testing procedures described further.

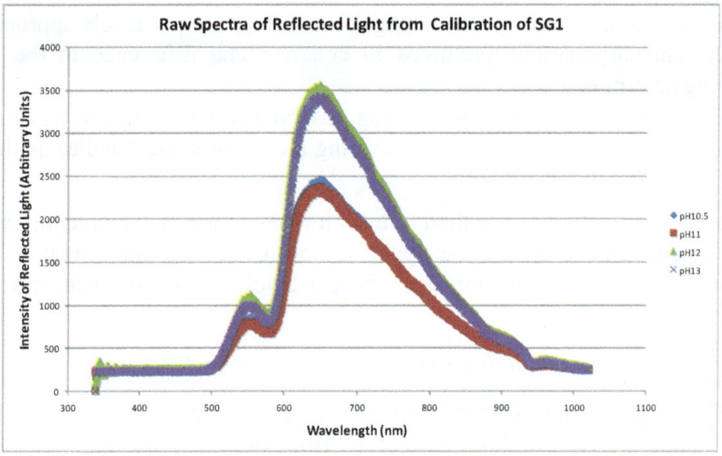

Fig. 17 Sol-gel spectrum after being in the three different pH levels with cresol red indicator

The calibration of the performance of the cresol red based sol gel sensor against the buffer solutions is shown in Figure 18.

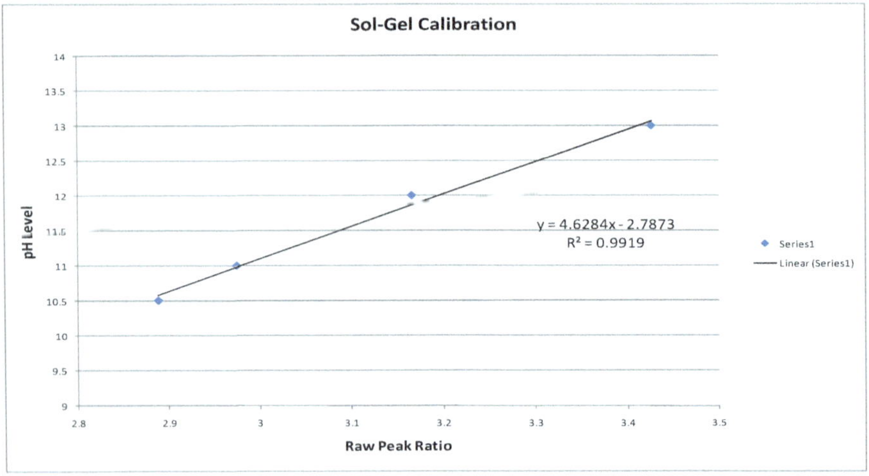

Fig. 18 Calibration plot of cresol red sol-gel using buffer solutions

The research carried out has shown that the key design issues to create an effective sol-gel for use as the basis of a sensor probe are as follows:

- the optimization of the sol-gel fabrication conditions (arising from the optimization and thus the most appropriate choice of chemical mix conditions) – this has been shown to be effective in producing sol-gels that are robust enough to withstand the high pH levels required to be used within a concrete environment.
- measurable indicator spectra being recorded – from pH levels appropriate to different carbonation conditions in concrete and difference in the spectra being determined
- this spectrum being capable of being observed using a commercial fiber optic bundle (for convenience over producing a custom made bundle) as the basis of the probe

The success of these tests has therefore been to demonstrate the potential with the sol-gel approach to create the type of sensor needed and opened up the opportunity to measure at more specific pH levels arising from the carbonated concrete.

(ii) Sensor B – commercial disc sensor

Commercial pH sensing systems using fiber optic technology are available from several manufacturers: in this case a probe from Ocean Optics [RFP200-UV/VIS] was chosen. However a critical factor is that these sensors have not been designed for use in the highly alkaline environment of concrete samples: concern about the durability of this commercial senor thus providing the initial drive of the work to create sol-gels which were potentially more durable during this research, to allow for measurements over a longer time scale.

The core component of the commercial sensor is a nylon disc that has a thymol blue indicator entrapped. However, it is not specified to operate beyond pH12 and as a result of this, the commercial software which comes with the sensor probes is designed to erase all data obtained should the level go beyond pH12. The aim in this work is, however, to measure pH values higher than this in concrete: thus it was important to evaluate the potential for use of this disc in these higher pH conditions and thus to extend its operation to try to make measurements into the higher pH region, should that be possible. This required the use of customized data processing and analysis techniques using spectral data captured, as the associated commercial software that was provided with the sensor could not be used. Thus the raw absorption spectrum obtained from the spectrometer was instead analyzed (in a similar way to which data were obtained from Sensor A) and the results reported were based on this approach. Each spectrum obtained (at a particular pH value) was normalized, with the resulting spectrum at a known pH value subtracted from the normalized spectrum produced when the disc was placed in deionized water and the change in the absorption spectrum recorded. This spectrum shows two peaks, both of which were examined to confirm the most repeatable data for a calibration. The result of subtracting the spectra at various pH levels from that for deionized water is as shown in Figure 19. The smaller peak at around 500 nm was selected for calibration purposes and the resulting calibration plot for Sensor B was created showing the pH value (from the buffer solutions selected) versus normalized peak intensity and shown in Figure 20.

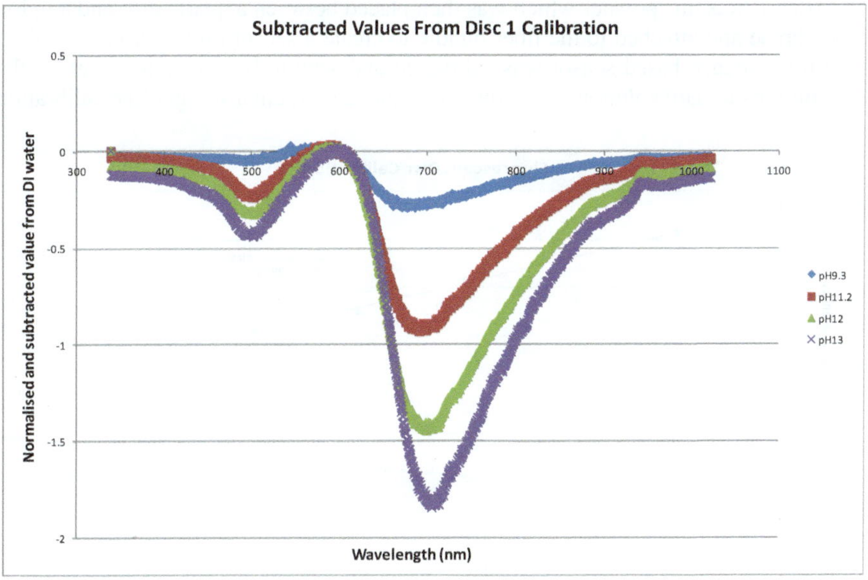

Fig. 19 Subtracted data used for calibration of commercial pH sensing disc

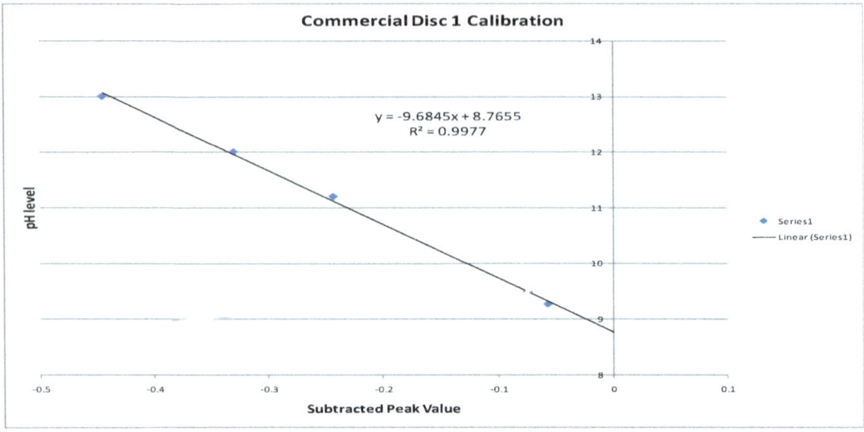

Fig. 20 Calibration plot for commercial pH sensing disc using buffer solutions

(iii) Sensor C – fluorescence-based sensor

Alongside the development of the sol-gel technique using absorption techniques, a fluorescence based sensor was developed. The sensor also works on the principle of the immobilization of an indicator dye: in this case to a solid substrate via covalent binding. This was chosen as it is a reliable way to immobilize the indicator as it is less likely to leach; however the chemistry involved is somewhat complicated and the approach was time consuming to develop. The detailed chemistry used to create the indicator is beyond the scope of this paper but in summary, the process begins with the hard bulk polymer containing the indicator which is ground up into a powder. It was this powder which was then placed between a quartz disc and a nylon membrane and attached to the fiber bundle to create a sensor probe. Prior to testing, the fluorescence based sensor was calibrated and seen to be responding well to the pH buffer standard solutions, as shown in Figure 21. Again a straight line calibration

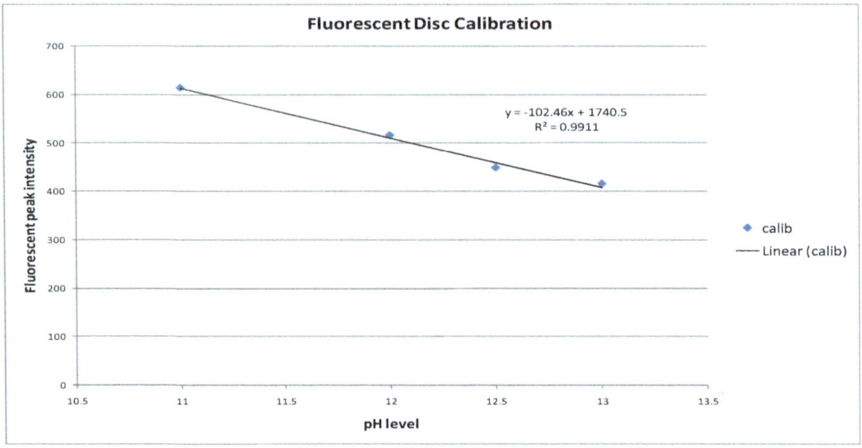

Fig. 21 Calibration plot for fluorescence disc using buffer solutions

was obtained and it was then used to investigate its response to the carbonated concrete in a similar way to Sensors A and B.

(iv) Sensor D – glass electrode pH meter

A commercial glass electrode pH sensor was used as supplied by Orion Instruments to provide a reference measurement where unknown values of pH were being measured.

ph monitoring from concrete samples. In order to investigate the performance of the sensors under conditions which represent structural monitoring situations, a series of samples arising from the carbonation of the cement mortar cubes was prepared and the response of each sensor, individually, was tested with reference to measurements made on the same samples using Sensor D, the standard glass electrode approach.

(a) Standardized tests on concrete samples

Prior to conducting the tests, three cubes were removed after 28 days and crushed as would be standard practice when evaluating the properties of a concrete mix. The results of this process were as detailed in Table 1 showing all samples had a similar and typical compressive strength. Given those results, the samples were shown to be representative and the pH tests described below were then conducted.

Table 1 28 day compressive strength test results

1	37.93 MPa
2	37.15 MPa
3	36.44 MPa
average:	37.17 MPa

(b) Response of pH sensors to carbonated cement mortar samples

Representative samples produced were subjected to measurement using each of the sensor systems and the results obtained are as detailed below. To achieve a good cross-calibration, for each of the sensors described data are taken under similar conditions. Measurements were taken regularly over a period of 6 weeks using samples from two different depths: 5 and 10 mm from samples which had been subjected to accelerated carbonation, as described above and thus for which the pH would be expected to change over the period of testing.

Then the time response of the sensors was investigated and to ensure that stable conditions were achieved, prior work enabled the following conditions to be set. For Sensor A, due to the long response time the active element was left overnight in the sample and a reading taken the next day. The standard laboratory system (Sensor D) and the commercial disc sensor (Sensor B) were found to require around 15-20 minutes to stabilize and so data could be obtained relatively quickly. The fluorescence sensor (Sensor C) required approximately 4 hours to stabilize, allowing typically 2 readings to be taken per working day at different pH values.

10.5 Cross Comparisons and Calibrations

(i) Sensor A: Sol-Gel based sensor developed in this work

A sol-gel sample from the test batch prepared which had successfully been calibrated using buffer solutions was incorporated in the probe arrangement and used to evaluate the performance of the concrete samples. The data obtained are shown in Figure 22 showing the response of Sensor A (compared to that using the same samples with Sensor D – the standard pH meter) after the different periods of carbonation of the samples over several weeks.

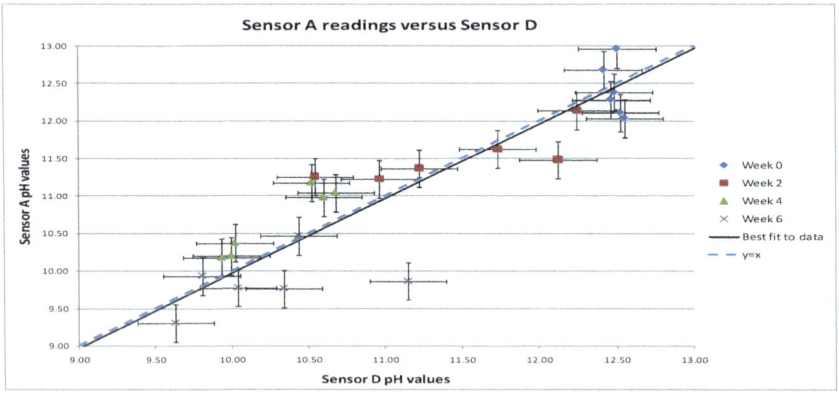

Fig. 22 pH readings obtained from Sensor A plotted against readings from Sensor D, best fit has been plotted alongside the ideal condition of Sensor A = Sensor D (y=x) for comparison

(ii) Sensor B: Commercial disc type sensor

A similar test was carried out using Sensor B and the measurement data from that series of tests on the concrete samples is shown in Figure 23.

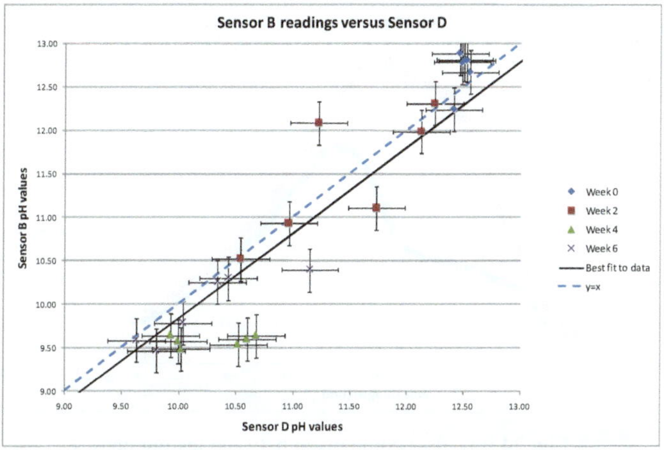

Fig. 23 pH readings obtained from Sensor B plotted against readings from Sensor D, best fit has been plotted alongside the ideal condition of Sensor B = Sensor D (y=x) for comparison

The data show a good level of agreement between the results of Sensor B and Sensor A (with respect to the response of Sensor D) prior to carbonation of the samples and also after 2 weeks of carbonation. In the third section of the testing phase (after 4 weeks) the fundamental shape of the spectrum being returned from the disc was found to be altered and Figure 24 shows an example of a spectrum returned during the first testing phase (week 0) compared to a spectrum taken from the third phase (week 4). These spectra were then normalised and referenced to a de-ionised water reading, which yielded data shown in Figure 25. This clearly is consistent with the drift in the calibration of Sensor B and may not have been evident from observation of the calibration data alone (such as would have been obtained from software set simply to measure the calibration peak intensity value alone). An attempt was made to recalibrate Sensor B by movement of the probe between the different pH solutions: this was seen not to be having any actual impact on the spectrum recorded and so it was decided to carry out a full recalibration before Sensor B was used in the fourth and final phase of the testing (at week 6 of the carbonation). This however yielded the same (imperfect) result and so it was decided to replace the disc. This new disc was calibrated (using known buffer solutions) in the intervening period (between weeks 4 and 6) and it was checked before its use that it was performing reliably. Hence there are two calibration curves designated for the commercial disc: the former is for the disc that failed by the end of week 4 of the tests and the latter is for the new disc used for the tests at week 6. As a consequence of using the new disc at week 6, the results from phase 4 of the testing saw a return of the close agreement of the readings from Sensor B with those from Sensor D (the standard laboratory pH meter), suggesting the limited lifetime of the disc sensor in this highly alkaline environment.

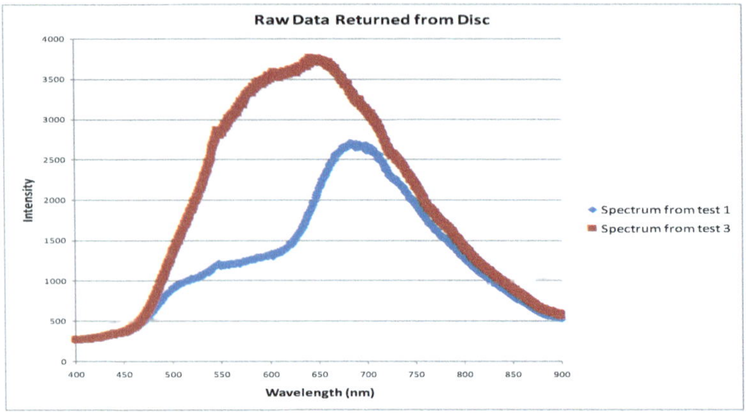

Fig. 24 Raw data comparison between testing phases

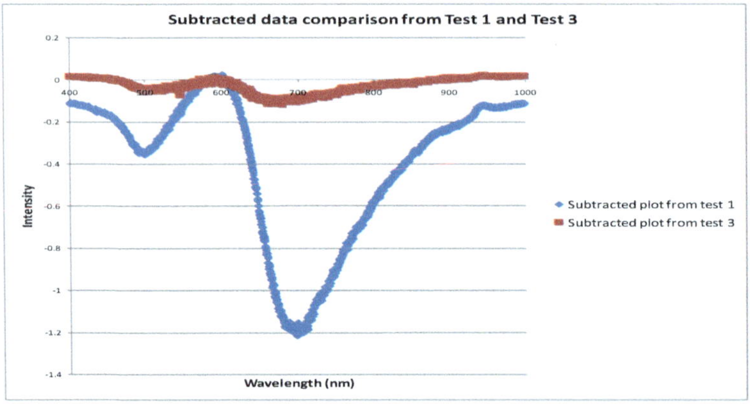

Fig. 25 Comparison of subtracted data plots for different testing phases

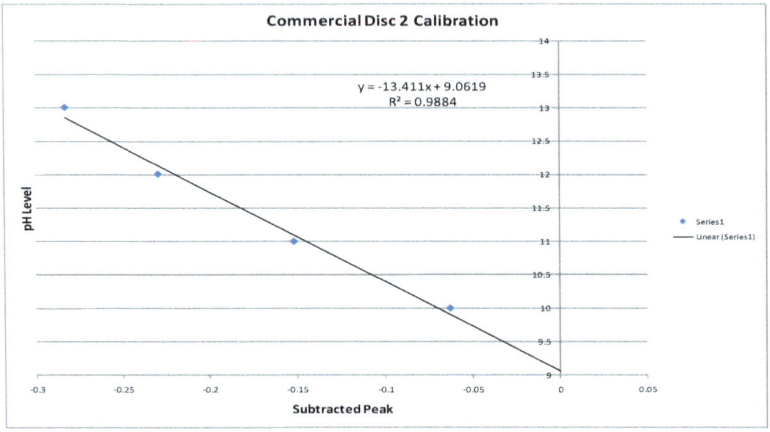

Fig. 26 Calibration plot for commercial pH sensing disc

(iii) Measurement using Probe C - Fluorescence based technique

As discussed earlier, prior to testing, the fluorescence based sensor was calibrated and seen to be responding well to the pH buffer standard solutions. This response was not repeated however once it was used with the sample solutions from the cubes. A further, successful calibration was undertaken (as shown in Figure 26) before use on the liquid samples but this again was not followed when using actual samples from the concrete. The shape and size of the fluorescence peak had altered (as is evident from the figure) and no further actions were able to bring this peak back to what was seen originally. Figure 27 shows a graph demonstrating the difference between the original fluorescence peak and a typical representation of the peaks being produced with the samples. As a result the data obtained which show the response of Sensor C against that of Sensor D can be seen to drift with time, as shown in Figure 28 and the expected calibration where y=x (as seen for Sensors A and B) was not obtained.

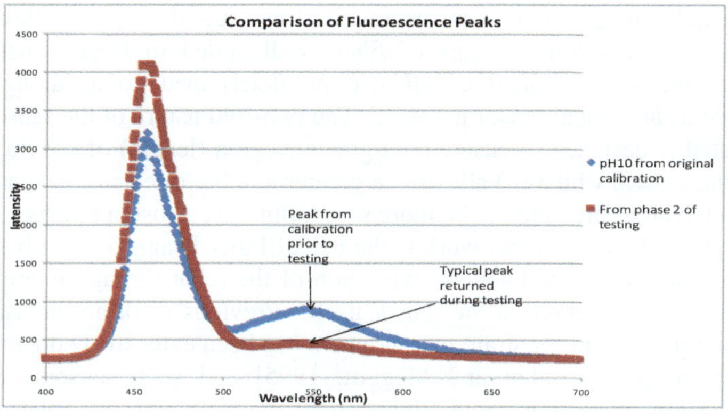

Fig. 27 Comparison of fluorescence peak during calibration and in testing

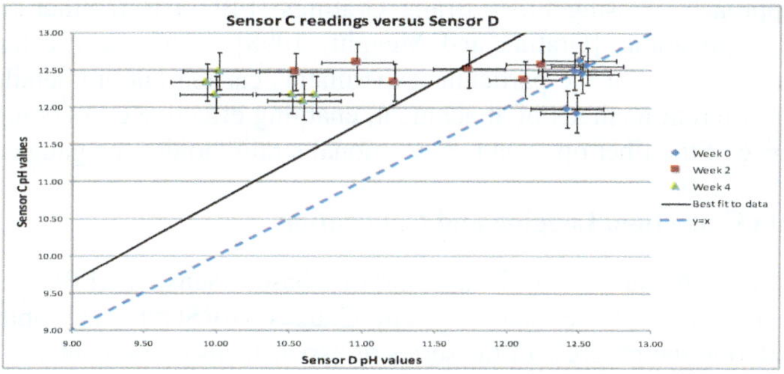

Fig. 28 pH readings obtained from Sensor C plotted against readings from Sensor D, best fit has been plotted alongside the ideal condition of Sensor C = Sensor D (y=x) for comparison

11 Corrosion of Steel Reinforcement Bars - Strain Sensing

Corrosion of steel reinforcement bars can produce waste products where the waste materials occupy between 2 and 6 times the volume of the original steel [Ervin et al, 2006], leading to localized strain and thus cracks and other defects as well as the loss in cross sectional area of the rebar, resulting in a degradation of the structural integrity.

Addressing this, the approach taken has been to use Fiber Bragg Grating-based (FBG) sensors, adapting an approach from their use in strain and temperature monitoring for other industrial monitoring applications [Grattan and Sun, 2000]. The FBG-based corrosion sensors are used with very little external protection, detecting corrosion-induced effects by monitoring the resultant strain on the reinforcement and including from the localized environment to indicate the onset of corrosion in the steel at a much earlier stage than is possible with familiar techniques such as visual inspection, thus being well suited to 'whole life' monitoring of a concrete structure. As in previous work by some of the authors [Grattan and Sun 2000] the sensors required can readily be multiplexed along what may be very long lengths of fiber, well suited to large structures, set accurately through placing the FBGs at pre-determined points along what is configured as an optical sensor network. The two-fold nature of the sensor system thus created is designed to ensure (i) a greater region (length) of coverage by the monitoring system whilst (ii) allowing a greater number of corrosion sensors to be placed in the areas predicted to be more susceptible to corrosion effects.

The approach taken in this work is the use of Fiber Bragg Grating-based strain sensors to monitor the volumetric expansion of the rebar through monitoring the increasing strain observed at the sensor itself. Previous work on the use of fiber Bragg Grating sensors for strain measurement has been extensively documented in the literature [e.g. Grattan and Meggitt, 1995] and such sensors have been developed for measuring rapid, dynamic changes to concrete platform steel bridges and composite structures [Gebremichael et al, 2005]. The application of these sensors to concrete structures has been discussed in some detail by a number of authors [e.g. KTV Grattan et al 2005].

The approach of using Fiber Bragg Gratings (FBGs) is familiar from other industrial applications [Grattan and Meggitt, 1998]. The specific numbers of gratings used in any of the particular experiments carried out are detailed below, as are the different methods of attachment, enabling effective cross comparison of performance of the fiber optic and conventional strain monitoring gauges.

11.1 Data Collection, Logging and Calibration

Data from both the Fiber Bragg Grating-based sensors (FBG) and from commercial Electrical Resistance Strain Gauges (ERSGs) were obtained and recorded during the progress of the series of experiments carried out and described below. A commercial geo-logger was used for data acquisition from the ERSGs and strain readings were continually monitored every hour. Similarly the wavelength shift data associated with the FBG-based sensor were recorded daily using an approach described previously [Grattan et al, 2007].

Representative Fiber Optic Sensor devices were calibrated *in situ* on rebars prior using a Nene tensometer testing machine where a sample reinforcement bar (to which was attached a fiber optic Bragg Grating based sensor) was put in direct tension. The displacement achieved was measured using the extensometer and from these data the calculation of the strain was obtained, thereby allowing for a linear graph of the wavelength shift of the Bragg Grating against the applied strain to be obtained. Further details of the calibration procedure are reported elsewhere by Grattan et al [Grattan and Meggitt 2000].

11.2 Experimental Aspects

The aim of the work was to conduct a series of sequential tests in which a number of different configurations of sensors under different, representative conditions were evaluated. A number of standard procedures, including the prior preparation of the rebars, the conditions for the accelerated corrosion of the rebars and the preparation of the various concrete samples used in this work were used, as discussed below.

(i) Accelerated corrosion – two approaches with 'rebars'

The rebars used were cleaned thoroughly with a wire brush prior to attaching the different strain gauges, to remove any existing corrosion products. Small flattened regions ('flats') were ground onto the bar to allow for the better attachment of the ERSG but this was not generally necessary for the FBG-based sensors used. Under normal circumstances corrosion of a rebar is a relatively slow process, taking often many years. In order to obtain data on a reasonable time frame for this laboratory-based study, using both FBG-based and Electronic Resistance Strain Gauge (ERSG) sensors, two different accelerated testing methods were employed.

In the first, exposed 'rebars' were used (not cast into concrete) to allow for easy non-destructive visual analysis of the effects seen. This was done using a specially constructed salt spray chamber, using a saline solution in an environment where the temperature and humidity was specially controlled. The salt solution added to the chamber consisted of 5kg of pure dried vacuum salt per 100 litres of water. The temperature in the chamber was set to 350C and the humidity to 85%. The spray was then set to activate every four hours for a half-hour period during the entire period of the tests.

In the second, the rebar was actually embedded in concrete slab(s), with or without the addition of chlorides to the concrete mix to accelerate the corrosion. This was done with the application of an electrical current – set to increase the rate at which corrosion occurs where an electrical loop was set up with the steel bar with the sensors attached being made anodic, (attached to the positive terminal of the power supply) with the negative terminal to a second, similar bar, embedded beside this main bar. Metal atoms move into the solution as positive ions and the excess free electrons move through the electrolyte to the cathode.

(ii) Preparation of the concrete samples

The concrete used was mixed in a 100kg mixer in accordance with the guidelines in BS1881: part 125 (BSI(1989)) and set in standard moulds for casting, taking particular care in pouring the concrete to avoid damage to the attached sensors. Samples were demoulded the day after casting and left to cure in air, prior to the application of voltage to accelerate the corrosion across the bars. Four distinct experimental programmes were carried out sequentially and building upon the results of prior work. This enabled different conditions to be examined and performance evaluated for the two different types of sensor systems. Four sequential test studies (denoted as Test A-D) were undertaken:

- Test A: both FBG and ERSG sensors were mounted separately on rebars (not encased in concrete) in a controlled, corrosion-inducing environment using a salt spray
- Test B: both FBG and ERSG sensors were separately mounted in 'identical' concrete slabs which both were subjected to electrically-induced accelerated corrosion
- Test C: both FBG and ERSG sensors were mounted in a single concrete slab (to which chlorides have been added to enhance the corrosion rate) on separate rebars and subjected to electrically-induced accelerated corrosion
- Test D: FBG-based sensors were mounted in a concrete slab (to which chlorides have been added to enhance the corrosion rate) and subjected to electrically-induced accelerated corrosion but using a different method of sensor attachment.

(iii) Initial Tests using a salt spray cabinet

In this arrangement, both the FBG and ERSG sensors used were mounted separately on rebars (but not encased in concrete) in a controlled, corrosion-inducing environment using a salt spray. For each sensor system, a 10mm diameter by 750mm long steel bar was used and cleaned before use with a wire brush. To one a fiber optic cable was attached, containing the 5 FBG sensing regions as follows and shown in Figure 29. The details of the sensors are as follows:

- FOS 1 – initial wavelength 1544.36 nm – not glued
- FOS 2 – initial wavelength 1539.96 nm – glued
- FOS 3 – initial wavelength 1536.27 nm – not glued
- FOS 4 – initial wavelength 1531.96 nm – glued but failed after being placed in the salt spray tank
- FOS 5 – initial wavelength not determined – not glued and failed to function from the start of the experiment

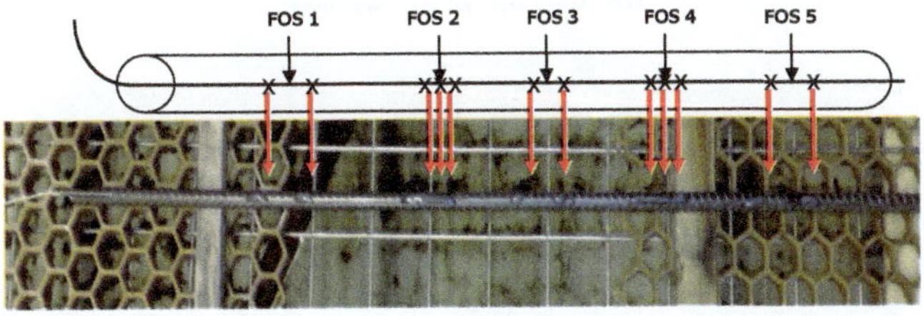

Fig. 29 Schematic layout of the placement of the FOS sensors (FOS 1-5) on the rebar

The FBG-based sensors were glued along the length of the raised edge of the bar, as is shown schematically in Figure 29 above. As can be seen the sensors were either covered with glue or else glue was applied to either side of the sensing region to hold it in place and in contact with the bar surface.

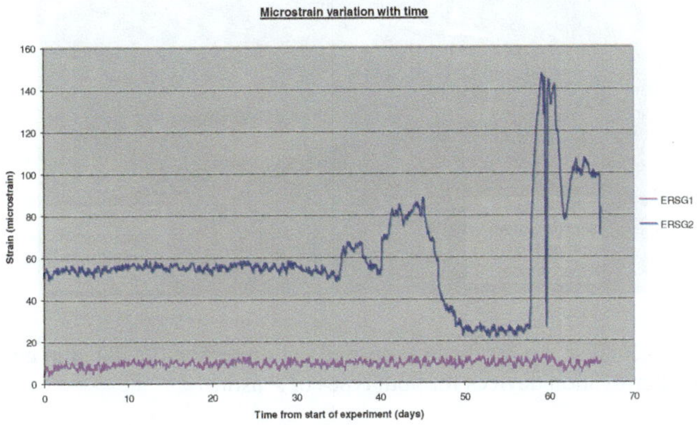

Fig. 30 Data showing strain (με) changes with time (days) from the two separate ESRGs used in the tests

For comparison, two ERSGs were fixed with 'superglue' and Araldite on either side on a similar separate steel bar (prepared initially as discussed above) and the strain readings were recorded and examined for signs of any variation arising from the corrosion process. Data from these sensors were logged (Figure 30).

Rusting was evident visually on the rebar onto which the ERSGs had been attached from 25 days after the start of the test but this produced no impact on the readings from the strain gauges. The bar was then left in the chamber for a longer period to investigate if there was any onset of corrosion and after ~35days, the strain level recorded in the top sensor (labelled ERSG2 in Figure 30) increased, this not being permanent as would have been expected from corrosion-induced strain – there were major fluctuations evident from the figure after which the strain reading returned to its previous level. The reading from the gauge on the underside of the bar did not vary and did not indicate any resultant strain arising from what was a (visually) obvious corrosion of the bar.

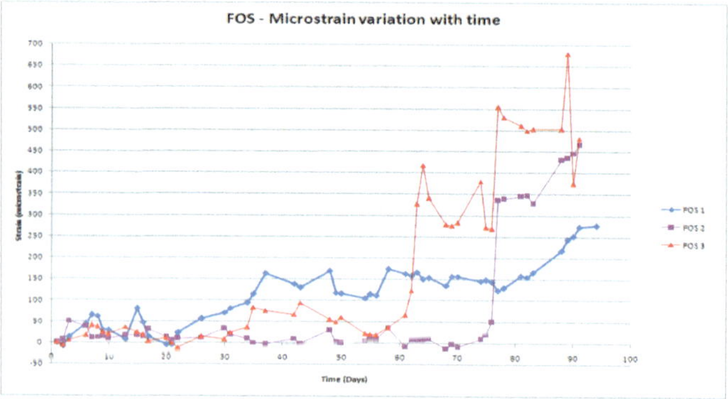

Fig. 31 Data showing strain (με) changes with time (days) from the three separate FBG-based sensors (FOS 1, 2 and 3) used in tests carried out

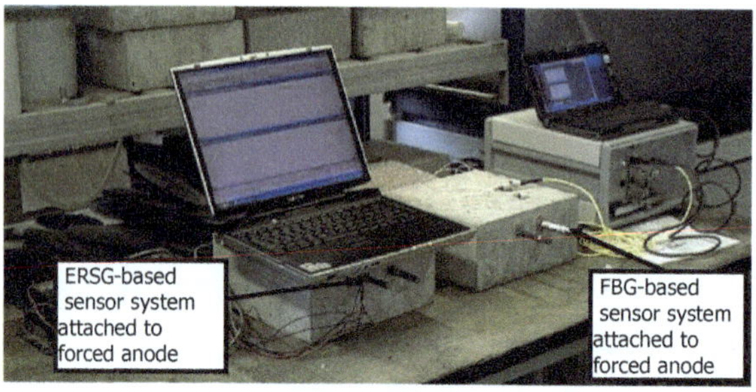

Fig. 32 Experimental set up for the tests carried out on sensors mounted in concrete blocks, showing the interrogation devices for both types of sensor.

For the FBG-based sensor system there was no support from the logged data for the visual signs of rusting which were evident until day 62, after which FOS 3 showed an increase in the strain level that was sustained until the end of the test. By day 76 a similar reaction was observed from FOS 2 where a dramatic rise in strain was observed that continued to increase for several days before stabilising/falling off. A rise of around 100με was observed for FOS 1 by approximately Day 37. However a larger change (or further increase) in the strain level was not observed until day 88. Data are shown in Figure 31.

(iv) FBG and ESRG sensors in two different but 'identical' concrete slabs

In this second arrangement both the FBG and the ERSG sensors were used in 'identical' concrete samples and subjected to an electrically-induced accelerated corrosion. A 12mm diameter by 400mm long rebar was allowed to protrude from the slab (to provide an electrical connection) and positioned at 67mm (concrete) cover (to the lower face of the slab). Both sets of sensors were mounted as discussed before, as shown in Figure 32. Two concrete blocks of identical dimensions (250mmx255mmx112mm) were created (using the same mix of concrete to avoid this having any influence) and demoulded the following day – one block containing FBG sensors and the other ERSGs attached to the rebar. The details for the concrete are given by Basheer [1994] and the mix ratios were as shown in Table 2.

Table 2 Characteristics of the Concrete used in the tests carried out

Ordinary Portland Cement	386 kg/m^3
Medium sand	636 kg/m^3
Coarse aggregate (20mm)	1158 kg/m^3
Water	212 Litre

Once the concrete has been allowed sufficient time to cure and the strain readings from the FBG-based sensors had stabilised (at day 23 after de-moulding), the accelerated corrosion process was begun. The voltage applied initially was 3V, but by day 56 a large electrical resistance was measured in both samples and the voltage was increased to 25V to accelerate further the corrosion process.

The sensor configuration for this test programme was as follows. The FBG-based sensor system used two sensors: labelled 'FOS 7 top' (facing the upper surface), the smaller of the two depths of concrete cover, and 'FOS 6 btm' facing the bottom surface (in Figure 4). Their specifications were:

- FOS 6 – initial wavelength 1543.88nm – glued
- FOS 7 – initial wavelength 1544.12nm – glued

For the ESRG devices, the sensors were labelled ERSG3, ERSG4 and ERSG5 and positioned with ERSG3 in the middle of the bar facing the upper surface, (similar in position to 'FOS 7 top') with ERSG4 attached to its side and ERSG5 facing the bottom (similar to 'FOS 6 btm').

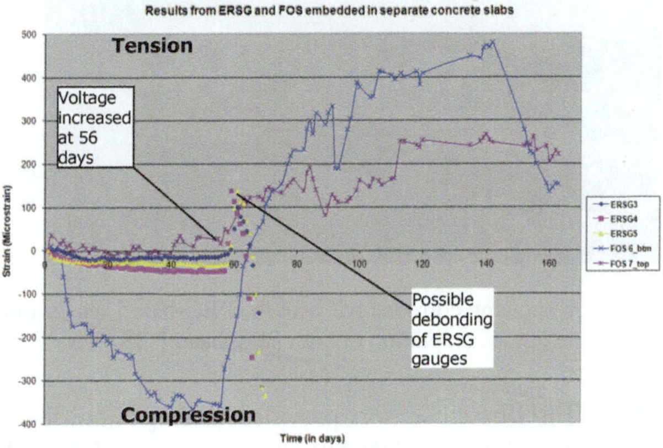

Fig. 33 Data showing strain (με) changes with time (days) from the three ESRGs and the two separate FBG-based sensors used in the tests

The test proceeded for a number of days but a substantial crack appeared in the block containing the ERSGs (due to the creation of corrosion waste products) and indicating that the accelerated corrosion was successful. Only minor cracks were seen in the other block containing the FBG-based sensors, event though the same concrete and conditions were used. Figure 33 shows the results obtained: the outputs from the ERSGs were extremely stable until the voltage was increased on day 23 – however by day 56 no indication of corrosion was seen. At day 56, the voltage was increased to 25V: shortly after there was a noticeable increase in the measured tensile strain which was followed by a huge apparent reduction to compressive strain, to an indicated value of -26,000με. This is clearly physically unrealistic and probably due to failure of the bonding of the ERSG to the sample. As it was not possible to draw any further conclusions from these erroneous data, the sample was split (and destroyed) to examine the sensors.

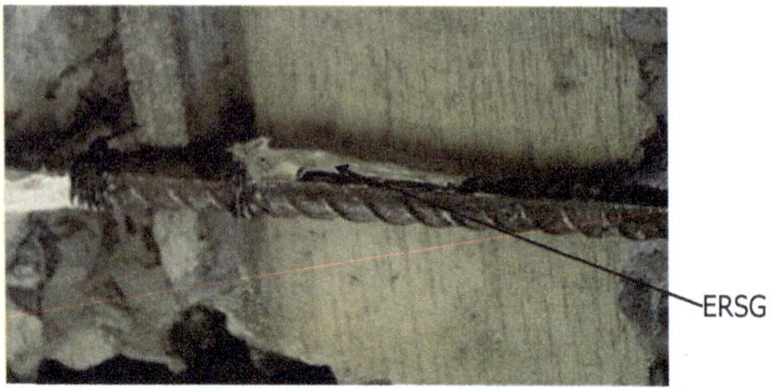

Fig. 34 (a) Photograph showing ERSG de-bonded from the rebar after the block was split open following completion of both ERSG and FOS tests

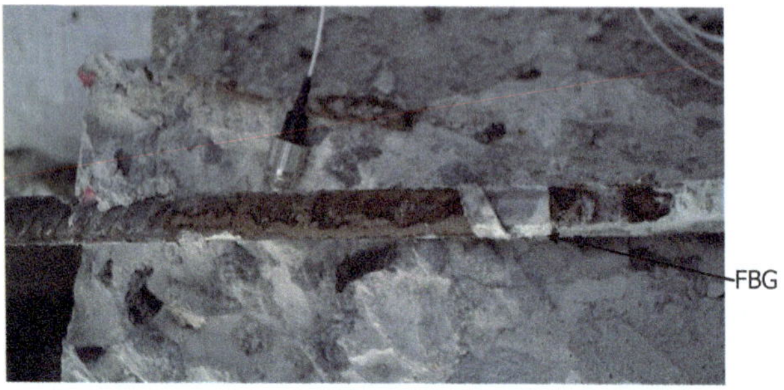

Fig. 35 (b) Photograph showing corroded bar with the FBG-based sensor in place following splitting of the concrete at the completion of both ERSG and FOS tests

By contrast, the FBG-based sensors provided readings until the end of the test (and were still functional at day 160) with no major cracks being observed in the block. In a similar way to the first sample, a sharp peak in the output readings was observed once the higher level of voltage was applied but, by contrast, readings from the FBG-based device were stable and 'realistic'. Some variation in the strain readings from the FBG-based sensors was observed: the measured strain from the sensor labelled 'FOS 6 btm' started to decrease at 140 days – probably due to de-bonding of this particular sensor (as occurred in the case of the ERSGs). The sample was split open for observation at the end of the test on day 160.

The rebars and the sensors were examined enabling two clear conclusions to be drawn (i) the ERSGs appear to have failed at a critical stage and thus (from this test) their durability under these conditions is questionable and (ii) the FBG-based sensors, whilst giving a noisier signal output, have demonstrated a clear difference between pre- and post-corrosion readings, showing that they were able to detect the strain-induced changes that have occurred to the rebar. The signal observed from the FBG-based sensors was noisier but able to give valuable data on the corrosion performance and this is the subject of on-going analysis.

Figure 34 (a) and (b) (for ERSG and FBG-based sensors respectively), showing the rebars themselves after splitting of the concrete slabs, indicate clearly that corrosion has occurred during the test and its effect on the bar had produced staining of the localised concrete area around it. This is consistent with the sharp drop in the strain signal observed from the ERSGs but a similar de-bonding could not be observed in FBG-based sensor.

The conclusion of these tests was that the experiment should be repeated, with both the ERSGs and the FBG-based sensors being attached to rebars in the same concrete sample.

(v) FBG and ESRG sensors in the same concrete block

In this approach, two 12mm diameter rebars were embedded in one concrete sample (to which chlorides (in the form of salt) have been added to enhance the corrosion rate) with two FBG-based and two ERSGs attached using superglue and Araldite. The experiment was conducted as before and the strain readings were allowed to stabilise before the corrosion acceleration voltage was applied, this time at day 118 after de-moulding of the concrete slab.

The rebar was positioned in a block of the same size as before in such a way that the black wire (to identify ERSG 6) and FOS8 (the first FBG-based sensor) were at the top of the sample and the brown wire (to identify ERSG7) and FOS9 (the second FBG-based sensor) were placed at the bottom. The depth of concrete cover was slightly smaller (by a few millimetres) towards the top of the sample.

The same mix proportions were used (see Table 2) but with the addition of chlorides to help accelerate corrosion (2% by the mass cement of chlorides (i.e. 8 kg/m^3)).

The results obtained from the FBG-based sensors are recorded in Figure 35, showing a large variation in the readings and a higher degree of compressive strain on the two FBG-based sensors than was observed previously. The sample was left to cure in air until day 76, when the block was wrapped in polythene sheeting to try and prevent moisture loss as this was a suspected cause of the compression effect being read by the two FBG-based sensors. On day 118 (after readings had been taken) 3V was applied with an increasing compressive strain (from FOS8 and FOS9) being indicated subsequently. The voltage was then increased to 25V on day 135 to continue to accelerate the corrosion process. It then became obvious that FOS8 had failed, as the signal recorded had dropped with a high level of noise, negating confidence in the data obtained from this sensor after day 153.

By contrast, Figure 12 shows that the ERSG readings remained fairly constant and did not vary substantially for the most part in comparison to the readings from FOS8 and FOS9 with no evidence of debonding of the ERSGs (the readings are consistent over the period).

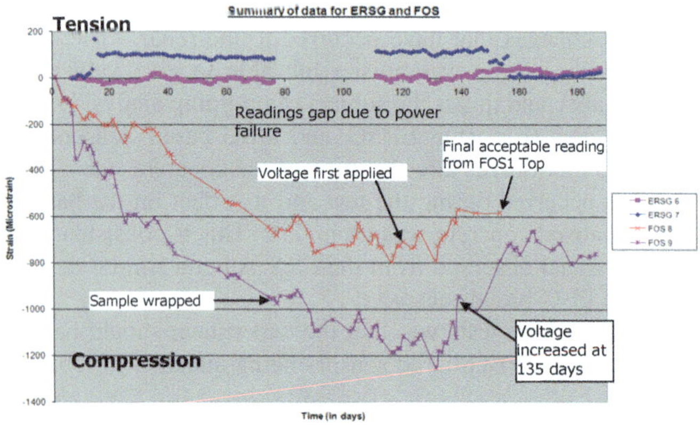

Fig. 36 Strain readings from the ERSG and FBG-based sensors. Positive strain data represent tension, negative values compression. (Strain data for the FBG-based sensors are derived using a calibration 1pm wavelength shift is equivalent to ~1.1$\mu\varepsilon$)

Unfortunately there is no indication of a response from the ERSGs to the increase in localised volume due to the corrosion. The data recorded, especially from day 150-160 from ERSG 7 on the underside showed a reduced strain, returning inexplicably to an almost zero position again – unlikely to be physically realistic. (The gap in the ERSG readings (between days 78 and 112) was due to a power failure – but subsequent readings showed that this did not have any influence on the measurements taken.

Analysis of the data showed that both the FBG-based sensors showed evidence of compressive forces, noting that the sample was wrapped to prevent excessive movement of water. By contrast, it was unclear why the results from the ERSGs were so different but being largely unchanged throughout the corrosion occurring doubt was cast on the veracity of the readings. One possible reason could lie in the gluing techniques used, leaving them less sensitive to strain effects. An obvious conclusion is that the sensors are not reliable in the environment of the wet concrete, failing to read the clear changes in strain – a large crack along the concrete slab was evidence of corrosion and after breaking open the sample, significant staining due to corrosion of the rebar was evident.

Thus the evidence obtained from a destructive test aligns with the evidence of compression obtained from the FBG-based sensors but not seen with the ERSGs.

(vi) FBG-based sensors alone

In the final programme of study the FBG-based sensors (which have successfully shown evidence of corrosion, validated in evidence from the destructive evaluation) were mounted in a concrete slab (to which chlorides have been added to enhance corrosion) and subjected to electrically-induced accelerated corrosion but using a different method of sensor attachment from before to enable a comparison of the attachment method to be carried out, especially in light of the failure of the ESRGs to show evidence of corrosion and to confirm the behaviour of the FBG-based. Here, by not gluing across the length of the FBG, the steel bar underneath is exposed as well and thus when the bar corrodes, the resulting strain values should vary from those previously recorded. In similar tests, strains give evidence of forces being imparted from localized corrosion regions that through their expansion press on the sensor: it was thus of interest to examine this method of attachment.

Two FBG-based sensors were attached to a steel rebar and embedded in a concrete block – labelled FOS 10 and FOS 11 and attached by glue applied to either side of the sensing region. Both sensors were facing towards the top surface of the concrete and an additional bar was embedded for electrical continuity. The sample was cured and the voltage was applied on day 21. The test specimen used was of similar dimensions but the concrete mix proportions differed, being designed for an accelerated corrosion environment, as given in Table 3 – the proportion of Ordinary Portland Cement and chlorides used was increased.

Table 3 Characteristics of the Concrete used to create the samples used in this programme

Ordinary Portland Cement	507.5 kg/m^3
Medium sand	647.5 kg/m^3
Coarse aggregate (20mm)	1010 kg/m^3
Water	215 Litre

The steel bars employed were 12mm in diameter and cut to a length of 750mm and a voltage (3V) was applied to the sample on day 21 (as before), and the onset and continuation of corrosion could clearly be seen.

Examination and cross comparison shows one sensor showing compression and the other tension. The 'compression dip' in the chart after the voltage is applied is common for both after which both show an increasing effect due to the corrosion products and associated strain. The readings from the two sensors vary in response to their respective positioning on the rebar. FOS 10 is placed under an increasing strain and shows a tension of 1700$\mu\varepsilon$ by day 50 – while FOS 11 is compressed and reaches a minimum of approximately 1200$\mu\varepsilon$, rising again towards day 50, the end of the test.

The results are what would be expected, even though FOS 10 shows a larger reaction to the corrosion of the bar than FOS 11. This likely arises as one sensor is in compression and the other in tension and the actual magnitudes of the readings depend naturally on the local conditions of the concrete immediately surrounding the sensor. As with previous test programmes, evidence of waste products seeping to the surface of the sample are seen, more so than from previous test programmes (this was a rapid corrosion test) and the visual evidence of the corrosion was clearly evident.

12 Summary and Future Prospects for Fibre Optic Sensor Systems in Structural Monitoring

This review has shown clearly the need for new and better sensing techniques for structural monitoring applications and has reported on the advantages and the use of fibre optic techniques for this application. The key conclusions of the work of the authors a reviewed below, together with some prospects for the future direction of research of this type

12.1 Sol-Gel Based pH Monitoring Techniques

Although sol-gel based techniques for pH monitoring have been reported in the literature for some 20 years, the research reported has focused on the optimization of the conditions for the creation of suitable sol-gels with the requisite stability and durability to survive the hard, very high pH environment of concrete. An optimized regime for the creation of a sufficiently durable and stable sol-gel into which a suitable pH indicator could be incorporated was developed and a suitable set of samples for mounting at the distal end of an a optical fibre to create a probe has been evaluated. Arising from the work, a number of broad conclusions can be drawn on the performance of the sensors developed:

- Sensors have been demonstrated which gave satisfactory readings of high pH values in buffer solutions when calibrated prior to the start of the experiments on the concrete samples and good performance was seen for *in situ* tests, validating the performance of these sensors
- Sensor A showed a good performance over the period of the experiments, yielding results which were consistent with Sensor D up to (and potentially beyond) week 6 of the accelerated carbonation tests. Giving confidence in the capability of the sensor is that the tests on the durability of the sol gel sample showed that after 24 months it remained intact and similar colour to a fresh sample, with no evidence of leaching.
- However, while Sensor B showed a good performance for several weeks, it failed before the end of the tests (it was replaced before week 6): when a new sensor disc element was introduced the sensor again worked well. This indicated that the durability of the sensor for this application was in question – as would be expected for a commercial probe not designed to be used at such high pH values and under these conditions
- Sensor C worked well in calibration but not in the environment of the liquid extracted from the concrete samples – this suggested that some interference was occurring and that a redesign of the fluorescence-based probe was required for use in this challenging environment.

Thus the research demonstrates the importance of the design and calibration of the sensors described: in particular their specific design for use in the harsh conditions seen in structural monitoring applications: only Sensor A showed the capability for the required longer term performance for *in situ* structural monitoring over extended periods, potentially stretching into years. The research demonstrates the validity of fibre optic sensors for this application, tailored to meet the demanding conditions, such as the high alkalinity and harsh materials in use, for the benefit of those seeking to carry out structural monitoring/testing.

12.2 Fibre Optic Strain Sensors for Structural Monitoring Applications

The research reported has shown that fibre optic sensors, widely used for strain monitoring in conventional environments can be used effectively in structural monitoring applications. Fibre optic strain sensors can be cross-compared and evaluated against conventional electrical resistance based sensors and also directly with strain measured using an extensometer. Thus fibre optic strain sensors have been specifically designed and tested both within and outside of the concrete environment to gauge the impact of the corrosion process on the steel bars being used as reinforcement. Results have been collected and analyzed showing the ability of the sensors to monitor the corrosion process in a manner that has, to-date, been found not to be possible with the conventional electrical resistance based strain sensors. Of particular importance was the packaging of such sensors – the research reported has shown that, for use in the concrete environment, they were found to be extremely robust and hardwearing in even the most challenging of conditions.

12.3 Summary of Results Obtained on Corrosion Sensing Using Fibre Optic Devices

In these tests fibre optic sensors were shown to be capable of sustaining measurements even when conventional sensors failed to perform in a satisfactory way. A series of sequential test programmes has been reported, extending over several long periods, stretching in one case up to 180 days (almost 6 months) and extending in total for over one year. Each of the tests carried out was designed to build upon the results of previous work and from the results conclusions on the response of both conventional (ERSG) and FBG-based fiber optic sensors to a range of extreme corrosion conditions, using materials and methods familiar to professional structural engineers, were drawn, as discussed below. The results have clearly shown that, using the salt spray cabinet, the ERSGs did not detect the expansion of the rebar due to what were visible corrosion waste products present and thus failed to be affected by the corrosion-induced strain. The reasons for this seem principally associated with either a lack of transference of the strain induced due to the expansion, difficulties associated with their method of attachment or the location of the ERSGs. The results are consistent with the glue initially holding the gauge no longer bonding correctly. By contrast, the results obtained from the FOS demonstrated the ability to measure strain and the differences in the corrosion signals from various areas of the bar under investigation.

From data obtained from the sensors encased in the concrete blocks and the samples split for inspection following the end of the tests to allow visual inspection, the FBG-based sensors were able to monitor the localized corrosion the rebar by detecting the changes in strain occurring and the strain effects of corrosion could also be distinguished from other induced changes in strain, such as that due to loading. Thus the research reported, through four sequential programmes over an extended period, has shown the value of the FBG-based sensors for monitoring both strains and compressions for applications of this type. A fuller evaluation and optimization of the adhesion methods, addressing even longer term tests and evaluating the impact of other external parameters, would be valuable.

12.4 Prospects for On-Going Research in the FOS Field for Structural Monitoring

The research reported in this chapter has shown both that there are weaknesses with conventional sensor techniques for many of the applications discussed and opportunities for new sensing techniques using fibre optic methods. The sensor devices using such methods, although in many cases development and enhancement is continuing in academic research laboratories, are available now from a number of commercial suppliers and will undoubtedly become more widely used by civil and structural engineers in the future. The research reported has shown that on-going work should be carried out on the optimization of the packaging of the sensors discussed, especially for internal structural monitoring, to determine the best packaging that can be developed to provide an optimum level of protection whilst also ensuring that there is sufficient sensitivity to detect the parameters required. In this way a range of different optical sensors can more easily be networked on a single optical cable, which could then lead to a simple, multi-parameter sensor system which could be tailored so that it is capable of installation in a variety of structures.

References

1. Al-Azzawi, A.: Fibre Optics: Principles and Practices. CRC Press, Boca Raton (2007); ISBN 0849382971
2. Andrade, C., Alonso, C.: On-Site Measurements of Corrosion Rate of Reinforcements. Construction and Building Materials 15(2-3), 141–145 (2001)
3. ASTM C: 1152, Standard test method for acid-soluble chloride in mortar and concrete, pp. 609–610 (1990)
4. ASTM C 876, Standard Test Method for Half-Cell Potentials of Uncoated Reinforcing Steel in Concrete (1991)
5. Badini, G.E., Grattan, K.T.V., Palmer, A.W., Tseung, A.C.C.: Developments of pH-sensitive substrates for optical sensor applications. In: Proceedings in Physics, vol. 44, pp. 436–442. Springer, Heidelberg (1989)
6. Bamforth, P.B., Price, W.F., Emerson, M.: An International Review of Chloride Ingress into Structural Concrete, p. 80. Thomas Telford, London (1997); ISBN 9780727729286

7. Basheer, P.A.M., Grattan, K.T.V., Sun, T., Long, A.E., McPolin, D., Xie, W.: Fibre Optic Chemical Sensor Systems for Monitoring pH Changes in Concrete. In: Proceedings of SPIE, vol. 5586. SPIE, Bellingham (2004)
8. Basheer, P.A.M., Russell, D., Andrews, R., McCarter, W.J.: Monitoring Internal Changes in Concrete During Carbonation and Chloride Ingress using a Covercrete Electrode Array. In: 11th Proceedings of Structural Faults and Repairs (2006a)
9. Basheer, P.A.M., Basheer, L., Long, A.E., Cleland, D.J.: Fifteen years of research on the assessment of durability of concrete using in situ air permeability and sorptivity measurements. In: 11th Proceedings of Structural Faults and Repairs (2006b)
10. Benmokrane, B., Debaiky, A., El-Ragaby, A., Roy, R., El-Gamal, S., El-Salakawy, E.: Laboratory and field performance of FOS sensors in static and dynamic strain monitoring in concrete bridge decks. In: Proceedings of SPIE, vol. 6176, pp. 617612–617638. SPIE, CA (2006); ISNN 0277-786X
11. Broomfield, J.P.: Corrosion of steel in concrete, 2nd edn. Taylor & Francis Group, Abington (2007); ISBN 0632052511
12. Brönnimann, R., Held, M., Nellen, P.M.: Reliability, availability, and maintainability considerations for fiber optical sensor applications. In: Proceedings of SPIE, vol. 6167, p. 61671B-1. SPIE, CA (2006); ISNN 0277-786X
13. Bungey, J.H.: Testing of Concrete in Structures, 2nd edn. Chapman and Hall, New York (1989); ISBN 9780415263016
14. Bungey, J.H., Millard, S.G., Grantham, M.G.: Testing of Concrete in Structures, 4th edn. Taylor & Francis Group, Abington (2006); ISBN 0415263018
15. Campbell, M.: Sensor Systems for Environmental Monitoring: Sensor technologies. Springer, Heidelberg (1997); ISBN 9780751404180
16. Climent, M.A., Viqueira, E., de Vera, G., López-Atalaya, M.M.: Analysis of acid-soluble chloride in cement, mortar, and concrete by potentiometric titration without filtration steps. Cement and Concrete Research 29, 893–898 (1999); ISSN 0008-8846
17. Cox, R N., Cigna, R., Vennesland, O., Valente, T.:(eds.) COST 509, Corrosion and Protection of metals in contact with concrete, EUR 17608 Part 2: Monitoring (1997)
18. Deeks, A.J., Hao, H.: Developments in Mechanics of Structures and Materials. In: Proceedings of the 18th Australasian Conference on the Mechanics of Structures and Materials. CRC Press, Boca Raton (2004)
19. Dhir, R.K., Jones, M.R.: Concrete repair, rehabilitation, and protection. Taylor & Francis, Abington (1996)
20. Doyle, J.F.: Modern experimental stress analysis: completing the solution of partially specified problems. John Wiley and Sons, Chichester (2004); ISBN 0470861576
21. Elsener, B.: Half-cell potential mapping to assess repair work on RC structures. Construction and Building Materials 15(2-3), 133–139 (2001)
22. Ervin, B.L., Bernhard, J.T., Kuchma, D.A., Reis, H.: Estimation of corrosion damage to steel reinforced mortar using frequency sweeps of guided mechanical waves. In: Proceedings of SPIE, vol. 6174, pp. 61740H-1 – 6174-15. SPIE, CA (2006); ISNN 0277-786X
23. Fuhr, P.L., MacCraith, B., Huston, D.R., Guerrina, M., Nelson, M.: Fiber optic chloride sensing: If corrosion's the problem, chloride sensing is the key. In: Third Pacific Northwest fiber optic sensor workshop, Proceedings of the Society of Photo-optical Instrumentation Engineers (SPIE), vol. 3180, pp. 92–104. SPIE, CA (1997); ISSN 0277-786X
24. Fuhr, P.L., Spammer, S.: Fiber Optic Sensors in the Waterbury Bridge. In: SPIE, vol. 3489, pp. 124–129. SPIE, CA (1998); ISSN 0277-786X

25. Gebremichael, Y.M., Li, W., Meggitt, B.T., Boyle, W.J.O., Grattan, K.T.V., McKinley, B., Boswell, L.F., Aarnes, K.A., Aasen, S.E., Tynes, B., Fonjallaz, Y., Triantafillou, T.: A Field Deployable, Multiplexed Bragg Grating Sensor System Used in an Extensive Highway Bridge Monitoring Evaluation Tests. IEEE Sensors Journal 5(3) (2005); ISSN 1530-437X
26. Geddes, C.D.: Optical thin film polymeric sensors for the determination of aqueous chloride, bromide and iodide ions at high pH, based on the quenching of fluorescence of two acridinium dyes. Dyes and Pigments 45, 243–251 (2000); ISSN 0143-7208
27. Glass, G.K., Wang, Y., Buenfeld, N.R.: An investigation of experimental methods used to determine free and total chloride contents. Cement and Concrete Research 26(9), 1443–1449 (1996)
28. Glass, G.K., Field, S.N., Green, W.K.: Non-destructive determination of the sheet resistance of conductive coating anodes on concrete. Anti-Corrosion Methods and Materials 47(1), 5–10 (2000); ISSN 0003-5599
29. Grahn, W., Makedonski, P., Wichern, J., Kowalsky, W., Wiese, S.: Fiber Optical sensors for in-situ monitoring of moisture and pH-value in reinforced concrete. In: SPIE, vol. 4480, pp. 395–403. SPIE, CA (2002); ISSN 0277-786X
30. Grattan, K.T.V., Meggitt, B.T.: Optical Fiber Sensor Technology. Chapman & Hall Publishers, Boca Raton (1995); ISBN 041259210X
31. Grattan, K.T.V., Meggitt, B.T.: Optical Fiber Sensor Technology, vol. 4. Kluwer Academic Publishers, Dordrecht (1999); ISBN 9780412825705
32. Grattan, K.T.V., Sun, T.: Fiber optic sensor technology: an overview. Sensors and Actuators 82, 40–61 (2000); ISSN 0924-4247
33. Grattan, K.T.V., Sun, T., Boyle, W.J.O., Gebremichael, Y.M., Basheer, P.M., Long, A.E.: Optical fibre sensor systems – new solutions for structural monitoring applications? In: Proceedings of SPIE, vol. 5826, pp. 412–424 (2005)
34. Grattan, K.T.V., Sun, T., Zhao, W., Basheer, P.M., Taylor, S., Grattan, S.K.T.: Challenges in Construction Monitoring using Fibre Optic Sensor techniques, Photon 06 Manchester, Invited paper (2006a)
35. Grattan, K.T.V., Sun, T., Zhao, W.: Fibre Optic Sensors: Principles & Practice. In: 11th Proceedings of Structural Faults and Repairs (2006b)
36. Grattan, K.T.V., Sun, T., Basheer, P.A.M.: Fibre optic sensors and their potential for structural monitoring. Concrete Platform, 77–91 (2007)
37. Grattan, S.K.T., Basheer, P.A.M., Taylor, S.E., Zhao, W., Sun, T., Grattan, K.T.V.: Corrosion induced strain monitoring through Fibre Optic Sensors. In: Third International Conference on Optical and Laser Diagnostics, ICOLAD 2007. IOP Publishing (2007); ISSN 1742-6596
38. Grote, N., Venghaus, H.: Fibre optic communication devices. Springer, Heidelberg (2001); ISBN 3540669779
39. Gu, P., Beaudoin, J.J.: Obtaining Effective Half-Cell Potential Measurements in Reinforced Concrete Structures, Construction Technology Update No. 18 (1998)
40. Hammond, D.S., Chapman, L., Baker, A., Thornes, J.E., Sandford, A.: Fluorescence of road salt additives: potential applications for residual salt monitoring. Measurement Science and Technology 18, 239–244 (2007); ISSN 0957-0233
41. Hannon, J.J.: Emerging technologies for construction delivery. Published by Transportation Research Board (2007)
42. Huber, C., Werner, T., Krause, C., Wolfbeis, O.S., Leiner, M.J.P.: Overcoming the pH dependency of optical sensors: a pH-independent chloride sensor based on co-extraction. Analytica Chimica Acta 398, 137–143 (1999); ISSN 0003-2670

43. Huber, C., Klimant, I., Krause, C., Wolfbeis, O.S.: Dual Lifetime Referencing as Applied to a Chloride Optical Sensor. Analytical Chemistry 73, 2097–2103 (2001)
44. James, S.W., Tatam, R.: Optical fibre long-period grating sensors: characteristics and application, Measurement Science and Technology 14 R49 - R61, Optical Society of America (2003); ISSN 0146-9592
45. Koch, G.H., Brongers, M.P.H., Thompson, N.G., Virmani, Y.P., Payer, J.H.: Corrosion Cost and Preventive Strategies in the United States, Technical report for the Federal Highway Administration, USA (2001)
46. Leng, J.S., Winter, D., Barnes, R.A., Mays, G.C., Fernando, G.F.: Structural health monitoring of concrete cylinders using protected fibre optic Sensors. Smart Mater. Struct. 15, 302–308 (2006); ISSN 0964-1726
47. McCarter, W.J., Brousseau, R.: The A.C. response of hardened cement paste. Cement and Concrete Research 20(6), 891–900 (1990)
48. McCarter, W.J., Emerson, M., Ezirim, H.: Properties of concrete in the cover zone: developments in monitoring techniques. Magazine of Concrete Research 47(172), 243–251 (1995)
49. McCarter, W.J., Ezirim, H., Emerson, M.: Properties of concrete in the cover zone: water penetration, sorptivity and ionic ingress. Magazine of Concrete Research 48, 149–156 (1996)
50. McCarter, W.J., Chrisp, T.M., Butler, A., Basheer, P.A.M.: Near-surface sensors for condition monitoring of cover-zone concrete. Construction and Building Materials 15, 115–124 (2001)
51. McCarter, W.J., Chrisp, T.M., Starrs, G., Basheer, P.A.M., Blewett, J.: Field monitoring of electrical conductivity of cover-zone concrete. Cement & Concrete Composites 27, 809–817 (2005)
52. McPolin, D., Basheer, P.A.M., Long, A.E., Grattan, K.T.V., Sun, T., Xie, W.: Fibre Optic Sensors for Monitoring Temperature, Chloride ingress and Carbonation in Cementitious Materials. Concrete Research in Ireland Colloquium (2005)
53. McPolin: Profiling of carbonation and chloride distributions in concretes and development of novel fibre optic sensors, PhD Thesis, Queen's University Belfast, United Kingdom (2005)
54. Majumder, M., Gangopadhyay, T.K., Chakraborty, A.K., Dasgupta, K., Bhattacharya, D.K.: Fibre Bragg gratings in structural health monitoring – Present stauts and applications. Sensors and Actuators A: Physical (2008); ISSN 0924-4247
55. Malhotra, V.M., Carino, N.J.: Handbook on nondestructive testing of concrete, pp. 10–15. CRC Press, Boca Raton (2004); ISBN 9780849314858
56. Measures, R.M.: Structural Monitoring with Fiber Optic Technology. Academic Press, London (2001); ISBN 0124874304
57. Meltz, G., Morey, W.W., Glenn, W.H.: Formation of Bragg gratings in optical fibers by a transverse holographic method. Optics Letters 14(15) (1989); ISSN 0146-9592
58. Méndez, A.: Fiber Bragg grating sensors: a market overview. In: Proceedings of SPIE, vol. 6619, Article 661905. SPIE, CA (2007); ISNN 0277-786X
59. Merzbacher, C.I., Kersey, A.D., Friebele, E.J.: Fiber optic sensors in concrete structures: a review. Smart Materials and Structures 5, 196–208 (1998)
60. Millard, S.G., Law, D., Bungey, J.H., Cairns, J.: Environmental influences on linear polarisation corrosion rate measurement in reinforced concrete. NDT&E International 34, 409–417 (2001) Paper 333

61. Moller, J.: Measurement of degree of carbonation in cement based materials, Concrete under severe conditions. In: Sakai, K., Banthia, N., Gjorv, O.E. (eds.) Environment and Loading, vol. 2. Chapman and Hall, Boca Raton (1995)
62. Mufti, A.: FRPs and FOSs lead to innovation in Canadian civil engineering Structures. Construction and Building Materials 17, 379–387 (2003)
63. Muller, N.J.: Desktop encyclopedia of telecommunications. McGraw-Hill Professional, New York (2002); ISBN 9780071381482
64. Naus, D.: International RILEM Workshop on Life Prediction and Aging Management of Concrete Structures. RILEM Publications (2000); ISBN 2912143195
65. Nawy, E.G.: Concrete Construction Engineering Handbook, pp. 5–10. CRC Press, Boca Raton (2008); ISBN 0849374928
66. Neville, A.M.: Properties of Concrete. John Wiley & Sons, Chichester (1996); ISBN 9780470235270
67. Newman, J.B., Choo, B.S.: Advanced concrete technology. Butterworth-Heinemann, Butterworths (2003); ISBN 9780750651035
68. Nilsson, L.O., Poulsen, E., Sandberg, P., Sorensen, H.E., Klinghoffer, O.: HETEK, Chloride penetration into concrete, state-of-the-art, transport process, corrosion initiation, test methods and prediction models, Report No. 53 (1996)
69. Othonos, A., Kalli, K.: Fiber Bragg Gratings: Fundamentals and Applications in Telecommunication and Sensing. Artech House, Boston (1999); ISBN 0890063443
70. Pal, S.: Characterisation and high-temperature sensing potential of fibre Bragg gratings in specialised optical fibres, Thesis, City University London, United Kingdom (2004)
71. Popovics, S.: Strength and related properties of concrete: a quantitative approach. John Wiley and Sons, Chichester (1998); ISBN 9780471149033
72. Ramachandran, V.S.: Concrete admixtures handbook: properties, science, and technology, p. 67. William Andrew (1995); ISBN 0815513739
73. Rasanen, V., Penttala, V.: The pH measurement of concrete and smoothing mortar using a concrete powder suspension. Cement and Concrete Research 34, 813–820 (2004); ISSN 0008-8846
74. Raupach, M., Schießl, P.: Monitoring System For The Penetration Of Chlorides, Carbonation And The Corrosion Risk For The Reinforcement. Construction and Building Materials Il(4), 207–214 (1997)
75. Raupach, M., Schießl, P.: Macrocell sensor systems for monitoring of the corrosion risk of the reinforcement in concrete structures. NDT&E International 34, 435–442 (2001)
76. Ren, L., Li, H.-N., Zhou, J., Li, D.-S., Sun, L.: Health monitoring system for offshore platform with fiber Bragg grating sensors. Optical Engineering 45 084401 (2006); ISSN 0091-3286
77. Richardson, M.G.: Fundamentals of Durable Reinforced Concrete, pp. 81–104. Taylor & Francis, Abington (2002);ISBN 9780419237808
78. RILEM CPC 18, Measurement of hardened concrete carbonation depth, Published by E & FN SPON, pp. 56–58 (1988); ISSN 1359-5997
79. RILEM TC 178-TMC: Testing and Modeling Chloride Penetratio. Concrete - Analysis of water soluble chloride content in concrete. Materials and Structures, 35, 586–588 (2002)
80. Robins, P., Austin, S., Chandler, J., Jones, P.: Flexural strain and crack width measurement of steel-fibre-reinforced concrete by optical grid and electrical gauge methods. Cement and Concrete Research 31(5), 719–729 (2001)

81. Sabnis, G.M.: Structural Modelling and Experimental Techniques. CRC Press, Boca Raton (1999); ISBN 9780849324697
82. Sakai, K., Banthia, N., Gjorv, O.E.: Concrete Under Severe Conditions 1: Environment and Loading. Taylor & Francis, Abington (1995); ISBN 9780419198703
83. Schiessl, P.: Corrosion of steel in concrete. Chapman and Hall, Boca Raton (1988); ISBN 9780412321009
84. Schießl, P., Raupach, M.: Monitoring System for the Corrosion Risk for Steel in Concrete. Concrete International, 52–55 (1992)
85. Tang, J.-L., Wang, J.-N.: Measurement of chloride-ion concentration with long-period grating technology. Smart Materials and Structures 16, 665–672 (2007)
86. Tennyson, R.C., Mufti, A.A., Rizkalla, S., Tadros, G., Benmokrane, B.: Structural health monitoring of innovative bridges in Canada with fiber optic sensors. Smart Mater. Struct. 10, 560–573 (2001); ISSN 0964-1726
87. Udd, E.: Review of multi-parameter fiber grating sensors. In: Proc. SPIE, vol. 6770. SPIE, CA (2007); ISSN 0277-786X
88. Villain, G., Platret, G.: Two Experimental Methods to Determine Carbonation Profiles in Concrete. ACI Materials Journal 103(4) (2006)
89. Xie, W., Grattan, K.T.V., Sun, T., Basheer, P.A.M., Long, A.E.: Fibre Optic chemical sensor systems for internal concrete condition monitoring. In: Proceedings of SPIE, vol. 5502, pp. 334–347. SPIE, CA (2004); ISSN 0277-786X
90. Zhan, C., Zhu, Y., Yin, S.: Fabricating harsh environment fiber Bragg gratings by ultrafast laser. In: Proceedings of SPIE, vol. 6314, p. 63141. SPIE, CA (2006); ISSN 0277-786X
91. Zhou, G.-D., Li, H.-N., Ren, L., Li, D.-S.: Influencing parameters analysis of strain transfer in optic fiber Bragg grating sensors. In: Proceedings of SPIE, vol. 6179, p. 61790R. SPIE, CA (2006); ISSN 0277-786X
92. Zhou, K., Chen, X., Zhang, L., Bennion, I.: Implementation of optical chemsensors based on HF-etched fibre Bragg grating structures. Meas. Sci. Technol. 17, 1140–1145 (2006); ISSN 0957-0233

Author Index

Batch number: 10755837

Printed by Printforce, the Netherlands